Subscribe to my free newsletter to access your complete skincare experience

Skincare Blueprint: Glow Up From Within

Access Skincare Routines Curated by a Board-certified Dermatologist

https://drtwl.substack.com

The skincare newsletter that offers an unparalleled learning experience from an internationally renowned skincare expert

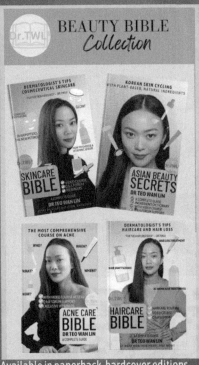

BEAUTY BIBLE
Collection

Available in paperback, hardcover editions

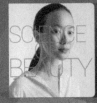

Dermatologist Talks: Science of Beauty

Dr. Teo Wan Lin

Asian Beauty Secrets by Dr.TWL

Dr. Teo Wan Lin

Listen to my podcasts

Welcome! I'm Dr Teo Wan Lin, a board-certified dermatologist and the host of leading beauty podcast Dermatologist Talks: Science of Beauty, which has collaborated with industry giants such as LVMH, Amore-Pacific and L'Oreal Paris amongst others for skincare education.

My published research includes work on the skin microbiome in top ranked dermatology journals like the Journal of the American Academy of Dermatology. I am also the author of "On Thoughts, Emotions, Facial Expressions and Aging", a key opinion piece on the intersection of philosophy, psychology and cosmetic dermatology in the International Journal of Dermatology by WILEY/Blackwell.

I created this skincare guide as a means to empower you with skincare knowledge that will radicalize the way you approach your self-care routine—mind, skin and gut (what the aesthetic industry really doesn't want you to know).

Welcome to the Beauty Library, a collection of beauty bibles on skincare, haircare, diet, holistic wellness, mind, skin and soul. I am excited to partner you on your beauty journey. I have a small request, do leave a review if you enjoyed the book, it goes a long way—I look forward to sharing more complimentary resources with you as well, just send me a message on my newsletter to connect!

Skincare Blueprint: Glow Up From Within
https://drtwl.substack.com

Ask A Dermatologist Community https://ask.drtwlderma.com

Follow me on Instagram & TikTok @drteowanlin
YouTube @drtwlderma where I share more skincare, haircare and beauty tips.

SKINCARE & COSMETIC INGREDIENTS DICTIONARY

Dr. Teo Wan Lin

Published by TWL Medical Pte Ltd, 2023.

Table of Contents

CHAPTER ONE

Introduction

Welcome to the Skin Masters Program, I am Dr. Teo Wan Lin, board-certified dermatologist and chief scientific officer of Asia's leading clinical skincare brand Dr.TWL Dermaceuticals. I created the Skincare and Cosmetic Ingredients Dictionary as a complete course for skin experts who desire true mastery of the art of skincare formulation. The teaching style is based on an optimised program developed with a workbook for an interactive learning approach that delivers results.

Unlike traditional teaching methods of skincare ingredients which focuses on rote learning and memorisation, this course takes a practical approach that allows you to demonstrate true mastery—critical in today's fast-paced world of beauty entrepreneurship. The beauty and wellness industry is estimated to be worth a whopping $571.1 billion in 2023 —and if you are seeking a share of the pie, whether as a beauty influencer, brand entrepreneur or an aesthetician, knowledge is the key to standing out.

Learning isn't just about remembering information—it's also about learning how to learn. And in today's world, knowledge alone isn't enough—information is just a click away with internet search engines. What's important instead is true mastery— in how you learn and apply knowledge acquired. You see, when it comes to personal branding and the business world, application of what you know is key—nobody cares what you know until they understand why they should listen to you. That's when expertise and certifications play a key role. The Skin Masters Academy was birthed out of a vision to empower beauty entrepreneurs—women who teach others to become beautiful, from the inside out.

Systematic foundation building begins with skin physiology
We begin with skin health. In this skincare course, I take you through step by step to build a solid foundation of skin knowledge—starting with skin physiology. As the author of key scientific papers in the skin microbiome and microclimate published in top journals like the International Journal of Dermatology and the Journal of the American Academy of Dermatology, I'll share with the the most up-to-date approach to understanding how skin works—literally from the inside out.

Created for true mastery
The handbook contains all that is required to get to an advanced level of skincare mastery based on the neuroscience-backed learning techniques that I have used throughout my academic career. Every visual included is created with a purpose—to keep your attention and spark new connections in your mind—the secret to creativity that's a must-have for every successful entrepreneur.

Ditch rote learning, learn only about skincare ingredients that the pros recommend
Study smart. Forget about traditional cosmetic ingredient dictionaries—in the age of cosmeceuticals, these long lists of meaningless synthetics are outdated. The Dr.TWL skincare ingredient dictionary was compiled based on a comprehensive analysis of over 100 bestselling skincare brands—both synthetic and botanical cosmeceuticals included. Distilled down to the core concepts, you will be learning about the latest actives that top cosmeceutical brands are incorporating into their skincare.

Content blueprints, speed guides for quick recap & reference
Learning can be fun—once you've discovered how to learn. That's true for me and has transformed me into a lifelong learner. I'll make sure it becomes your reality. This is why I have created this book not just as a collection of foundational notes, but also one that includes an entire section dedicated to learning aides—cut-out flash cards, mind map style worksheets as well as

a bullet point summary after each lecture that reinforces what you have learnt. Included with the book purchase are module-specific video workshops as well as special community access where I'll answer your questions.

You will also get a $200 off discount code to the full online cosmetic formulation course with all 10 modules plus the complete Skin Masters Program that comes with video instruction based on the textbook material. I'll also be answering your questions on a students only Q & A platform.

Divided into 10 modules, the Skin Masters Program introduces must-know skincare actives in the context of skin physiology & functions, taught by a board-certified dermatologist.

CHAPTER TWO

How to Use the Textbook

As a standalone or a companion textbook to the Skin Masters Program, maximise your learning with the following guide:

Register for an account with your Amazon order receipt number in the comment section. Your account will be verified within 24 hours following which you will gain access to the accompanying video workshops, including an important introductory session which will help guide your learning journey.

Access Dr.TWL's online learning portal*

- Video workshops
- Self-test flashcards
- Community Q & A with Dr.TWL

What you'll learn
- A-Z all-you-need-to-know comprehensive guide to state-of-the-art cosmeceuticals
- Shortform notes for quick recap & mastery
- Emphasis on knowledge application focused on skin concerns
- How to create custom formulated skincare safely & effectively, sourcing raw materials (small business, DIY beauty)
- Synthetic cosmeceuticals vs botanicals (function, subtypes, skin penetration, clinical studies)
- Master the gold standard* retinoid family of actives for all skin types without harming the skin barrier
- Core syllabus with detailed notes and course workbook (worksheets)
    - Hyaluronic acid

- Polyglutamic acid
- Vitamin C
- Niacinamide
- Ceramides
- Retinoid alternatives
- Resveratrol
- Peptides
- Hydroquinone & alternatives: kojic acid, arbutin
- Novel ingredients based on latest dermatological research
- Specialised syllabus organised according to skin function
  - Sensitive skin & barrier repair: amino acids, aquaporin mediators
  - Acne & rosacea: microbiome friendly botanicals
  - Pigmentation: bacterial ferment filtrates
  - Natural Moisturising Factors (NMF), Coenzyme Q10, Vitamin U
- Ethnobotanical dictionary (principles of Eastern, Ayurvedic ethnopharmacology & application to modern cosmetic formulation)

Additional Topics Covered
- How to choose skincare ingredients for your skin type
- Dermatologist's guide to ingredient mixing & pairing
- Customising the ideal skincare regimen on a rotational basis for maximum efficacy
- Navigating ingredient safety in pregnancy & breastfeeding
- Formulation secrets to success

Make beauty your business*
- Starting a skincare line (partner selection, social media marketing, templates & brand-building)
- Becoming a beauty brand owner, influencer (personal branding, social media post content creation, building a loyal audience)

Syllabus Outline

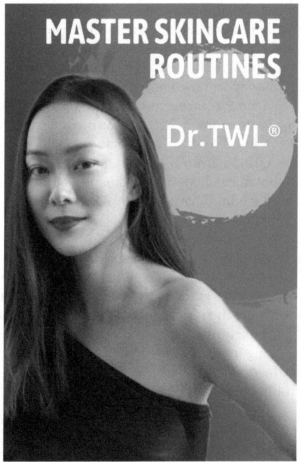

SECTION 1
SKINCARE ROUTINE STEPS FOUNDATIONAL COURSE
This section provides a complete foundational course in advanced skincare routines—you'll learn about the purpose

behind each skincare routine step, the science as well as how skincare can alter underlying skin physiology. This is an essential part of the course which puts the study of skincare active ingredients into perspective and its correct context. I wrote this book with a goal in mind—to help you achieve true mastery of skincare and cosmetic formulation; including in depth-knowledge about active ingredients which you will familiarise yourself with. Unlike traditional skincare ingredient dictionaries, it isn't just about a reference book which in the era of the internet is rendered quite obsolete. What you want instead, is a handbook that teaches you the art and science of cosmetic formulation—it is the practical mastery that matters in the age of social media and personal branding.

- Master the science and art of skincare routines
  - Understand how skincare routines affect local skin physiology
  - Tailoring each step to suit specific skin conditions i.e. acne, rosacea, sensitive skin
  - Choosing active ingredients for oil control, pigmentation

After gaining mastery of foundational skincare routines, you are now well equipped to learn about modifications such as the 2 and 3-step protocols incorporating facial device technologies. In addition, you will learn about specific skincare layering techniques used by dermatologists in a clinical setting tailored to optimise the skin microenvironment.

Foundational skincare routines
  - 7 STEP
  - Modifications (home devices)
    - 2-STEP
    - 3-STEP
- Double cleansing
- Moisturiser layering techniques
  - Serums

13

- Lotions/emulsions
- Cream
- Mist

In the next segment, you will focus on advanced skincare techniques such as exfoliation and face masking in a professional setting, based on the latest advancements in cosmeceuticals and biomaterial engineering. There is a link for you to download skincare planner templates for client/personal use (register at https://www.twlskin.com/dictionary/ for access). Take this opportunity to customise the templates as practice to chart your skincare journey based on the new knowledge you have acquired.

Advanced master course material for skin experts
- Skin treatments
  - Exfoliation
    - Mask peels
    - Microdermabrasion
    - Chemical peels
  - Masking
    - Traditional sheet masks
    - Gel masks
    - Novel biomaterials I.e. polysaccharides
  - Developing a customisable mask system (video lecture access)
  - Combining technologies into skincare routines
    - Radiofrequency protocol
    - Skin hydration analyzers
    - Copper peel microdermabrasion
  - Download skincare planner templates for client/personal use

SECTION 2
Section 2 is when we lay the groundwork for in-depth understanding of cosmeceuticals. You will first learn about the

framework dermatologists use to assess effectiveness of active ingredients before moving on to a discussion on the core cosmeceuticals you must know. In our discussion of the retinoid family for instance, you will acquire specialised skills dermatologists use to monitor, prevent and treat side effects such as retinoid dermatitis—this includes advanced skin cycling techniques, how to check for skin barrier damage and identifying early warning signs. We will then cover in a comprehensive manner the other key cosmeceuticals to know such as natural moisturising factors for barrier repair, synthetic, botanical antioxidants, retinol alternatives such as sea buckthorn, bakuchiol and oligopeptides. You will also learn about novel actives used for the treatment of hyperpigmentation such as bacterial ferment extracts as well as tyrosinase inhibitors .

All these will be recapped individually in mini-segments when we introduce case studies from my own skincare line—as I spill the formulation secrets behind each best-selling product.

The section concludes with notes on functional dermatology which puts all you have learnt in context; you will understand the critical role skincare plays in altering the skin exposome— the most accurate skin aging model based on the science behind inflammaging. There are also some finer points we will cover such as tailored actives with quasi-drug effects when it comes to treatment of acne, sensitive skin conditions like eczema and also how to assess efficacy of eye creams. I will also be clarifying misconceptions about the use of fragrances in skincare.

- Introduction to cosmeceuticals
- Function, subtypes, skin penetration, clinical studies
- Synthetic cosmeceuticals vs botanicals
- Core syllabus
  - Master the retinoid family
    - Skin cycling techniques
    - Respect the barrier

- Warning signs
  - Natural Moisturising Factors (NMFs)
  - Hyaluronic acid
  - Polyglutamic acid
  - Green Tea extract (EGCG)
  - Vitamin C
  - Niacinamide
  - Ceramides
  - Retinoid alternatives
  - Resveratrol
  - Peptides
  - Hydroquinone
  - Hydroquinone alternatives: kojic acid, arbutin
  - Salmon Roe DNA
  - Soy isoflavones
- Concepts in functional dermatology
- Skin exposome and inflammaging
- Advanced actives for specific skin concerns
  - Eczema/sensitive skin
    - Fermented functional actives
  - Acne
  - Anti-aging
  - Eye creams
  - Notes on the use of fragrances in cosmeceuticals

SECTION 3

By Section 3, you are ready to understand how custom formulation works. In the accompanying video workshop, I'll take you behind the scenes of my apothecary, where I personally coach our pharmacy technicians on the art and science of custom compounding. You will receive a complete step by step guide to formulating skincare cocktails, including my list of 7 key cosmeceuticals you should include that sets you up for success.

To put what you have learnt into context, I will cover 2 key frameworks:

We first go in-depth into the Skincare Plus Accelerate Program, a clinical protocol I developed that maximises the efficiency of skincare routines by intentionally breaching the skin barrier—without damaging the protective wall.

Second, we will do a case study on what I consider the key formula to master—the gold standard anti-aging serum formulated without traditional cosmeceuticals such as retinol or acids. Instead, we will apply our newly acquired knowledge on retinol alternatives to create a highly effective anti-aging serum formula for universal skin types.

Ethnobotanical dictionary:
- ○ Overview
- Principles of ethnopharmacology
- Application to modern cosmetic formulation
- Guide to formulating skincare cocktails: how customised formulas work
- ○ Best practices for compounding
- Dr.TWL Skincare Plus Accelerate Program
- Case study of gold standard anti-aging serum with retinol alternatives

SECTION 4

We now jump right into the learning methods, backed by neuroscience—incorporating both visual and auditory tools—that will be key to your mastery of every single skincare ingredient you will ever come across. The database of skincare actives and cosmeceuticals is ever-evolving—as the highly competitive aesthetic industry churns out more scientific research; it seems almost impossible to keep up. What I have done for you in this course is to compile a list of cosmeceutical actives identified from an analysis of over 300 prominent cosmetic brands; as the basis to jumpstart your lifelong learning journey as skincare expert/beauty entrepreneur. I will be introducing the 2 methods of learning I have found most effective—flash cards and concept maps. I have prepared for you additional learning material in the form of digital flashcards as well as bonus blank templates for concept maps within the workbook itself. I have also included audio guides and bullet style lecture notes as learning aides (register at https://www.twlskin.com/dictionary/ for access).

2 Systems of Learning
☐ Must-know actives curated from analysis of over 300 skincare brands/product formulations
☐ Bullet style lecture notes

- Set A ingredients
  - Flash learning method
- Set B ingredients
  - Flash cards with audio guide
- Which is my best learning style?

SECTION 5: Course Workbook
Next, we take a breather—in the form of a fun workbook I have designed for you to create your own skincare bible. You will find blueprints and protocols designed infographic-style that serves as a visual recap of all that we have covered in the earlier sections. Each page has margin space intentionally demarcated for you to scribble your own notes as well as to compile lists of actives you come across. Not forgetting speed guides for common skin disorders and my home facial protocols that will serve as a handy reference for your career as a skin expert.

- Cleansing
- Toning (updated perspective)
- Moisturiser layering techniques
  - Serums
  - Lotions/emulsions
  - Cream

- ○ Mist
- Skin treatments
  - ○ Exfoliation
  - ○ Masking

Speed guides
- Acne
- Pigmentation
- Sensitive skin
- Rosacea
- Perioral dermatitis
- Dull skin

Facial protocols
- Instant glow facials
- 7-Phase medifacial system

SECTION 6: Skin Expert Mastery

We are now at the very last section of the course, which is when we conclude with the review and consolidation stage. I have prepared here 2 styles of lecture notes: bullet-style and prose style upon which you will create your very own learning materials using the techniques we have gone through in the earlier chapters. You will utilise concept maps, worksheets and flashcard templates in the workbook to create your own summaries of what you have learnt. These will be important references as you continue on your lifelong learning journey—I encourage you to continually review and add on to your set of notes; this exercise will help cement your knowledge base—a critical skill set for a skincare professional.

Review/consolidation
- Concept maps
- Mind maps
- Worksheets
- Flashcards
- Checklists

BONUS LEARNING TOOL: CHECKLIST GUIDE

Use this checklist to guide your learning. Checklists are an underrated learning tool—they serve as a form of reinforcement which is essential to the learning process. They are especially helpful for keeping track, staying motivated and as summaries of what you have learnt. Bearing in mind that these are merely sample templates to give you an idea of how to create your own learning checklists—you can continue to build on this.

Check against each box when you are done with each subtopic. After completing each subsection, jot down in the space provided some notes to help jog your memory. Recommended revision/learning timelines provided as a guide.

1. INTRODUCTION

The importance of learning how to learn. The way our minds consolidates information follows a certain timeline. The note taking space is best utilised this way:
- Write down only keywords
- Keywords serve to jog your memory of the entire concept
- Analyse the material when studying to find similarities and differences
- Write down your analysis rather than copying wholesale as per rote learning
- Important timelines for long term memory
  - DAY 1, 2 (keywords)
  - WEEK 1, 2 (make comparison tables based on your analysis)
- Limited space due to publishing constraints, if you require more writing space, add on with post-it stickers
- ***TIP: Get the accompanying course notebook to create your own mini skincare bible with this method***
- ☐ How to navigate the book
- ☐ Tips on maximising your learning experience
- ☐ Guide to learning tools for skincare ingredients

☐ Flash card system, charts, mind-map

MY GOALS:

2. SKINCARE ROUTINE STEPS
☐ Definitions to know
☐ Mechanism of action
☐ Applied skin anatomy & physiology

MY NOTES (ON FIRST DAY OF STUDY)

MY NOTES (ON SECOND DAY OF REVISION)

MY NOTES (1 WEEK LATER)

MY NOTES (1 MONTH LATER)

3. CORE SKINCARE INGREDIENTS ACCORDING TO PRODUCT/STEP

- ☐ Cleansers
- ☐ Toners
- ☐ Serums
- ☐ Moisturiser
- ☐ Face mist
- ☐ Face essence
- ☐ Face masks
- ☐ Exfoliants
- ☐ Textiles

MY NOTES (ON FIRST DAY OF STUDY)

MY NOTES (ON SECOND DAY OF REVISION)

MY NOTES (1 WEEK LATER)

MY NOTES (1 MONTH LATER)

SECTION A: IN-DEPTH MASTERY

4. COSMECEUTICALS
    ☐ Definitions

- ☐ Scientific basis
- ☐ Core syllabus
- ☐ Active ingredients to know

MY NOTES (ON FIRST DAY OF STUDY)

MY NOTES (ON SECOND DAY OF REVISION)

MY NOTES (1 WEEK LATER)

MY NOTES (1 MONTH LATER)

5. ETHNOBOTANICAL DICTIONARY

☐ Important plant actives to know

MY NOTES (ON FIRST DAY OF STUDY)

MY NOTES (ON SECOND DAY OF REVISION)

MY NOTES (1 WEEK LATER)

MY NOTES (1 MONTH LATER)

6. SYNTHETICS
- ☐ Biomimetic actives
- ☐ Application to skin physiology & structure

MY NOTES (ON FIRST DAY OF STUDY)

MY NOTES (ON SECOND DAY OF REVISION)

MY NOTES (1 WEEK LATER)

MY NOTES (1 MONTH LATER)

7. SPOT TREATMENT
- ☐ Science of targeted skin treatment
- ☐ OTC actives
- ☐ Prescription actives

MY NOTES (ON FIRST DAY OF STUDY)

MY NOTES (ON SECOND DAY OF REVISION)

MY NOTES (1 WEEK LATER)

MY NOTES (1 MONTH LATER)

SELF-TESTING & KNOWLEDGE APPLICATION (FLASHCARD SYSTEM)

8. SKINCARE FOR SENSITIVE SKIN & ECZEMA
   ☐ Focus on actives

☐ Flashcard Set A

9. SKINCARE FOR ACNE, ACNE SCARS
☐ Focus on actives
☐ Flashcard Set B

10. SKINCARE FOR ROSACEA
☐ Focus on actives
☐ Flashcard Set C

11. SKINCARE FOR HYPERPIGMENTATION
☐ Focus on actives
☐ Flashcard Set D

12. SKINCARE FOR PHOTOAGING
☐ Focus on actives
☐ Flashcard Set E

SECTION B: CONSOLIDATION & MEMORY TECHNIQUES (MIND MAP)

In this section, you will create your own 1-page learning map for all 5 core modules we have covered in Section C using the Dr.TWL method:
☐ Skeleton: framework for quick recap
☐ Color coding: speed reading trick
☐ Organic lines & squiggles: for neuroplasticity
☐ Details: fill in the fine details
☐ Self-testing

SECTION 1

Foundational Skincare Routines

download textbook resources and printables*

*https://www.twlskin.com/dictionary/ register account and receive download access in your welcome email

CHAPTER THREE

Skincare Routine Steps Foundational Course Material

Master the Science & Art of Skincare Routines

The complete foundational course with each step broken down based on ideal product formulation, skin science and tips on practical application. Learn how to tailor specific steps in the skincare routine to suit different skin types and choose active ingredients to tackle skin concerns such as acne, hyperpigmentation, oily skin, wrinkles and skin sensitivity.

By the end of this chapter you should be able to master the following in the context of every skincare step. Use this checklist as your revision guide.

Learning goals:

- ☐ Learn how to build a purposeful skincare routine for yourself/your client
- ☐ Navigating different options available
- ☐ Choose actives tailored to individual concerns

Skincare Fundamentals

The following is applicable for both day and night skincare routine steps. For night time skincare, you may omit sunscreen, and also add on application of a sheet mask and eye cream. Targeted treatment of spots such as with prescription creams containing retinol/retinoids or hydroquinone should also typically be applied at night in order to reduce the risk of photosensitivity.

Why skincare layering is a must for all skin types

A common question that's asked is if the use of multiple skincare products can be avoided. Here's why you won't find an all-in-1 skincare product that can replace the need for skincare layering.

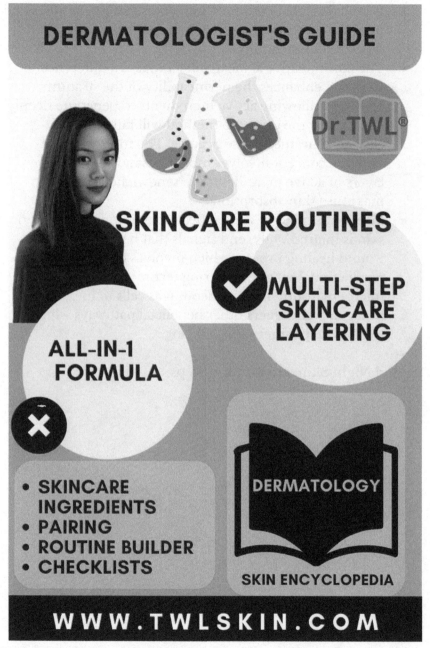

You can't get the same benefits without layering skincare because

- It's the dose that counts. When you separate the steps and products, you are effectively increasing the dose delivered in each step
- The cummulative skincare effect makes a difference. Layering enhances the permeability of the stratum corneum, allowing active ingredients to penetrate deeply. This is why the one-step method will fail. Also why cleanse-tone-moisturise is passé. The most effective skincare concept involves moisture sandwiching, when layers of active ingredients are sandwiched in order to maximise skin absorption.
- Mimics the natural wound healing environment. When skin is injured, cells send signals that help kickstart the wound healing process which involves collagen production. Using the layering technique recreates this microenvironment that encourages cells to increase collagen and triggers other beneficial pathways which work to help target signs of aging.

Day and Night Skincare Routine Steps

SKINCARE ROUTINE STEPS

 Dr.TWL® **DOUBLE CLEANSING**

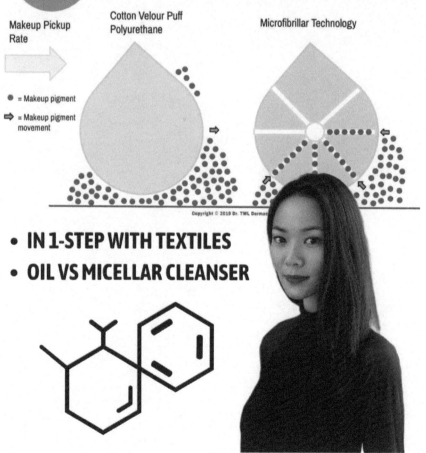

- IN 1-STEP WITH TEXTILES
- OIL VS MICELLAR CLEANSER

Double cleansing

Double cleansing is a 2 step process which involves first removing makeup and sunscreen, followed by a second cleanse. The first cleanse focuses on oil soluble pigments, sebum, grime whereas the second step is focused on removing the residue. The primary goal of cleansing is to restore the healthy skin microbiome—a balance of good and bad germs. However, it is equally important to respect the skin barrier. An ideal double cleansing regimen should not strip the skin of moisture. Rather, it should cleanse skin and restore moisture levels.

SKINCARE ROUTINE STEPS FOR SENSITIVE SKIN

Dr.TWL®

• GENTLE MAKEUP REMOVAL

☐ Learn how to build a purposeful skincare routine for yourself/your client

Cleansing is the single most important step in any skincare regimen which is also the most misunderstood—the goal is not to degrease or cleanse away bacteria. Rather it is a step that helps to

- rebalance sebum levels (remove excess)
- maintain a healthy microbiome (balance of good and bad bacteria

When it comes to microorganisms, it is the competition between the good and bad that determines if a harmful skin condition such as infections occur. For instance, in the case of acne, it is not merely bacteria that drives the disease. Cutibacterium acnes is present on healthy and acne-prone skin, but it is only in the latter group that it drives excess inflammation that leads to comedone (whitehead/blackhead) formation.

☐ Navigating different options available

The three main categories of facial cleansers are:
- Foaming surfactants
- Oil/emulsion "milk" cleansers
- Micellar cleansers
- Foaming surfactants

SKINCARE ROUTINE STEP 1
MAKEUP REMOVAL

Dr.TWL®

- **MICELLAR FORMULATION**
- **HYDROPHOBIC (WATER-HATING) AND HYDROPHILIC (WATER-LOVING)**
- **PURE OIL CLEANSERS**
- **MILK CLEANSER**

Choose amino acid or botanical-based surfactants. Honey, soy and botanicals which contain saponins (soap-like compounds) are natural emulsifiers, which means it creates a foamy texture. Foam cleansers are preferred for those with combination/oily skin but care must be exercised to avoid those high in laureth sulfates (sodium or ammonium) as these chemical surfactants dehydrate skin and disrupt the skin barrier. The key here to note is that virtually all foaming facial cleansers contain laureth sulfates, even those which are dermatologist recommended for sensitive skin—it is the concentration and the formulation that matters.

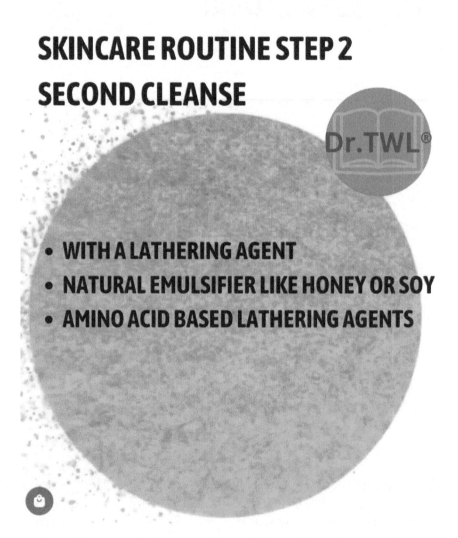

SKINCARE ROUTINE STEP 2
SECOND CLEANSE

- WITH A LATHERING AGENT
- NATURAL EMULSIFIER LIKE HONEY OR SOY
- AMINO ACID BASED LATHERING AGENTS

For instance, our pharmacy's Miel Honey Cleanser contains only a low dose of laureth sulfates compared to commercial cleansers yet it retains remarkable foaming properties—because of the addition of honey which is a natural emulsifier. It is ultra-gentle and leaves skin feeling hydrated because it contains other actives designed to repair the skin barrier while cleansing skin. The Honey Cleanser is formulated as an ideal foaming cleanser should include hydrating ingredients such as natural moisturising factors, glycerin and anti-inflammatory botanicals like Artemisia.

- Oil/emulsion "milk" cleansers
- Micellar cleansers

Both are designed for efficient removal of makeup, often referred to as the first step of the double cleanse. The commonest match for skin types is: sensitive/combination skin—milk cleansers; combination/oily skin—-micellar cleansers. In my dermatology practice however, I find that almost all micellar cleansers cause skin irritation/dryness regardless of the brand. For all problem skin, including acne-prone oily skin types, micellar formulations involve increased contact with chemical surfactants and also friction that is induced when a textile (cotton pad usually) is used to physically wipe off the makeup residue. This is why I stick to recommending milk cleansers for ALL SKIN TYPES, in the context of the double cleansing model. The Le Lait Milk Cleanser includes additional camphor which has a soothing and calming effect on the skin barrier. The oil in water texture means that it leaves a sticky residue on skin which further acts as a protective barrier that prevents skin irritation/dryness with the second cleanse.

☐ Choose actives tailored to individual concerns
Here are some active ingredients included in cleansers which are recommended for treatment of problem skin:
- Artemesia vulgaris (anti-inflammatory, anti-flaking)
- Honey/soy (natural emulsifiers, natural antibacterial effect)

- Amino acids/Natural moisturising factors (serine, histidine)
- Humectants (glycerin)
- Camphor (calming, soothing)

Skincare Routine Step 1 Makeup removal
There are two options for makeup removers. The first is a micellar formulation. The second, an oil-based cleanser or an emulsion, sometimes known as a "milk" cleanser. I will go through the pros and cons of each but first let us define some terms.

Micellar water works by hydrophobic (water-hating) and hydrophilic (water-loving) properties of a micelle. The makeup residue is attracted to the water-hating aspect, this is best thought of as a ball that is wrapped up which continues to roll on skin grabbing the residual pigment and dirt. To remove the ball which is a micelle, you use a cotton pad. Friction or rubbing is inevitable and this can be harsh for sensitive skin.

Pure oil cleansers are often too greasy, my choice is an emulsion or a milk cleanser. Milk cleansers are oil in water formulations, the oil component dissolves makeup pigments and removes excess sebum. The "like for like" principle here is that oil soluble pigments are dissolved in a similar substance—an oil in water emulsion.

The benefits of an emulsion are that it is less greasy than pure oil formulations. It is also effective as a humectant if formulated with moisturising ingredients. When you physically rub off the makeup on a cotton pad, the oil component protects your skin. It acts as a barrier between the cotton pad and skin, hence reducing friction unlike with micellar solution.

Skincare Routine Step 2 Second cleanse with a lathering agent

This step is best paired with a natural emulsifier like honey or soy, or similar botanical emulsifiers. The process of generating a foam can help improve the cleansing experience, so users feel thoroughly cleansed. However, using chemical lathering agents like laureth sulfates can strip the skin of natural moisture and cause dysregulation of oil production. This can sometimes lead to the oily dehydrated skin phenomenon. Amino acid based lathering agents are also gentler on skin.

Skincare Routine Step 3 Serum Application

SKINCARE ROUTINE STEP 3

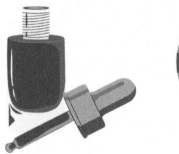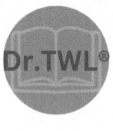

• SERUM APPLICATION

• MULTI-WEIGHTED MOLECULAR HYALURONIC ACID
• STABILISED FORMS OF VITAMIN C
• L-ASCORBIC ACID, SODIUM ASCORBYL PHOSPHATE OR MAGNESIUM ASCORBYL PHOSPHATE

☐ Learn how to build a purposeful skincare routine for yourself/your client

Serums must be taught as must-haves in a basic skincare routine. It's not an optional step. The reason is because it makes a critical difference in skin quality vs just using a moisturiser alone. There are 2 main factors involved:

- Concentration of actives is higher in serums
- Certain actives like vitamin C are only stable in serum form
- Hyaluronic acid is an example of an active that has a dose-dependent effect i.e. the higher the dose the greater the efficacy—which makes serums the ideal vehicle for delivery

☐ Navigating different options available
Here's what I would recommend in terms of serums for

Basic skincare routines:
- Vitamin C
- Hyaluronic acid

These are the must-haves in a foundational skincare routine. Vitamin C boosts the skin's natural antioxidant reserve which is an essential part of healthy skin functions i.e. collagen production, fighting free radical damage etc. Hyaluronic acid is part of a set of molecules known as natural moisturising factors that help skin regulate moisture levels and maintain healthy barrier functioning.

Advanced skincare routines:
- Ferulic acid
- Resveratrol
- Peptides
- Botanical actives for anti-inflammatory effect

Details of each are covered in the ingredient dictionary subsection.

☐ Choose actives tailored to individual concerns
Serums are an effective method of topical delivery and can be thought of as adjunct treatments for various skin conditions. They are the most effective way cosmeceuticals (AKA quasi-drugs) are delivered to skin. The actives are chosen for the ability to penetrate the stratum corneum and also have clearly defined cell targets—so we know exactly how cosmeceutical

49

actives work. Here are some actives ideally delivered in serum form, especially when paired, possess therapeutic effects for the following skin conditions:

- Acne
  - Vitamin C + Camellia sinensis (Green tea extract EGCG)
  - Antioxidant boost with this pair reduces lipid peroxidation in acne-prone individuals
  - This creates an environment that discourages growth of acne causing bacteria
  - Lipid oxidation occurs when sebum on skin is oxidised by environmental O2, which causes increased inflammation
  - This inflammation drives whitehead/blackhead formation i.e. comedone formation
- Rosacea
  - Gingko biloba
  - Camellia sinensis (Green tea extract EGCG)
  - Aloe vera
    - Aloe, aloe emodin, aletinic acid, choline, choline salicylate
  - Allantoin (comfrey plant)
- Eczema/sensitive skin
  - Hyaluronic acid
  - Polyglutamic acid
  - Natural moisturising factors i.e. free amino acids that strengthen the skin barrier
  - Ceramides (most efficiently incorporated in cream form although also possible in serums)

Serums deliver high concentrations of water soluble actives such as hyaluronic acid and vitamin C. The reason why an all-in-1 skincare cream does not work well is because the entire process of skincare layering creates a moist skin healing environment, which is not achieved with the traditional cleanse-tone-moisturise regimen. Important skincare actives to look for:

Multi-weighted molecular hyaluronic acid has benefits because it can act on multiple layers of skin and activate different targets.

Stabilised forms of vitamin C include L-ascorbic acid, sodium ascorbyl phosphate or magnesium ascorbyl phosphate. L-ascorbic acid is acidic and can cause irritation to sensitive skin. For this reason, I usually recommend vitamin C serum formulations based on the latter ascorbyl phosphate compounds. Sodium ascorbyl phosphate also is effective at lower concentrations.

The effects of vitamin C are as follows:
- Skin brightening
- Antioxidant environment to fight free radical stress caused by environmental damage (UV, air pollution)
- Treatment of acne (reduces skin inflammation by inhibiting lipid peroxidation in acne-prone, oily skin)

The power twins: hyaluronic acid and vitamin C
These are the foundational concepts you should familiarise with. We will revisit these 2 actives in greater detail in the ingredient dictionary section.

SKINCARE ROUTINE STEP 4

 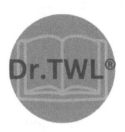

• EMULSION/LOTION

- **LIGHTWEIGHT**
- **OIL-IN-WATER TEXTURE**
- **FEELS COMFORTABLE ON SKIN THROUGHOUT THE DAY**
- **QUICKLY ABSORBED**

The equivalent of a day moisturising cream is a lotion formula which is lightweight, feels comfortable on skin throughout the day and is quickly absorbed. The oil-in-water texture is the ideal day moisturiser because it maintains effectiveness while reducing any uncomfortable sticky sensations. Some important active ingredients like ceramides and also water soluble actives like plant antioxidants show increased absorption when in an oil vehicle. The oil-in-water formula is hence ideal.

☐ Learn how to build a purposeful skincare routine for yourself/your client

When discussing emulsion/lotion type moisturisers, the focus should be on

- Cosmetic acceptability when applied under makeup i.e. there should not be pilling
- Non-greasy/sticky texture is especially important for those living in humid climates
- These are ideal for combination/oily skin types. Dry skin types should consider using a cream moisturiser.
- Technique of application to reduce skin pilling
  - Damp skin right after cleansing this increases absorption
  - Allow 1-2 minutes for full absorption, massage excess in neck/décolleté area before applying foundation/concealer

☐ Navigating different options available

- For those with extremely greasy skin, they may feel more comfortable skipping moisturisers altogether. While the traditional advice has been to always use a moisturiser, even if you have greasy skin—it needs to be interpreted in today's context of cosmceutical skincare. Moisturisers can also come in the form of face mists and serums, which are inherently water-based and also contain skin barrier repairing actives such as hyaluronic acid, polyglutamic acid and glycerin. All of which are considered effective moisturisers and can help to regulate oil production. In the case of oily-dehydrated skin, the problem usually is with
  - Overcleansing i.e. with harsh astringent cleansers
  - Use of acne creams that irritate skin i.e. benzoyl peroxide

      o   Not using serum/water-based moisturisers to help rebalance sebum production

This checklist can help you determine if there are any mistakes in your client's skincare routine.

☐ Choose actives tailored to individual concerns

Emulsions or lotions are highly versatile carriers of cosmeceutical actives that directly treat skin conditions. Our pharmacy's prescriptive series specifically utilises an oil-in-water vehicle to deliver skincare actives for concerns such as hyperpigmentation, acne and rosacea. Refer to the custom formulation section for details on how cosmeceuticals can be implemented in emulsions as targeted treatments.

SKINCARE ROUTINE STEP 5

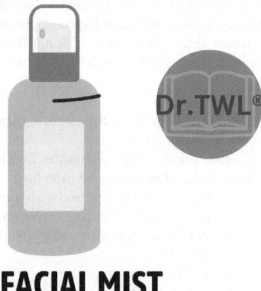

FACIAL MIST

- **HYALURONIC**
- **POLYGLUTAMIC ACID**
- **HYGROSCOPIC MOLECULES**
- **PREVENTS TRANSEPIDERMAL WATER LOSS**

Many consider this to be optional, but it is actually a key step to increase penetration of all the skincare actives. The concept of sheet masking is really wet occlusion therapy which means applying products on damp skin and creating a moist microclimate enhances skincare absorption. The outermost layer of skin known as the stratum corneum naturally impedes absorption of skincare actives, enhancing permeability is hence an important principle in effective skincare routine steps.

The ideal facial mist should contain hyaluronic and polyglutamic acid, as these are hygroscopic molecules that help trap moisture under the surface of skin. Ultimately this prevents transepidermal water loss, which is a key problem in dehydrated skin.

☐ Learn how to build a purposeful skincare routine for yourself/your client

Facial mists are highly versatile. Besides providing on-the-go skin hydration, facial mists can be used for

- Cleansing when paired with a micellar textile i.e. microfibre makeup remover pad
- Part of the moisture sandwich model of layering skincare
- Used as makeup primer
- Sets makeup
- Aerosol method improves even skin distribution—preferred cosmetic effect vs cream/lotion textures which can appear cakey

☐ Navigating different options available

There are 2 main categories you should be aware of:

- Thermal spring water-based facial mists
  - These were what I call the classic face mists which touted the benefits of thermal spring water with its mineral rich content for sensitive skin. The downside is that it is after all just water, which evaporates. The additional minerals have been proven in studies to exert a calming effect on sensitive skin conditions such as eczema and is likely to be beneficial for overall skin cell functioning.
- K-beauty style facial mists

- Considered the most efficient types of face mists
- Contain a mixture of water soluble humectants
- Tested for staying power on skin i.e. does not evaporate as per thermal water type face mists
- Optical effects contribute to the highly coveted glowing, glass-skin complexion

☐ Choose actives tailored to individual concerns

Face mists are ideal for efficient delivery of a synergistic blend of multiple botanicals and synthetics in a water vehicle. For instance the Mineral Booster from our pharmacy boasts over 17 different actives from amino acids, botanicals (discussed in ethnobotanical dictionary) and traditional humectants. Further customisation can be done by adding water-soluble actives such as

- Papain/bromelain enzyme peels
  - For oily, acne-prone skin
- Centella asiatica
  - For hyperpigmentation
- Grape seed oil
  - Stabilises skin, tightens pores
- Yeast peptide
  - Antiaging, brightening
- Green tea
  - Acne, pigmentation, scars
- Arnica montana
  - Redness, flaking
  - Anti-inflammatory

Small doses of 0.01-0.05% of each are effective when incorporated in a standard base of a facial mist—based on clinical experience, though the doses are small, the results are highly satisfactory to patients.

SKINCARE ROUTINE STEP 6

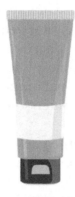
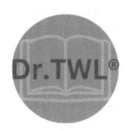

SUNSCREEN (ALWAYS APPLIED LAST)

- **SPF 50, BROAD SPECTRUM**
- **COMPATIBLE WITH NATURAL SKIN COLOR (FOR ASIANS AND OTHER SKIN OF COLOR INDIVIDUALS, A WHITE-CAST IS UNPLEASANT AND WILL AFFECT COMPLIANCE. I.E. INSUFFICIENT PRODUCT USE CAN LEAD TO LOWER SUNPROTECTION)**
- **LIGHTWEIGHT, EASILY ABSORBED, COSMETICALLY APPEALING TOR REAPPLY**

For the day skincare routine, I will usually wait 2-3 minutes for the facial mist to fully absorb before applying sunscreen. The ideal sunscreen formula should possess the following properties:

- SPF 50, broad spectrum
- Compatible with natural skin color (for asians and other skin of color individuals, a white-cast is unpleasant and will affect compliance. I.e. insufficient product use can lead to lower sunprotection)
- Lightweight, easily absorbed, cosmetically appealing tor reapply

☐ Learn how to build a purposeful skincare routine for yourself/your client

Sunscreens are a non-negotiable aspect of skincare routines. However, one must bear in mind the following

- Sunscreen does aggravate certain dermatological conditions
  - Acne, oily skin types may find their symptoms worsening with particularly greasy sunscreens
  - Perioral dermatitis also known as a hormonal acne lookalike is actually specifically triggered by application of sunscreen
  - Sensitive skin/eczema will be aggravated by sunscreen application
    - Most sufferers also have sweat allergy which is why when they sweat, itch and stinging results
    - Symptoms are pronounced with chemical sunscreens i.e. when sweat mixes with chemical sunscreen components

☐ Navigating different options available

It is critical that we present the various options of sun protection to the client
- Traditional physical sunscreen

These are based on zinc oxide, titanium dioxide which are ideal for those with sensitive skin/eczema. However, they also tend to be rather cakey in appearance and match skin tones poorly, especially when it comes to skin of color.
- Chemical sunscreen

Chemical sunscreens include avobenzones, octinoxates and oxybenzones. These are usually combined with physical sunscreen components in a broad spectrum sunscreen that confers broad protection against UVA and UVB rays. UVA are regarded as the most damaging when it comes to photoaging, whereas UVB rays account for skin immunosuppression and is blamed for the production of cancerous cells.
- UPF Textiles

In my paper "Diagnostic and management considerations of maskne in the era of covid-19" published in the Journal of the American Academy of Dermatology, I introduced the concept of biofunctional textiles that simultaneously treat the skin microbiome and also over UV protection with a UPF 50 rating. These ratings are traditionally applied to sun protective clothing. When worn as a face mask, this can also be a useful intervention for those who do not tolerate sunscreens due to any of the above dermatological conditions.
- Oral sunscreen

Based on polypodium leucotomos, oral sunscreens slow down the rate of sunburn by boosting the skin's antioxidant reserve. Generally recommended as an adjunct to topical sunscreens and not used alone.

☐ Choose actives tailored to individual concerns
Additional photoprotection

Multifunctional sunscreens are now regarded as the gold standard formulations. Essentially, the latest research sunprotection goes beyond traditional sunscreen agents—the key is in the array of botanicals that boost the skin's natural antioxidant capacity. This means that when UV rays generate surface free radicals, these are rapidly neutralised before it causes skin damage.

Anti-wrinkle peptides

Sunscreens are also the ideal vehicle to incorporate novel botox alternatives such as acetyl hexapeptide and oligopeptides.

Plant adaptogens

Desert plants like aloe and purslane boast an unusually high content of bioactives that enhance skin resilience i.e. the ability to fight off damaging free radical stress.

SKINCARE ROUTINE STEP 7

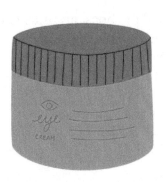
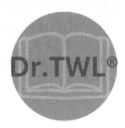

• KEY ACTIVES IN EYE CREAMS

- **4% NIACINAMIDE (SKIN BARRIER REPAIR AND SKIN LIGHTENING)**
- **PHYTOCERAMIDES (ANTI-INFLAMMATORY, SKIN BARRIER REPAIR)**
- **OLIGOPEPTIDES (ANTI-WRINKLE EFFECT)**

For daytime, oily and combination skin types will do well with the day moisturiser lotion alone. However dry skin types should use a moisturiser cream formula containing ceramides both day and night. In the case of a day skincare routine, the cream should be used before sunscreen. Ideally, it should be left on to be absorbed for 3-5 minutes to minimise sunscreen or makeup pilling.

For night time, all skin types including oily and combination skin will benefit from using a ceramide based moisturiser. It is also important to use a targeted eye cream to reduce fine lines and wrinkles. The key actives in eye creams can include
- 4% Niacinamide (skin barrier repair and skin lightening)
- Phytoceramides (anti-inflammatory, skin barrier repair)
- Oligopeptides (anti-wrinkle effect)

These actives are covered in detail in the ingredient subsection.

Night Skincare Routine Step: Targeted treatment
Actives like prescription retinoids, hydroquinone and OTC retinol are to be used at night. This is to reduce the risk of sun sensitivity. Generally, retinoids can be used over an entire area, avoiding the part around the eyes and lips as the skin is more sensitive. Hydroquinone is a bleaching agent which should only be used on pigmented spots or as per physician's directions. For details of targeted treatment with OTC cosmeceuticals, ***refer to Chapter Ten on custom formulation best practices.***

MODIFICATIONS OF SKINCARE ROUTINES WITH HOME DEVICES
- **2-STEP**
- **3-STEP**

Back when I was a teen in the nineties, cleanse-tone-moisturise was the mantra of the day. By the time I became a dermatologist in the 2010s, there were serums, face oils and sheet masks. Today, Korean skincare routines have exploded in popularity, thanks to K-beauty's ambassadors—the K-Pop stars and the glass skin they sport. The elusive glowing skin popularised by K-beauty when K-pop fever swept the globe also sent those in the scientific community investigating. Soon, dermatologists also realised that the glow they sported was for real. The standard skincare routine now averages about 5 steps, though I wager the ideal one that incorporates all the elements of skincare layering stands at 9 steps at the least.

It's important to take into account individual preferences when tailoring a skincare routine—truth be told, most would find the idea of a 2-3 step routine appealing. Advancements in skincare devices have made possible integration of office technology into home skincare routines. The result? Steps that promise professional results.

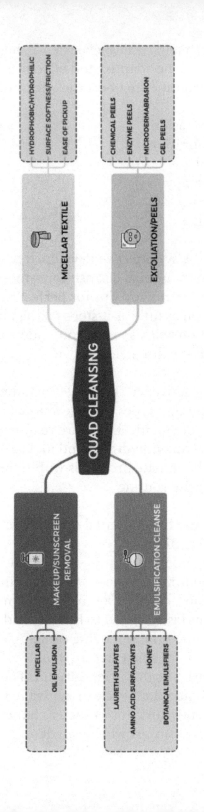

QUAD CLEANSING

MICELLAR TEXTILE
- HYDROPHOBIC/HYDROPHILIC
- SURFACE SOFTNESS/FRICTION
- EASE OF PICKUP

EXFOLIATION/PEELS
- CHEMICAL PEELS
- ENZYME PEELS
- MICRODERMABRASION
- GEL PEELS

MAKEUP/SUNSCREEN REMOVAL
- MICELLAR
- OIL EMULSION

EMULSIFICATION CLEANSE
- LAURETH SULFATES
- AMINO ACID SURFACTANTS
- HONEY
- BOTANICAL EMULSFIERS

Based on my research and clinical experience, here are the top technologies which can be adapted and effectively incorporated into home skincare routines to boost the effects of cosmeceutical skincare:

- Microdermabrasion
- Hydrodermabrasion
- Microcurrent
- LED light therapy
- Radiofrequency
- Sonic cleansing

I've compiled here the systems I've developed based on modifications of the traditional cleanse-tone-moisturise skincare routine steps. These are my top tips for perfecting skincare routine steps based on as little as 2-steps taking under 3 minutes each time. This section will also help you understand why I have omitted toners from the discussion above.

They are tailored for universal skin types including dry, combination and oily skin types, with additional tips on how to identify your skin type. An ideal skincare regimen can repair your skin barrier, leaving it hydrated and looking healthy. But first, we begin with the innate problems within the cleanse-tone-moisturise routine

- **Cleansing is the fundamental skincare routine step that must never be missed**

Single step cleansing does not completely remove makeup and pollutants. If pressed for time, those with dry skin should just use an emulsion cleanser. This is a milky solution rather than a lathering cleanser, and is designed to hydrate and repair the skin barrier at the same time removing oil soluble makeup pigments. Those with dry skin can skip double cleansing and avoid micellar cleansers as this dries out skin. Those with combination skin should double cleanse, ideally with a lathering cleanser based on gentle surfactants such as honey and soy, instead of SLS-laden cleansers which can damage the skin barrier. Those with oily skin should use a hydrodermabrasion or microdermabrasion device with their cleanser, this will increase the effectiveness of the cleansing skincare steps.

- **Toning is an outdated concept—Korean skincare routine steps replace toners with hydrating facial mists, lotions and essences that repair the skin barrier**

Don't use any toners that contain acids or alcohol. In the past, toners were regarded as astringents which dry out skin. This is a no-no for sensitive and dry skin types. K-beauty toners are more like facial mists/essences. These contain botanicals like rice bran extract, broccoli extract, purslane that are anti-inflammatory. Look for moisturising actives like glycerin, hyaluronic acid and polyglutamic acid.

This is based on the latest science about the skin barrier. Importantly, dermatologists have discovered that even those with oily skin can have a dehydrated skin barrier. The key function of a toner is to rebalance, and that does not mean to remove surface oil. Rather the korean beauty approach is to incorporate synergistic extracts which help to create the ideal skin microenvironment. For those with oily skin, water alone has an astringent effect—the same reason why wet compresses are recommended by dermatologists for oozing wounds, and why your skin feels refreshed by water cleansing. Alcohol always damages the skin barrier and must be avoided.

Some toners incorporate salicylic acid and glycolic acids, but as leave-on skincare products, they should be avoided if you have dry skin. For combination and oily skin users, it can be helpful but some users also develop skin sensitivity after some time. Enzyme peels based on bromelain and bakuchiol are gentler and are used in K-beauty formulations.

- **Moisturising is key in any skincare regimen—here are my modifications to the traditional skincare routine steps based on K-beauty**

This is the second most important step in a skincare regimen after cleansing. If you adopt the same approach of skipping toner and replacing it with a facial mist instead, you are already hydrating your skin. However, to repair the skin barrier fully, layering is an important concept. Skincare layering means to use products in a sequence to increase effectiveness of the ingredients and actives. Typically, serums go first, followed by lotions, emulsions and moisturising creams and mists. This is based on the texture of each skincare produc. The main principle being the most lightweight ingredients go first. As a dermatologist, I have been recommending the following for my patients with different skin types:

How a new approach to skincare routines can work on harnessing skin resilience
Skin resilience is about strengthening the skin barrier and enhancing the skin's immune functions

Dry skin: moisturise with serums, lotions, facial mists but if you have only time/patience for 1 step, use a palm-sized amount of moisturiser each time and allow it to fully absorb before leaving the house. Just massage any residue onto your neck and body. Repeat at night, this is the concept of a "sleeping mask" which really is just a moisturiser..

Combination skin: I recommend using a facial mist throughout the day to help balance the skin moisture levels especially over areas that tend to be dry, for instance the cheek area. The above mentioned sleeping mask method should be helpful for hydrating skin once to three times a week.

Oily skin : It is possible to skip traditional cream or lotion moisturisers especially in tropical, summer climates. Opt for hydrating water based serums and facial mists instead. However, I would definitely use a ceramide-based cream moisturiser once a week to fully repair the skin barrier with lipids. This is an often overlooked component in skincare routine steps for those with oily skin.

Here's the science behind the specific steps of a skincare routine that targets the commonest skin complaint—dullness. Also the aspect of skin that is most readily addressed by correcting your skincare routine, what I call the 3 physiological pillars of glowing skin:

- Skin cells are renewed
- Skin cells are energised
- Skin barrier is hydrated

Understanding these 3 processes are critical to crafting the optimised minimalist skincare routine. For instance, my bare-bones skincare routine includes the following

- I double cleanse and add on gentle exfoliation with a hydrodermabrasion tool
- I use skincare serums that contain botanical actives and ubiquinone
- I always use a moisturiser after cleansing

EASY HACK: I avoid air conditioning when I sleep—that dries out the skin barrier due to transepidermal water loss—the biggest enemy that we are always trying to address with humectants and emollients used in skincare.

HOW THE STEPS IN SKINCARE ROUTINES ADDRESS SKIN PHYSIOLOGY
- Cell renewal

Dull skin is caused by dead skin cells retained at the surface. That's also one of the causes of acne, a phenomenon known as follicular hyperkeratosis.
- Cell energy

That's why skin dullness is associated with ageing skin. When cell activity slows down with biological aging, so does cell energy. Using serums and creams with botanical actives can help stimulate cell energy. For example, CoEnzyme Q10 also known as ubiquinone works by enhancing cell energy

- Barrier hydration

If you suffer from dry or sensitive skin, you'll probably observe that your skin looks dull. That's really because the skin barrier is damaged. The layers of skin at the surface are held together by ceramides, and when that is defective, it can cause flaking, scaling and redness. That has nothing to do with dead skin cells and you definitely shouldn't exfoliate—it will only make it worse. Rather you need to hydrate with ceramide-based moisturising creams.

UNDERSTANDING THE FOUNDATIONS OF MINIMALIST SKINCARE REGIMENS

BASICS OF SKINCARE FORMULATION

OVERVIEW
CLEANSING STEP

- Triple cleanse in 1 step by adding on gentle exfoliation with a hydrodermabrasion tool

Hydrodermabrasion is the use of focally directed vacuum pressure to increase absorption of skincare and also physically exfoliate dead skin cells. Pore vacuums are simple hacks for larger systems used in professional settings. If you are a therapist, you may wish to invest in a portable, countertop system* that is much more cost-efficient—the secret is really in the medifacial solution that's used rather than the device itself which merely delivers mechanical effects on skin.

MAKEUP REMOVER
The ideal makeup remover is one that

- Is gentle on skin i.e. beeswax
- Dissolves makeup rapidly and easily
- No need for vigorous rubbing/friction with cotton pad

- "Milk" emulsion formula (hydrating) vs micellar
- Repairs skin barrier damage i.e. hyaluronic acid, glycerin
- Contains antioxidants that can heal photodamaged skin (sage leaf, camellia sinensis, macadamia seed)
- Anti-inflammatory, skin soothing agents i.e. camphor, menthol, argan oil
- Biomimetic amino acids i.e. methionine, adenosine, oligopeptides
- Vitamins, mineral rich (niacinamide, sea water, vitamin E)

HYDRATING/MOISTURISING STEP
- Choose skincare serums that contain botanical actives and ubiquinone
- Use right after cleansing *without drying skin*

BONUS TIP: Avoid air conditioning when sleeping—that dries out the skin barrier due to transepidermal water loss.

Consumers are spoilt for choice when it comes to skincare products. Here's how to make your advice as a skin expert stand out:

- HIGH YIELD ACTIVES:
  - Botanicals (refer to ethnobotanical dictionary) with 3-in-1 effects i.e. antioxidant, anti-inflammatory and antimicrobial
  - Synthetic mimics of naturally occurring compounds i.e. peptides, Coenyme Q10/ubiquinone
- APPLICATION TECHNIQUE
  - Use a palm-sized amount of a ceramide-dominant moisturiser directly on wet skin without patting dry. Leave to absorb for at least 15 minutes before application of makeup
- CONCENTRATIONS TO CHOOSE
  - Hyaluronic acid: choose a concentrated hyaluronic acid serum 1-1.5%
  - Vitamin C:
    - L-ascorbic acid average 15-20%

- Sodium ascorbyl phosphate 1-5% (suitable for sensitive skin)

MOISTURISER LOTION Day vs Night
Do you really need 2 separate moisturisers?
The essential differences between a day and a night moisturiser:
Day:
- Lightweight, easily absorbed
- Invisible under makeup (good cosmetic effect)
- Enhance UV-protection with antioxidants i.e. botanical filters (hyssop, brassica, jojoba seed, artemisia vulgaris, arnica montana)
- Harmonise skin microbiome to reduce problem skin (acne, rosacea, sensitive skin flare-ups)
  - lactobacillus +soybean
  - lactobacillus + punica gunatum
  - lactobacillus +pear juice ferment
  - lactobacillus + barley seed
- Holy grail for holistic skin barrier repair 'P's
  - Phytoceramides (shea butter, capric triglyceride, niacinamide)
  - Polyglutamic acid
  - Portulaca oleracea
  - Peptides
  - Panthenol
Night:
- Richer texture for enhanced absorption
- Focus on skin repairing actives

DERM TIP:
Normal/combination/oily skin: You can use the same moisturiser for day and night. Apply a much larger amount i.e. palm-sized and use a reusable sheet mask made of polysaccharides for wet occlusion therapy.

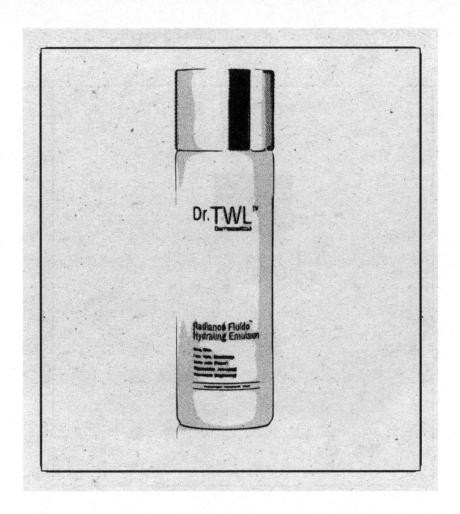

CASE STUDY: The Radiance Fluide was formulated as a *versatile day-night moisturiser*, functioning also as an effective sleeping mask.

EXERCISE: Components of a functional sunscreen

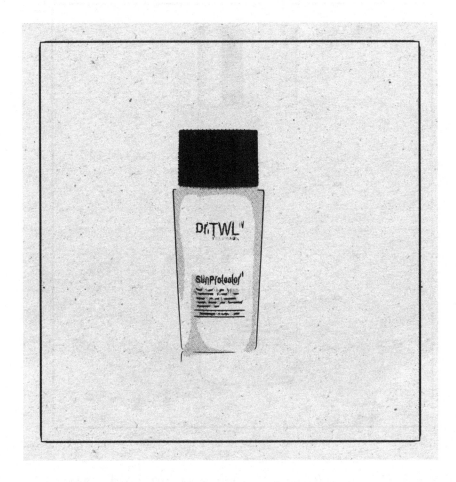

What is in a dermatologist-recommended sunscreen?
- Broad spectrum protection with balance of physical and chemical sunscreen components
- Physical sunscreen (zinc oxide, titanium dioxide)
- Chemical sunscreen (methoxycinnamate)
- Functional ingredients to build skin resilience
    - Barrier repair (glycerin, sodium hyaluronate)
    - Antioxidant, anti-inflammatory botanical trio (portulaca, aloe, chamaecyparis obtusa)

- Anti-wrinkle: acetyl hexapeptide-8 (topical botox), hydrolysed collagen
- Microbiome-stabilising: oligopeptide

EXERCISE: What's in a dermatologist-recommended facial mist?

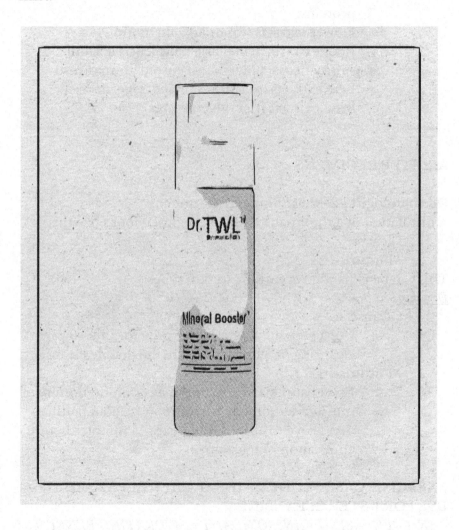

- Mineral rich microbiome balancing deep sea water
- Moisturising actives (humectants)
  - Polyglutamic acid

- Amino acid pentad (serine, histidine, methionine, arginine, lysine)
    - Sodium hyaluronate
- Multifunctional botanicals (antioxidants, anti-inflammatory, barrier repair damage)
    - Protein triad (hydrolysed corn, wheat, soy proteins)
    - Flower extracts (rosemary, chamomile)
    - Root extracts (scutellaria baicalensis, paeonia suffructicosa, polygonum cuspidatum, carrot)
    - Leaf extracts (brassica, spinach, sage, licorice)
    - Seed extracts (rice, glycine max)

A. 2 STEP REGIMENS

Dermatologist's 2-Phase Skincare Routine
A distillation of a minimalist skincare regimen looks like this:
1. Cleanse
2. Moisturise

This can be expanded according to skin types:
Dry skin:
- Cleanse
    - Use a creamy milk cleanser only for one-step cleansing of all makeup (skip the double cleanse)
- Moisturise
    - Use a palm-sized amount of a ceramide-dominant moisturiser directly on wet skin without patting dry. Leave to absorb for at least 15 minutes before application of makeup

EXERCISE: CASE STUDY OF IDEAL MILK CLEANSER TO USE FOR 1-STEP CLEANSING
3-IN-1 CLEANSING + ANTIOXIDANT + HYDRATING BENEFITS

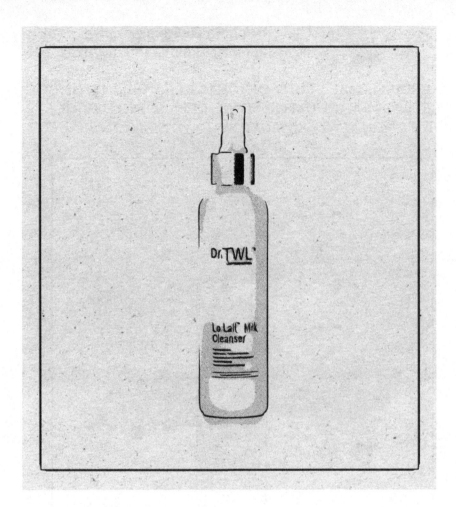

Combi/normal/oily skin:
2 steps possible for daytime routine (skipping makeup removal)

- Cleanse
  - Foaming cleanser only for one-step cleansing use with a handheld pore vacuum
    - *Choose dermatologist-recommended gentle cleanser* with hydrating properties & antioxidants
    - Apply appropriate amount of cleanser on damp skin

- ■ Glide the pore vacuum over oily parts of face, skipping areas that feel dry/irritated

EXERCISE: CASE STUDY OF IDEAL CLEANSER TO USE WITH PORE VACUUM OR SONIC CLEANSING DEVICE
3-IN-1 CLEANSING + ANTIOXIDANT + HYDRATING BENEFITS

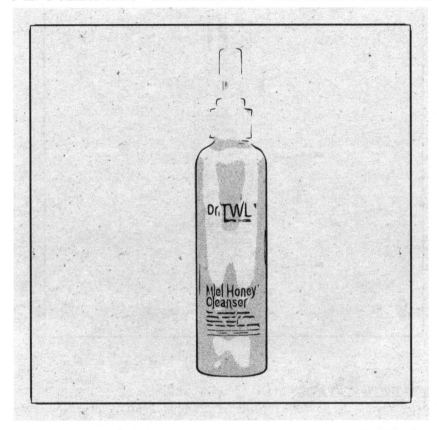

N.B. There are 2 main types of sonic cleansing devices: the spatula style which is used in clinics offering the korean medifacial and the silicone brush head which is marketed mainly for home use. I would recommend the spatula style for the following reasons:
- *Hygiene and ease of use*
- *Less skin irritation on sensitive skin*
- *Choose dual function settings reverse blade models which allow*
  - ○ *Cleansing*

o   *Infusion*

The concept that underpins the 2-PHASE systems is this: utilising home devices to

- Physically exfoliate/cleanser
- Increase antioxidant active absorption from specifically formulated cleansers via transdermal delivery

   In a single optimised cleansing step

Throughout the day, the client/patient can be encouraged to use a hydrating facial mist which is also a quick way to refresh skin while hydrating it.

EXERCISE: CASE STUDY OF IDEAL FACIAL MIST FOR ALL SKIN TYPES
3-IN-1 CLEANSING + ANTIOXIDANT + HYDRATING BENEFITS

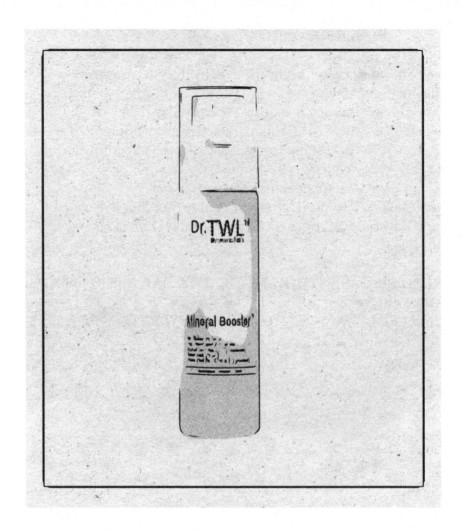

B. 3-STEP REGIMENS
Dermatologist's 3-Phase Skincare Routines

The psychology behind a 3-PHASE VS 2-PHASE routine is this: it is a valuable upgrade for your client who has learnt how skincare routines can be optimised with the help of home devices. It's also much more appealing for them when they realise that by choosing multi-functional skincare products, they can "hack" perceived "cumbersome" skincare steps while still retaining the benefits of layering skincare. *(The 2-step regimen is really 3-steps if you include the facial mist which is an on-the-go product that appeals to most.)*

By this time, it's easy to incorporate HIGH YIELD steps that will increase client satisfaction instantly.

4 MAIN TYPES OF FACE MASKS

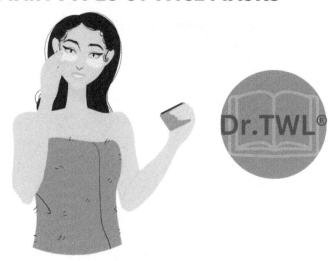

STEP #2 MASKING

- **SHEET MASKS (REUSABLE OR ONE-TIME DISPOSABLE)**
- **LEAVE ON GEL MASKS (HIGH DOSE ANTIOXIDANTS LIKE VITAMIN C, SKIN BARRIER REPAIR ACTIVES LIKE ALOE, GLYCERIN)**
- **DRY MASKS (POLYMERS LIKE SILICONE, HYDROCOLLOID THAT CREATE AN ARTIFICIAL MICRO-CLIMATE AROUND SKIN)**
- **TEXTILES (FACE MASKS, PILLOWCASES ENGINEERED FROM NOVEL NANOMATERIALS LIKE COPPER THAT EXERT ANTI-AGING EFFECTS ON SKIN).**

DR.TWL'S HIGH YIELD STEPS & ROUTINE SECRETS
- Specialised sheet masks

Sheet masking is overrated—for traditional sheet masks, it's essentially no different from applying a well formulated face essence or moisturiser and increasing skin absorption by applying a wet layer on top. The key here instead, is to show clients how the same step of sheet masking can be hacked to double the results in half the time spent:

Sheet masking mini masterclass: how to hack the step

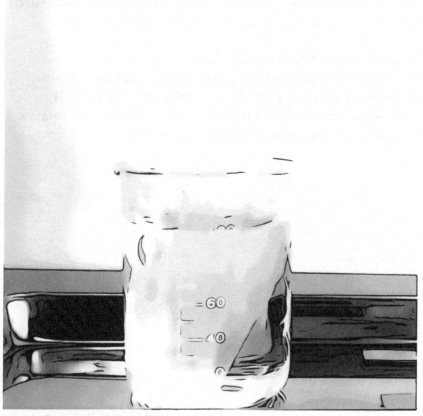

Access demonstrative video workshop
https://www.twlskin.com/dictionary/

1. Use a polysaccharide material
Polysaccharides are valuable materials that attract moisture to the skin and can be processed to create a textile—i.e. woven as a reusable sheet mask that is also 100% biodegradable. The science behind this is the creation of little mini-reservoirs that form a

microclimate around the individual pores to harmonise skin functions—sebum regulation, aquaporin activity etc.

2. Consider the shelf-life of sheet masks
As the polysaccharide is separately packed and freeze-dried in sterile conditions, it has a longer shelf-life of 5 years compared to typical 2 years for wet sheet masks. As a business owner, this poses a challenge when you are manufacturing the masks—high MOQ and short shelf lives are important considerations.

3. Customise essences for your client
The additional benefit is that you can customise facial essences to be paired with the mask with our proprietary mask bar system—the customisation process also has certain advantages when it comes to rapport building and client retention.

WEEKLY SKINCARE ROUTINE

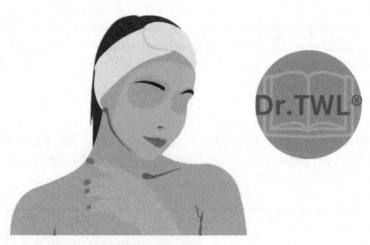

STEP #2 MASKING

- **CREATING A MICRO-CLIMATE AROUND YOUR SKIN THAT ENHANCES SKIN HEALING AND STIMULATES BENEFICIAL PROCESSES LIKE COLLAGEN PRODUCTION AND CELL TALK**
- **WET OCCLUSION THERAPY WHICH INCREASES THE ABSORPTION OF SKINCARE ACTIVE INGREDIENTS BY IMPROVING EPIDERMAL PENETRATION. I.E. THE ABILITY OF THE COSMECEUTICALS TO CROSS THE SKIN BARRIER IS IMPORTANT FOR EFFICACY.**

EXERCISE:
HOW TO DEVELOP SKINCARE ROUTINES CUSTOMISED FOR SPECIFIC SKIN CONCERNS

The Upgrade

By now you would have acquired the key principles of a minimalist skincare routine based on the incorporation of home device technologies. Then next step is to modify steps your client is already familiar with for the extra benefits. This can be done at the 2-4 week mark, which allows sufficient time for the first skin cycle to full display results of a well-planned, efficient cosmeceutical regimen.

1. Dry Skin: Skin Flooding System
Recommended for those with dry skin on a daily basis and up to three times a week for those with combination skin to optimise barrier function.

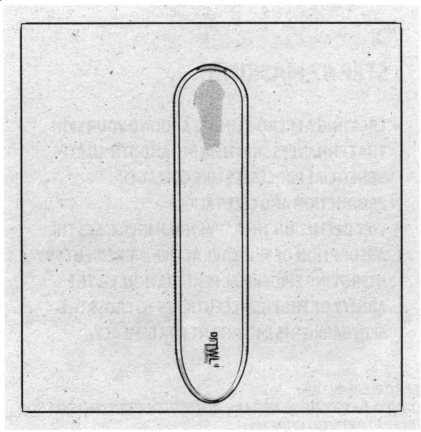

Radiofrequency

Hand-held radiofrequency devices are the ACTUAL best kept secrets I believe—sonic cleansers are overhyped. A well developed radiofrequency tool can deliver all the functions of sonic cleansers when it comes to cleansing, and much more for increasing cosmeceutical absorption and directly stimulating collagen production.

This is the number 1 tool I recommend for increasing skin moisture levels—apply your moisturiser, the polysaccharide material functions as a barrier between the device and your skin, turn on the moisture delivery mode and let it do its job.

Radiofrequency delivers immediate results when it comes to increasing skincare absorption—so this means it is a guaranteed immediate improvement in skin hydration levels.

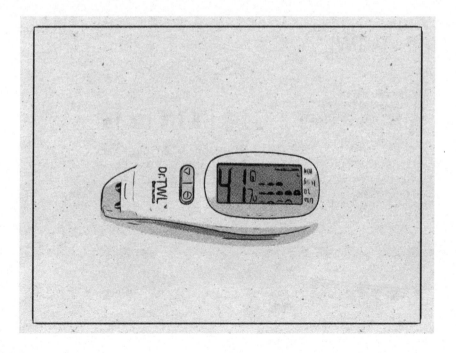

Skin hydration analyser

For those with dry skin, I also recommend a skin hydration analyser which uses biocapacitance analyses to measure hydration levels of the stratum corneum. An example of improvement in skin moisture levels before/after moisturiser treatment is shown here. You can also ask your client to tabulate this as a way to track skin progress.

2. Combination Skin: Skin Rebalancing System

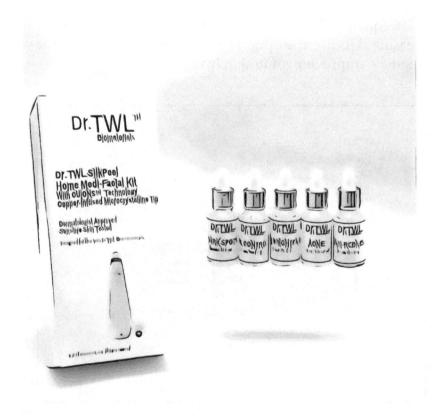

Combination skin is the easiest to manage in theory, though in my experience most are dissatisfied with the lack of "glow" or perceived levels of skin radiance. The quickest and most gratifying upgrade would be with a microdermabrasion set—a handheld kit which features a microcrystalline handpiece that's used with a protective gel to resurface skin.

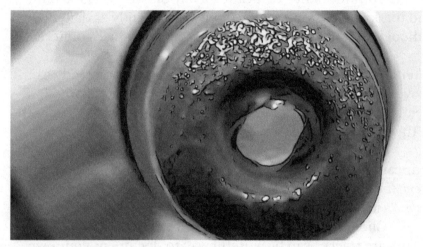

Handpiece made of microcrystalline oxide with barrier gel for skin protection, infusion of peptides.

Microcrystalline copper oxide is what we use which is suited even for sensitive skin—the additional benefits include the release of copper ions which are shown to stimulate collagen production on its own. The protective gel in this case is a peptide-based gel mask with high doses of vitamin C. Together, an "instant' glow result is achieved with immediate delivery of antioxidants and removal of dead skin cells.

3. Oily Skin: Skin Harmonising System
Oily skin does have slightly different requirements such as sebum regulation and perhaps even addressing acne flares. I would recommend starting with the same skin rebalancing

system as per 2. However, I would emphasise gentle exfoliation techniques *daily* such as the mask peel which is covered in detail in the next chapter.

The science of the weekly treatment routine
This chapter so far has focused on the fundamental steps of skincare routines, the next part goes in depth into what I consider "treatment" routines which are best thought of as a weekly commitment—dedicating a day or two for exfoliation and masking. Masking can be done as frequently as daily, although that would also depend on the individual's preference.

After completing this foundational section, you are ready to move on to the next set of advanced course material on cleansing, exfoliation and masking which are covered in-depth in the next chapter.

Skincare routine planners: client engagement tip
complimentary template download at
https://www.twlskin.com/dictionary/ with purchase verified account
 • Client engagement strategy/self-motivational
A skincare tracker can be a useful way to document your own skincare journey or as a way to review your client's progress.

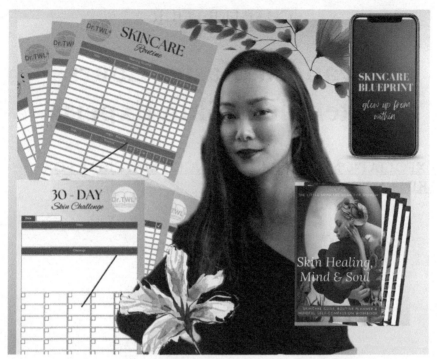

A self-care journal that includes a skincare routine planner may be a useful way to track your skin healing journey. Printable digital skincare planners with templates, skincare routine steps checklists and motivational prompts can be a part of your daily self-care routine.

CHAPTER FOUR

Advanced Master Course Material for Skin Experts

EXFOLIATION MASTERS ADVANCED MATERIAL FOR SKIN EXPERTS

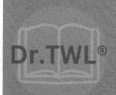

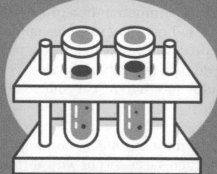

Types of at-home face peels

- **Traditional peels: acid/retinol i.e. AHA, BHA, lactic acid, retinol peels**
- **New generation water/jelly peels, gel peels, mask peels**
- **Microdermabrasion (microcrystalline copper)**
- **Hydrodermabrasion**

DERMATOLOGIST RECOMMENDED SKINCARE ROUTINES

Exfoliation is the removal of dead skin cells from the top most layer of skin, but most importantly, a process that encourages cell renewal. It's also important to understand the skin cycle here, the entire process from new skin cells moving to the surface and shedding it takes about 27-28 days. Exfoliation helps remove the dead skin cells to reveal younger, brighter and more radiant skin.

It is also one of the most misunderstood steps in skincare routines. Decades ago, facial scrubs with abrasive beads were marketed as a cure for flaky, dull skin.

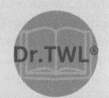

4

WAYS TO GET NATURALLY GLOWING SKIN

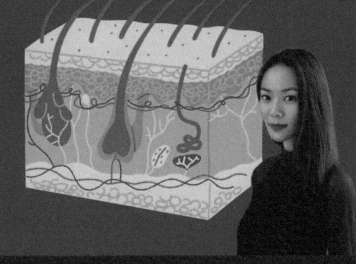

WWW.TWLSKIN.COM

There are several issues here. Firstly, skin cells actually "exfoliate" naturally—at its own time. The movement of skin cells from bottom layers to the surface, is also known as cell differentiation, which occurs during the skin cycle. The trouble is with aging, the skin cycle lengthens. The layer known as the stratum corneum accumulates dead skin cells—that's when skin looks dull.

There are two main types of exfoliation.
- Physical exfoliation

Using granules or abrasive beads which I don't recommend, especially for sensitive skin or those with active inflamed acne.
- Chemical exfoliation

With AHAs, BHAs and lactic acids exfoliate microscopically and can improve skin irregularities.

SKINCARE TIPS FOR GLOWING SKIN

SKINCARE ROUTINE STEP	EFFECTS
CLEANSING	REMOVE DEAD SKIN CELLS. FOR SKIN RENEWAL
MOISTURISE	• HYDRATE STRATUM CORNEUM • DERMIS PLUMPNESS
EXFOLIATE	• CHEMICAL/ENZYME PEEL • MICRODERMABRASION

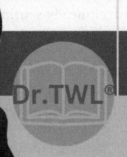

Dr.TWL®

SKIN MASTERS ACADEMY
NEXT LEVEL SKINCARE ROUTINES

Exfoliation can take place in the following settings:
- Professional

Dermatologists' offices or at the aestheticians'
- Home based kits

When it comes to chemical exfoliants, the most important aspects that distinguish between the two are the
- Concentrations used
- Length of time
- Type/depth of peel

Depending on regulations where you live, acid concentrations of 20% or more must be administered only by medical professionals. This is due to the risk of chemical burns and irritation to the mucosal areas such as the eyes and lip areas. Glycolic acid peels typically need to be neutralised by a separate agent, which means it must be done by a trained skincare professional. The discussion here is limited to superficial chemical peels with glycolic, lactic and salicylic acids—medium/deep chemical peels are beyond the scope of this course.

Good to know cosmeceutical active

Polyhydroxy acid: Exfoliant. Known to be as effective as AHAs but less sensitizing. Chemically and functionally similar to AHA but larger in molecular size, limiting potential to penetrate the skin. Found to be compatible with clinically sensitive skin, including rosacea and atopic dermatitis.

DERM'S PRO TIP: For salon/home kit chemical peels, the key is to choose the lowest possible concentration that does not irritate skin and also a formulation that has moisturising effects on skin to reduce the risk of irritant contact dermatitis—there is no point inducing any sort of visible "peeling effect" when you are performing a chemical peel because it simply means the skin barrier has been disrupted. K-beauty skincare routines developed by dermatologists for instance recommend using low concentrations of glycolic, lactic and salicylic acid peels in rotation, up to 3 times a week in those who tolerate it. It is far better to do superficial peels, using lower concentrations and upping the frequency than stage a "all-out" peel and telling the client to wait it out. By the time you see visible skin irritation, it's a sign that the barrier has been damaged—that's not the purpose of exfoliation.

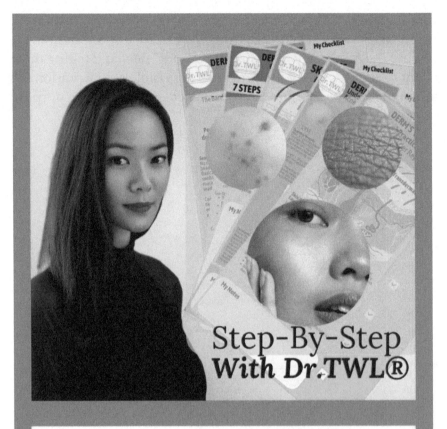

Step-By-Step
With Dr.TWL®

SKINCARE ROUTINE GUIDE
HOW TO INCORPORATE
Face Peels

WWW.TWLSKIN.COM

Alternative home peel kits

The ideal home peel kit is one that

- Has no/minimal risk of skin irritation
- Easy to use/apply
- Delivers quick results for instant gratification

These are the 5 top skin concerns that peels address

- Skin dullness
- Uneven skin tone
- Textural irregularities
- Oily-dehydrated skin
- Acne, whiteheads, blackheads

Designing a customisable home peel kit for your client
Components:

1. Packaging

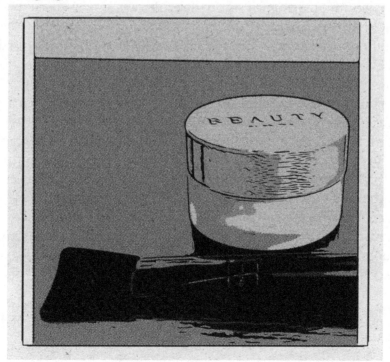

- Reusable glass jars:

We use reusable glass jars with a bamboo lid for our customisable mask peel series for first purchases as the mask peel is in a dehydrated powder form. Subsequent orders can be in the form of refills in ziplocks packed securely. This minimises packaging waste. Glass is also ideal for protecting and storing the powder concentrates which are used in our formulations.

2. Selection of 3 out of 5 peels for addressing
   ☐ overall skin microclimate
       ☐ Anti-pollution
       ☐ Barrier harmonising
   ☐ specific skin concerns
       ☐ Pores
       ☐ Dull skin
       ☐ Fine lines/wrinkles

3. Device/tool pairing for optimal results
   - Skin cryotherapy tool

Cryotherapy tools aka skin icing are available in the form of ice globes or actual ice holders made from food grade silicone. Cryotherapy works by reducing local skin inflammation by vasoconstrictive effects on the blood vessels—this translates into reduced skin redness and swelling. Skin icing is not recommended for those suffering from eczema as cold contact can further exacerbate skin barrier damage. The key is avoiding frostbite, as that itself can damage healthy skin. The ideal cryotherapy tool is one made from a metal alloy—-the one we incorporate in our pharmacy is impregnated with zinc nanoparticles. Used right after a mask peel treatment, it instantly reduces the appearance of enlarged pores. The zinc particles also control excess sebum production.

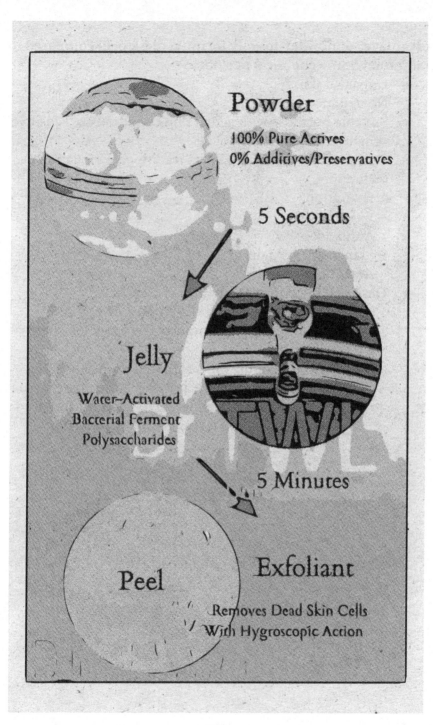

Powder

100% Pure Actives
0% Additives/Preservatives

5 Seconds

Jelly

Water–Activated
Bacterial Ferment
Polysaccharides

5 Minutes

Peel

Exfoliant

Removes Dead Skin Cells
With Hygroscopic Action

103

Advantages of powder-to-jelly formula mask peel compared to traditional home chemical peel kits:

- Universal skin types
- No irritation
- Suitable for those with actual skin conditions i.e.sensitive skin, rosacea, hormonal acne
- Delivers 5-in-1 skin benefits vs traditional exfoliation techniques:
  – Hydration
  – Exfoliation
  – Antioxidant
  – Skin barrier repair
  – Anti-inflammatory
- Designed for skin-rebalancing i.e.
  - Prolonged contact with skin vs conventional chemical peels <10 minutes increases transdermal delivery
  - Peel off formula means there is no risk of overexfoliation i.e. the polysaccharide base forms a natural fibre that adheres to excess oil and dead skin cells without damaging the skin barrier

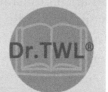

7

Causes of skin dullness

- **Free radical induced**
- **Retention hyperkeratosis**
- **Dehydrated skin**
- **Loss of collagen/elastin**
- **Antioxidant depletion**
- **Cell senescence**
- **Inflammaging**

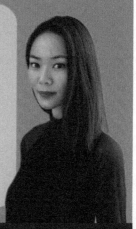

WWW.TWLSKIN.COM

Let's get to the root cause of dull skin. We all desire skin radiance, translucency, elasticity and clarity but we must begin by understanding one thing- dull skin is caused by a combination of factors both at the level of the epidermis and the dermis.

Here are the 7 causes of dull skin:

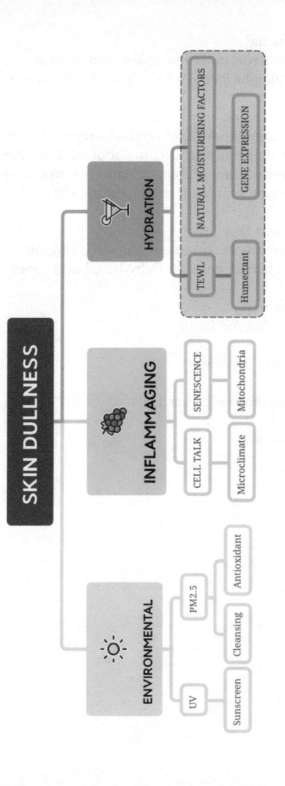

Environmental
1. Oxidative stress caused by free radical damage
External aging factors: PM2.5 pollutants, UV damage.

Epidermal factors
2. Accumulation of dead skin cells aka retention hyperkeratosis
Besides causing dull skin, accumulation of dead skin cells leads
to formation of mini whiteheads known as microcomedones
which subsequently result in whiteheads and blackheads.

3. Dehydrated skin
Water loss to the environment, impaired ceramide production
causes skin barrier damage. Dehydrated skin appears dull.

Dermal factors
4. Loss of collagen/elastin

5. Antioxidant depletion

6. Cell senescence affects cell talk

7. Inflammaging

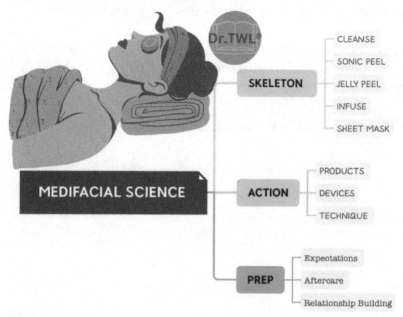

Notes

Everyone knows about traditional acid peels, I'm sharing this program because it has significant advantages for use in a home/aesthetician setting. The program is also based on novel biomaterials such as plant polysaccharides which directly target the skin microclimate and microbiome. I developed this home exfoliation program as an efficient method of tackling all 7 causes of dull skin with the goal of achieving quick results and providing long-term maintenance without the fuss of visiting a doctor's office:

1. Weekly Microdermabrasion

Copper Peel: Microcrystalline copper peel stimulates collagen production, ensuring more youthful, plump-looking skin.

2. Daily Peel Off Gel Mask/Mask Peel: 100% natural origin plant polysaccharides bind to superficial skin cells, excess sebum for gentle & effective exfoliation

3. Oily/Acne Skin Microneedle Treatment:

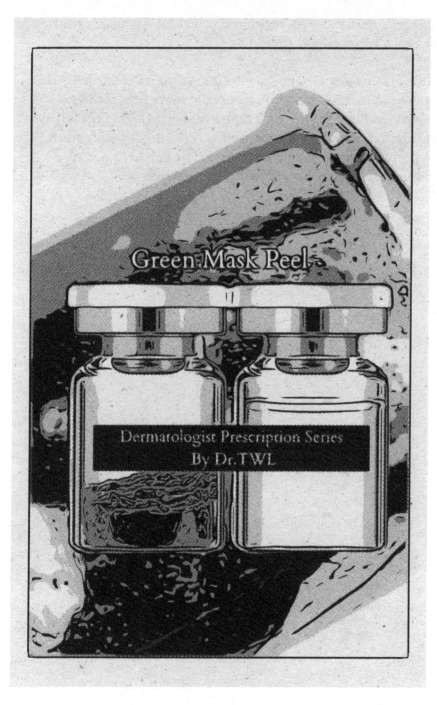

Spongilla spicules are packaged in vacuum sealed vials and rehydrated to form a jelly mask for application.

100% freshwater sponge spicules AKA Spongilla Lacustris is known as nature's living microneedle mask peel for ultra-fine microneedling treatment. There are specific benefits such as regulating oil production as well as reducing inflammation, hyperpigmentation and acne scars. The key here is gentle exfoliation while respecting the skin barrier.

FACE PEELING

 Peel Off Gel Mask

How it works:

- **GEL COMPONENTS ACRYLATES (CARBOMERS) AND CELLULOSE**
- **ABSORB SEBUM AND MOISTURE**
- **FIBRE FORMATION: CLINGS TO SUPERFICIAL CORNEOCYTES**

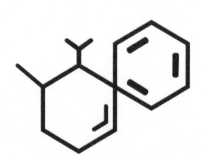

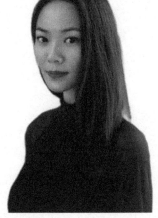

Key actives in the 360 Exfoliation Program
A. Mask peel
The polysaccharide actives

- [ ] create multiple mini-reservoirs within which the antioxidants and humectants deeply penetrate the deeper layers of skin.
- [ ] unique skin micro-climate creates ideal milieu for cell talk

DERM'S PRO TIP
Cell communication is the key to skin health. The cell signals weaken with age and environmental stress, leading to development of abnormal skin texture and signs collectively described as photoaging. The multi-active botanical essences in the home face peel kit re-create the ideal skin microenvironment to reawaken skin cells.

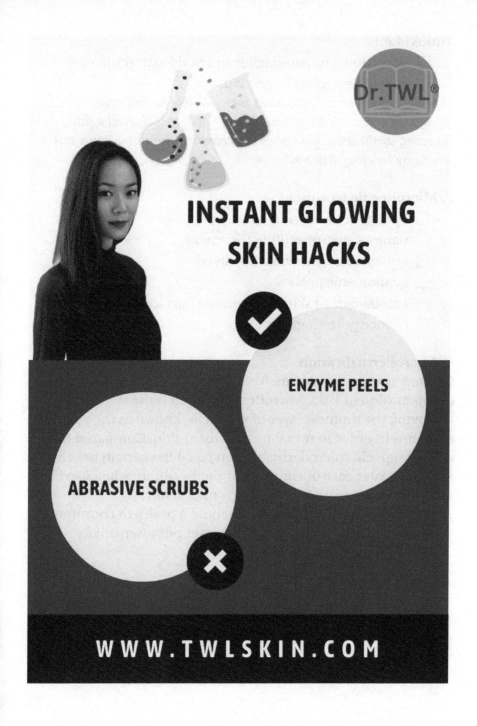

Antioxidants
- [ ] slows down inflammaging and build skin resilience
- [ ] encourages microbiome balance

Chronic, low-grade inflammation is responsible for cell aging throughout the whole body. Most of this is due to biological aging. However, application of targeted cosmeceuticals can slow down this process by building skin resilience

B. Microneedle treatment
- [ ] Spongilla Lacustris freshwater sponge
- [ ] nature's microneedling treatment
- [ ] enhances cosmeceutical delivery
- [ ] adaptogenic peels
- [ ] exfoliate dead skin cells without surface irritation
- [ ] reduce pore clogging

C. Microdermabrasion

Created as a gentler alternative to chemical peels and dermabrasion in 1985. Microdermabrasion is the technique of removing the topmost layer of skin cells, known as the stratum corneum in order to reveal more radiant skin. Compared to chemical peels, microdermabrasion facial has certain benefits such as greater ease of control and predictability when used in skin of color. Pigmented skin tends to develop post-inflammatory hyperpigmentation, a problem common with chemical peels which also increases photosensitivity.

FACE PEELING

 ## Peel Off Gel Mask

Benefits:

- **PREFERRED PHYSICAL EXFOLIATOR VS. TRADITIONAL EXFOLIATORS WITH ABRASIVE BEADS**
- **NO PHOTO SENSITIVITY**
- **TOLERATED BY SENSITIVE SKIN TYPES**

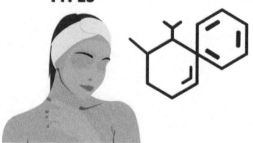 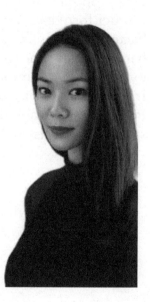

SKIN EXPERT FAQ MASTERY
The terms *mask peels, peel off mask, face peels* are used interchangeably throughout.

What are peeling masks?

Peeling masks with a gel like texture rely on carbomer technology for gentle skin exfoliation. It is an ultra-gentle method of exfoliation because it automatically adjusts to your skin's sebum levels. This means that unlike retinol/AHA based peels, it does not carry any risk of damaging the skin barrier.

Can I wash my face after using a peeling mask?

Yes. This is the best method to get rid of any residue on skin. If you are using the jelly exfoliant, any remaining residue can readily be dissolved and absorbed onto the skin after rinsing with water. It is not necessary to use a face cleanser after the peel off mask.

What type of peeling masks are suitable for sensitive skin?

100% pure polysaccharide gels can be formulated from cosmetic grade xanthan gum and sodium alginate. These are available in powder form commercially. As derivatives of brown algae and bacterial ferment, both naturally enhance the skin's natural barrier repair functions by upregulating aquaporin gene expression. Most importantly, there should be no acids nor irritating retinols in formulations for sensitive skin. Polysaccharides are ideal for sensitive skin because of its skin stabilising effects.

FACE PEELING MASK

 ## Peel Off Gel Mask

What are the benefits of gel peel?

- **GENTLER ON SKIN**
- **SAFE FOR SENSITIVE SKIN TYPES**
- **USED DAILY**
- **IMMEDIATE RESULTS**

W W W . T W L S K I N . C O M

How often can I use peeling masks?
Depending on the manufacturer's recommendation and presence of potentially skin irritating actives i.e. inclusion of

traditional acid/retinol peels in formulation. For pure polysaccharide based formulations such as those in our pharmacy that target specific skin concerns, the ideal frequency is at 1- 3X weekly.

Why incorporate face peels into your skincare routine?
- Brighten dull skin
- Increase translucency
- Reduce pore-size
- Even out irregular skin tone
- Smoothen surface irregularities

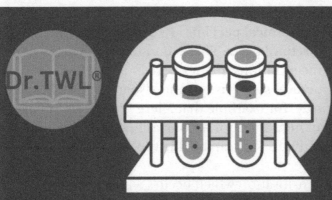

EXFOLIATION METHODS

01 **ENZYME PEELS**

02 **MICRODERMABRASION**

03 **JELLY PEELS (POLYSACCHARIDE)**

04 **SONIC CLEANSING**

05 **HYDRODERMABRASION**

DERMATOLOGIST RECOMMENDED SKINCARE ROUTINES

What are the disadvantages of traditional chemical peel kits?
Traditional home chemical peel kits are based on glycolic, lactic, salicylic acid and retinol peels. These tend to be limited by the relatively low concentrations (higher percentages of actives must be used under medical supervision) and also unpredictable side effects. It is not true, for example that allergy develops quickly. You may tolerate these acids for as long as several years and one day develop sensitivity. This can be due to 2 main reasons:

- Delayed sensitisation which occurs with prolonged usage
- Damaged skin barrier as chemical peel/retinol based exfoliants disrupt the bonds between the superficial skin cells i.e. corneocytes

Why home face peels based on novel biomaterials such as polysaccharides may have advantages over traditional chemical peels?
- Skin harmonising actives
- Self-regulating: barrier-respecting jelly exfoliation technology
- Adjusts to your skin's moisture and sebum levels

Ingredients of natural origin such as brown algae and bacterial ferments are packed with antioxidants and release additional nutrients for skin compared to traditional acid peels.

SKINCARE ROUTINE STEPS

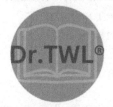 **HOME FACE PEEL**

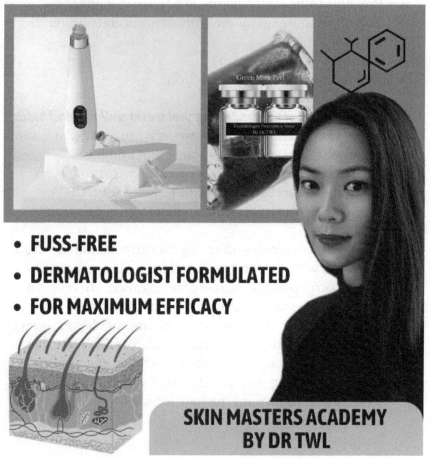

- **FUSS-FREE**
- **DERMATOLOGIST FORMULATED**
- **FOR MAXIMUM EFFICACY**

**SKIN MASTERS ACADEMY
BY DR TWL**

Are at home face peels for acne effective?

Acne is caused by a combination of factors including genetics, hormones and inflammation which drive comedone formation. The skin environment plays a part too. For instance, increased bacterial counts i.e. Cutibacterium acnes is associated with acne flares. Occlusion effects such as wearing of face masks or application of comedogenic cosmetics also worsens acne.

How at home face peels for acne work:

- Increasing skin cell turnover
- Prevents follicular plugging aka "pore clogging"
- Enhanced antioxidant environment Inhibits bacterial growth
- Removal of excess sebum
- Regulation of sebum production

A specific type of microneedling peel works well for blackheads

Spongilla Lacustris, also known as nature's microneedling treatment is a freshwater sponge that enhances cosmeceutical delivery. Our pharmacy formula is an adaptogenic peel fortified with ginseng root, CICA (centella asiatica), forsythia and Dennettia Tripetala.

The delicate spicules on spongilla extract exfoliate dead skin cells without surface irritation. It also combines a novel cosmeceutical delivery mechanism whereby the microneedles enable penetration of the actives past the skin barrier the stratum corneum into the deeper layers of skin where anti-inflammatory actives like forsythia, dennettia tripetala work. The exfoliating effects also reduce pore clogging, which is really due to retention of dead skin cells around the hair follicles.

What ingredients should I look for in a peel off mask that targets hyperpigmentation and dark spots?
Centella asiatica and scutellaria baicalensis specifically target melanin formation. To note the microneedling mask can also be used to increase delivery of active ingredients.

CHEMICAL PEELS

Skin Peeling Factors

- **DURATION OF APPLICATION**
- **CONCENTRATION**

- **NEED FOR NEUTRALISATION**
- **PERFORMED MONTHLY, LOWER CONCENTRATIONS WEEKLY**
- **NEED TO ADJUST BASED ON TOLERABILITY**

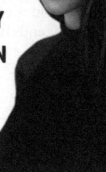

How can mask peels help oily skin?

Oily skin isn't just associated with acne, it is also quite uncomfortable for sufferers. A common complaint is that of the oily-dehydrated skin phenomenon. Mask peels can address this by targeting 2 important physiological pathways:

- Regulating sebum production with glycerol, mannitol and sodium hyaluronate
- Absorbing excess sebum with natural plant polysaccharides that form the carbomer-fibre that peels off when the gel is removed

What are the side effects of mask peels?

Depending on the specific formulation, some commercial labels include retinols/acids which can cause skin irritation. If you have sensitive skin, choose dermatologist formulated mask peels without acids/retinols. In such formulas, actives are generally selected based on tolerability, unlike traditional face peels or chemical peels which can cause sensitisation.

MICRODERMABRASION

Microdermabrasion was created as a gentler alternative to chemical peels and dermabrasion in 1985. We've come a long way since. It is the technique of removing the topmost layer of skin cells, known as the stratum corneum in order to reveal more radiant skin. Compared to chemical peels, microdermabrasion facial has certain benefits such as greater ease of control and predictability when used in skin of color. Pigmented skin tends to develop post-inflammatory hyperpigmentation, a problem common with chemical peels which also increases photosensitivity.

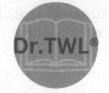

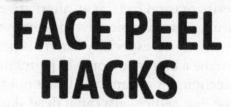

FACE PEEL HACKS

- Brighten dull skin
- Increase translucency
- Reduce pore-size

- Even out irregular skin tone
- Smoothen surface irregularities

The wrong way to exfoliate

The traditional idea of getting rid of dead skin—literally by scrubbing it off is unfortunately not how skin works. By scrubbing skin down like one does sandpapering wood, skin actually gets irritated.

The correct way to exfoliate without chemical peels

Microdermabrasion facial is an alternative to chemical peels. Gentle microdermabrasion avoids common chemical peel related side effects, especially when deeper peels are performed. There can be a better outcome in pigmented skin types, when correct techniques are applied.That's not the end of the story. When the dust settles (just call it dead skin)—she actually decides to grow new skin cells. But it's not what we wanted. Instead of fresh, baby soft skin, you get layers of thickened, dark skin. What dermatologists term at first as post-inflammatory hyperpigmentation (PIH for short) becomes lichenification—the development of a tree bark-like skin texture.

How microdermabrasion affects the skin cycle

The core principles of microdermabrasion facial relate to the natural skin cycle. As skin cells move up from the bottom layers of skin i.e. the stratum basale, they differentiate. By the time it reaches the top most layer, we refer to these cells as the corneocytes. The superficial skin cells reside in the stratum corneum. When one grows older, the skin cells are retained for longer periods of time and this causes dull skin. Microdermabrasion utilises crystal/diamond resurfacing technology to remove superficial dead skin cells, thereby enhancing skin radiance. Combining two principles i.e. vacuum assisted topical delivery and crystal/diamond skin resurfacing in order to enhance absorption. However there are some significant limitations to traditional microdermabrasion, it was quite messy and required eye protection as salt crystals were involved and in the crystal-free systems aka diamond microdermabrasion systems the procedure still required skill operators in-office. The procedure also took quite a significant chunk of time—30-60 minutes.

How microdermabrasion compares with chemical peels in-office

Glycolic, lactic and salicylic acids are must-haves in a dermatologist's office setting. For a good reason—these actually do exfoliate in a way that doesn't damage skin barrier the way physical scrubs do. Except that thw downsides are real
Sun sensitivity occurs commonly with chemical peels. As does skin irritation i.e. redness, flaking—as a result of a disrupted skin barrier. The concentration of the peel acid, the duration it's left on skin affects how intense the effects are. Hence, higher concentration peels (the most effective) must be performed under medical supervision.

Chemical peel acids work at a microscopic level, which means it specifically dissolves the bonds between the surface skin cells known as corneocytes. The result is the appearance of renewed, softer and smoother skin.

New generation microdermabrasion facial systems

In the mid 2010s, Korean medi-facials took off with vacuum only skin resurfacing techniques which focused on minimal epidermal disruption and maximum antioxidant delivery. Hydrodermabrasion is the technology widely used in Korean medifacials. The key difference with this microdermabrasion facial technology is that it does not use any abrasive handpieces at all, compared to traditional counterparts. Instead, vacuum pressure is utilised to enhance skincare absorption. This is a closed loop system which requires a filter. The system also utilises a vortex handpiece which focuses vacuum pressure optimally at the level of the stratum corneum. Sufficient pressure is generated to enhance cosmeceutical absorption. Effective resurfacing occurs with salicylic acid—the gentlest of chemical peels.

Microcrystalline copper peel

Dr.TWL Biomaterials Copper Peel System was launched in 2020 as a revolutionary copper oxide based microcrystalline handpiece with the ability to exfoliate, infuse and repair the skin barrier all at once. Designed for use with a gel mask, it delivers a suite of benefits in a single application:

- ☐ Peptides for anti-wrinkle effects
- ☐ AMPs as a natural microbiome stabiliser
- ☐ Propolis for anti-inflammatory, antioxidant shield
- ☐ Adaptogens for skin resilience

This novel microdermabrasion facial handpiece features microcrystalline copper oxide instead of the traditional aluminium oxide or diamond tip. The result is an even distribution of microcrystals that is gentler on skin and enhances skincare absorption.

CLEANSING MASTERS ADVANCED MATERIAL FOR SKIN EXPERTS

The concept of face masks are twofold:
- Creating a micro-climate around your skin that enhances skin healing and stimulates beneficial processes like collagen production and cell talk
- Wet occlusion therapy which increases the absorption of skincare active ingredients by improving epidermal penetration. I.e. the ability of the cosmeceuticals to cross the skin barrier is important for efficacy.

There are 4 main types of face masks
- Sheet masks (reusable or one-time disposable)
- Leave on gel masks (high dose antioxidants like vitamin C, skin barrier repair actives like aloe, glycerin)
- Dry masks (polymers like silicone, hydrocolloid that create an artificial micro-climate around skin)

- Textiles (face masks, pillowcases engineered from novel nanomaterials like copper that exert anti-aging effects on skin).

I recommend using leave on gel masks together with reusable sheet masks made of polysaccharide for ideal results. Dry masking can be implemented simply by switching to biofunctional textiles for your pillowcase for instance.

CLEANSING MASTERS ADVANCED MATERIAL FOR SKIN EXPERTS

In this subsequent section, we go into the technical details of the single most important step of the skincare routine which you absolutely must master—cleansing. I've included the information in FAQ style for practical purposes. As a skin expert, you must become familiar with the answers to these advanced questions on the topic of double cleansing.

How does micellar water work?
Micellar water contains micelles that soak up oil, dirt and pigment. How they do it is by trapping and dissolving the impurities, so it can be wiped off easily. The simplest way to imagine this is as a ball. The outside of the ball holds the water loving tails, whereas the centre of it is oil-loving, water hating which eats up the makeup, oil and dirt—which you can then wipe off with a cotton pad.

Micellar textile

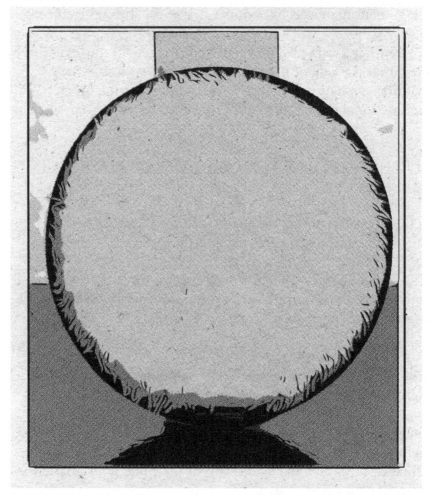

TYPE 1: Ideal for makeup removal with water alone. Longer fibres, ultra soft and fluffy texture for efficient pigment pickup.

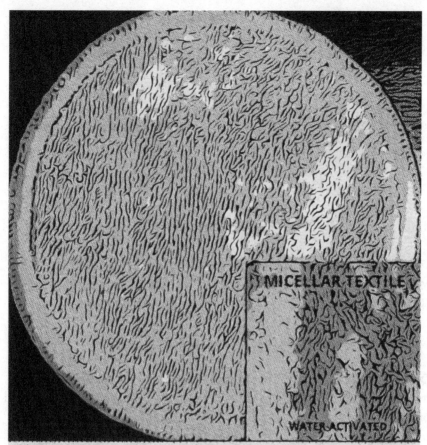

MICELLAR TEXTILE

WATER-ACTIVATED

MICELLAR EXFOLIATING PEEL PAD

TYPE 2: No visible fibres, shorter, woven as single piece with light texture for gentle exfoliating effects when wet. Suitable as "water exfoliation" step for hypersensitive skin unable to tolerate acids.

- Here's a hack, certain textiles like microfibres can be engineered to achieve a similar effect without the use of micellar surfactants

- Why is this beneficial? The micelle in this case is a textile, which means it does not contain surfactants unlike traditional cleansers that will disrupt the skin barrier.
- But you still need water to activate the effect as a solvent. Here's the huge benefit, you can use water based hydrating mists to cleanse on-the-go, touch up your makeup throughout the day without the use of makeup wipes.

What does micellar water do for skin?
Essentially, it attracts the pigments, dirt and sebum in a micelle that is physically rubbed off with a material like a cotton pad.

What are the disadvantages of micellar water
Micellar water contains surfactants that are drying for skin. Heavy makeup pigments like eyeliner and eyeshadow require quite a lot of cleanser to remove, skin may be irritated by excessive rubbing with the cotton pad material as well.

Do I need to wash my face after using micellar water?
It is advisable. The surfactant residue on skin is meant to washed off, not left on skin. The differences between leave on and wash off products are that leave on products are moisturising, whereas wash off products tend to contain irritating ingredients such as detergents.

Oil cleanser or micellar water?
I recommend oil based cleansers for removing makeup—especially if you have dry, sensitive skin. Here's why

PROS OF MILK I.E. OIL CLEANSERS
- Milk cleansers are really "oil cleansers" that are not as greasy as pure oil formulations. They are really oil in water mixtures known as emulsions.
- The like dissolves like principle: the key benefit is that oil cleansers are the most effective at dissolving makeup

pigments, especially difficult to remove mascara, eyeliner, heavily pigmented eye makeup.

- Leave a hydrating layer on skin that acts as a humectant, preventing trans-epidermal water loss. Depending on formulation, the residue can also include photoprotective antioxidants and soothing actives like camphor.

CONS OF MICELLAR CLEANSERS

- Contains additional surfactants that can disrupt the skin barrier
- Friction is required to physically remove the micelle complex that contains the dissolved dirt and makeup pigments. This is bad for the skin barrier.

Should I use makeup wipes?
It's not necessary. Wipes contain the highest concentrations of detergents to dissolve makeup pigments quickly and effectively with just a single wipe and that usually also disrupts the skin barrier. Because makeup wipes are usually used on-the-go when there is no access to water, what happens is that there is also a residue left on skin. And remember, surfactants are meant to be wash-off products, not leave on—that's bad for the skin barrier.

SECTION 2

Cosmeceuticals
(Core Syllabus)

download textbook resources and printables*

CHAPTER FIVE

Cosmeceuticals & the Retinoid Family

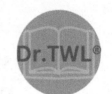

EVIDENCE-BASED
SKINCARE ROUTINES

COSMECEUTICALS
QUASI DRUGS

PRESCRIPTION
CREAMS

WWW.TWLSKIN.COM

What is a cosmeceutical? What qualifies as a cosmeceutical?
There are 3 important criteria that must be fulfilled when it comes to active ingredients, according to Dr Albert Kligman, widely considered the father of cosmeceuticals.

- Penetrates the stratum corneum, delivered in sufficient concentrations to reach skin targets, over the duration of application
- Known, specific biochemical mechanism of action on human skin cells
- Published, peer-reviewed, double-blind, placebo-controlled statistically significant clinical trials to back up claims

Why choose cosmeceuticals?
- Can be non-prescription
- Clinically proven to be effective

This offers added convenience to consumers who do not have to visit a physician for a prescription cream.

This section goes into the core cosmeceuticals you must master. When you study each ingredient, bear in mind the 3 principles we've discussed. You should be able to confidently talk about each ingredient in the context of the Kligman criteria.

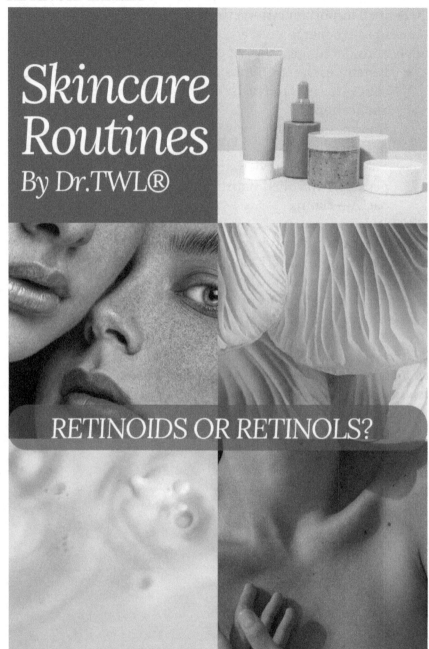

Skincare
Routines
By Dr.TWL®

RETINOIDS OR RETINOLS?

Retinoids were long considered by dermatologists as the gold standard in anti-aging skincare. For a good reason too—they are considered the primary cosmeceutical prescribed in dermatologists' offices for decades. Retinol actives act on multiple pathways in the skin. The benefits include collagen stimulation, increased skin cell renewal and treatment of hyperpigmentation. The results? Almost too good to be true. Radiant, glowing skin that's plumped and elastic. The trouble is, retinoid side effects are real too.

For a complete understanding of the topic, we will discuss the following:
- Types of retinoids (what is relevant to skincare routines)
- What are the 4 types of retinoids?

The retinoid family of chemical compounds includes Vitamin A also known as retinol, derivatives of which are—retinaldehyde, retinoid acid and retinyl esters, amongst other synthetic versions of retinoids. Retinoids are essential to various biological processes.

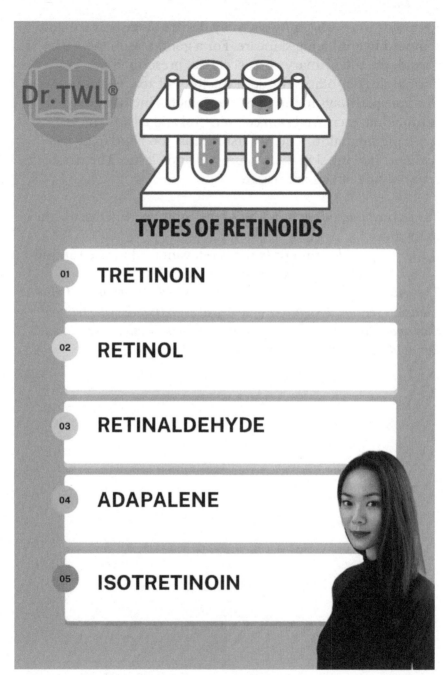

TYPES OF RETINOIDS

01 **TRETINOIN**

02 **RETINOL**

03 **RETINALDEHYDE**

04 **ADAPALENE**

05 **ISOTRETINOIN**

Retinoids for beginners, are they worth it?
The reason retinoids are recommended by dermatologists are:

- *Retinoids treat comedonal acne*
- *Retinoids help reduce scarring and post-inflammation hyperpigmentation (PIH) by regulating cell turnover*
- *Retinoids before and after:*
- *Retinoids are known to enhance skin glow aka the "retinoid glow" which is due to the multiple actions on the epidermis and dermis. Namely, cell renewal rates, enhancing collagen formation for a tighter and more lifted appearance of skin.*
- *Retinoids stimulate collagen production and targets aging skin processes*

For purposes of skincare, we only need to recognise the following main classes of topical retinoids. Based on chemical structure, the earliest generation of retinoids also known as first generation topical retinoids are namely: retinol, retinaldehyde and tretinoin. These are also listed in order of activity from weakest to the most potent. The fourth topical retinoid is known as adapalene which is a third generation retinoid, also known by its trade name adapalene. Isotretinoin is the oral form of retinoid that is prescribed for cystic acne treatment, commonly referred to by its trade name accutane.

- **Retinoids vs Retinol, Benefits & Side Effects**

Over the counter vs prescription retinoids

For over the counter retinoids, these are retinols and retinaldehyde found in skincare products. The AMORE PACIFIC group actually owns the patent to the gold standard retinol ingredient, which is a retinaldehyde derivative that is gentler on skin. Prescription retinoids adapalene and tretinoin have higher potency. Dermatologists usually recommend application of prescription retinoids with a ceramide-dominant moisturiser to reduce irritation. OTC retinol formulations are usually formulated with hydrating ingredients which further reduce its irritation potential. However, the way retinols and retinoids work is that even with great care it can disrupt the skin barrier due to its irritation potential. This can be an immediate reaction, or more commonly a delayed reaction which is due to skin sensitisation. Skin hardening is a phenomenon whereby skin develops tolerance to irritating actives like glycolic acids, retinols, retinoids. This is also the reason dermatologists advise gradual increase in concentration or frequency of use for prescription retinoids.

There are 2 ways to increase the dosage of topical tretinoin, which is the commonest type of prescription retinoid:

1. Starting at 0.01%, 0.025%, increasing to 0.05% then 0.1% Most individuals, especially skin of color cannot tolerate concentrations of higher than 0.05% without photosensitivity and irritation. Always use with cream moisturisers, ceramide dominant formulations recommended).

2. Increasing frequency of application This can mean beginning with a EON regimen for 1 week. Upping it to nightly the following week. Depending on reactions observed, the EON regimen can be further tailed down to twice a week. Any reaction that persists on a twice a week regimen would indicate a need to stop retinol/retinoid product because of intolerance to avoid further side effects,

I would combine both methods 1 & 2 for those with sensitive, dry skin conditions.

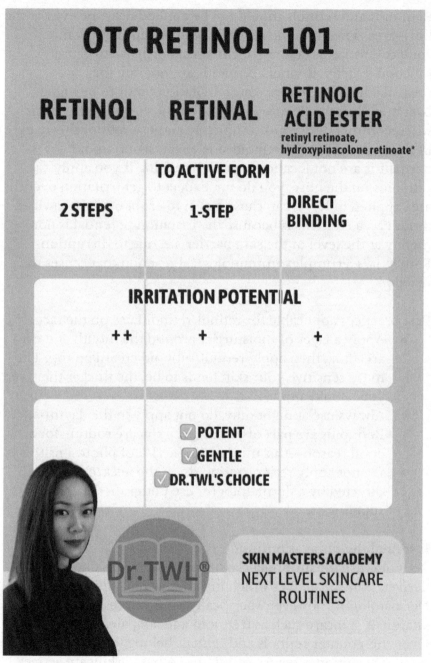

OTC RETINOL 101

RETINOL	RETINAL	RETINOIC ACID ESTER retinyl retinoate, hydroxypinacolone retinoate*
	TO ACTIVE FORM	
2 STEPS	1-STEP	DIRECT BINDING
IRRITATION POTENTIAL		
++	+	+
	☑ POTENT ☑ GENTLE ☑ DR.TWL'S CHOICE	

Dr.TWL®

SKIN MASTERS ACADEMY
NEXT LEVEL SKINCARE
ROUTINES

- Where to apply retinoids (location specific concerns)

Retinoids and retinols should not be applied near the eyes or the lips—areas known as the mucosa. Besides causing irritant contact dermatitis (a form of chemical burn), it can cause mucosal toxicity. Retinols/retinoids are not safe for breastfeeding/pregnancy states. Irritation tends to be higher over areas like the flexures, sides of the nose, neck area—which I will recommend to avoid completely and use retinol alternatives like peptides instead. Retinoid side effects like retinoid dermatitis are not location specific, meaning if you apply retinoids on the nose, you do not expect to get irritation over the area applied only—it can cause a rash to erupt over the jawline, mouth area etc. This is because the irritation potential is not merely at the level of the skin barrier, i.e. due to disruption. Rather, it is a complex immunological reaction that causes the reaction.

Best practices applicable for retinol/retinoid use on the face:
- Apply a layer of moisturiser around the mouth and eye area first, then apply retinol/retinoid cream on top. The more sensitive your skin tends to be, the thicker the layer you should apply.
- Always use at night only, do not apply in the daytime. Retinoids are part of your night skincare routine for a good reason—this minimises the risk of photosensitivity
- Do not apply retinol/retinoids on the neck/chest unless directed by a dermatologist, use under medical supervision

Is retinal the same as retinoid
Retinoids are the umbrella classification term for all vitamin A derived skincare actives which includes retinal and retinol. Dermatologists however, specifically refer to prescription vitamin A skincare such as tretinoin and adapalene as retinoids. Over-the-counter retinols and retinals belong to the non-prescription category of Vitamin A based skincare actives.

Is 0.1% retinal strong?

The concentration of retinal matters. Too low, it doesn't work. Too high and it causes skin irritation.
Dermatologist-recommended OTC skincare typically contains between 0.01 to 0.1% retinal.

Here's an overview of how it works:
Retinoic acid is the form of Vitamin A that is active in skin.

SINGLE STEP CONVERSION

Retinal is directly converted to retinoic acid in a single step
I.e. Retinal—>Retinoic acid

Whereas **retinol** requires 2 stages of conversion to reach its bioactive state
Retinol—>retinal—>retinoic acid

DR.TWL'S TOP PICK FOR SENSITIVE SKIN & ACNE

Retinyl palmitate requires 3 steps of conversion to become retinoic acid.
This is the least potent of OTC retinoids and is also the ideal option for those with extremely sensitive skin who still want to incorporate retinol into their skincare routines. While it is a milder form of retinoid, it does have the same effects of
- Enhancing your skin cell renewal rate
- Boosting collagen production
- Minimise fine lines/wrinkles
- Smoothening skin texture
- Brightens skin
- Antioxidant protection

Retinyl palmitate is converted by enzymes in the skin.

Some key features to note about retinoid family
Ingredient pairing:
- Vitamin C, E, Ferrulic Acid

- Botanical antioxidants

To avoid concurrent use:
AHA, BHA (salicylic acids)
All can cause heightened sun sensitivity

Based on this concept, we understand that retinal is in fact a more efficient active than retinol itself. It acts faster and you get results quicker. This also translates into enhanced skin cell renewal rates but it also means higher irritation risks.

Retinoids for truncal acne
Body acne is often a combination of fungal folliculitis known as pityosporum folliculitis and acne vulgaris. It tends not to respond to topical therapy only and requires oral antibiotic treatment. However, chemical peels with glycolic salicylic and lactic acids up to 20% concentrations can be used twice a week (depending on formulation and manufacturer's recommendations) as adjunct treatment. An effective way to manage truncal/body acne is with LED light therapy. The machine design ought to be one that can wrap around the entire body, i.e. those with a strap design.

Key retinoid benefits
- What retinoids do
- How retinoids work by targeting skin physiology

Retinoids target skin receptors known as nucleic acid receptors. The easiest way to remember retinoid benefits is a mnemonic I designed:
Alteration (changes the skin surface)
Biosynthesis of GAG (glycosaminoglycan)
Cell differentiation
Compaction of stratum corneum
Collagen stimulation
Deposition of GAG
Epidermal thickening

Growth
Immune modulation

- **What is the "retinoid face"?**

Retinoid use has been associated with a "rosy glow". Let me break down for you what's really happening:

1. Compaction of stratum corneum so skin appears thicker
2. Enhanced cell renewal rate: skin appears more radiant
3. Stimulates collagen: fuller, tighter, more lifted appearance

- How to incorporate retinoids into your skincare routine
  1. Night skincare routine Note of caution: retinoids should only be used in your night skincare routine. This is because of photosensitivity side effects—meaning that redness, flaking, swelling which are all signs of skin inflammation triggered by retinoids. UV exposure worsens retinoid dermatitis, what dermatologists specifically consider retinoid induced photosensitivity is an interplay of UV damage, immune alterations and disrupted skin barrier function.

  2. Use sunscreen religiously and practice sun avoidance This means using a SPF 50 broad spectrum sun screen. Wear a broad rimmed hat if you are outdoors but honestly, just get out of the sun if you are using retinoids

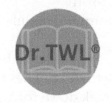

ANTIAGING SKINCARE ROUTINES FOR SENSITIVE SKIN

RETINOL ALTERNATIVES i.e. peptides, bakuchiol

Retinols, retinoids

WWW.TWLSKIN.COM

3. Consider retinoid alternatives *My number 1 choice

My preference is for bakuchiol, a plant derivative with equivalent physiological mechanisms and skin targets as retinol/retinoids but without the irritation side effects. This is because of the anti-inflammatory properties of the extract. It also hydrates the skin barrier, unlike retinols which disrupt the skin barrier.

- Introduction to retinoid relevant Tik Tok trends, skincare trends

Skin cycling was the term introduced in 2023 to describe a skincare regimen that alternates retinoids, acids and moisturisers with off days prescribed.

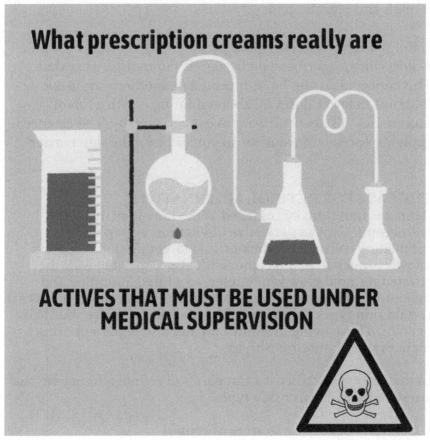

Here's how it applies to retinoid use:
1. Cut down dose of retinoid by lowering frequency i.e. apply it less frequently
When you cycle, essentially it means alternating the days you apply retinoids with moisturisers. This means your skin has time to recover from any irritation caused by retinoids.

2. Minimises irritation potential of acids
By prescribing a regimen that alternates the use of glycolic acids, salicylic acids, retinoids and moisturisers, you will reduce chances of skin irritation. Ultimately, this means the moisturiser gets to repair skin barrier function in between usage of retinoids, retinols and glycolic acids.

3. Emphasise moisturiser therapy
Skin cycling prescribes a dedicated day to moisturising skin. This concept can also be re-invented in another way: using retinoids in lower doses by always diluting it with a ton of moisturiser. It's how you want to explain it really. The essence is applying enough moisturiser so you can heal the skin barrier.

THE CASE FOR RETINOL ALTERNATIVES
Retinol is traditionally regarded as the holy grail of OTC cosmeceuticals. As a derivative of vitamin A, it works by stimulating collagen production and targeting skin receptors known as nucleic acid receptors. It's also associated with the coveted retinoid glow which refers to a lifted, plumped and tightened skin appearance. However, one major downside is that certain skin types do not tolerate it well, i.e. sensitive skin, skin of color. Those living in sunny climates also experience much higher rates of photosensitivity.

In this section, we discuss 7 categories of retinol alternatives that are suited for sensitive skin types.

1. Naturally occurring sources of retinol
The best retinol face serum is found in nature's actives

The brassica oleracea genus includes crucifierous vegetables such as broccoli, cauliflower and cabbage. These are natural sources of Vitamin A found in food. Applied on skin, the body possesses the ability to convert it via a two step process to reach its active retinoic acid stage.

Retinol—>retinal—>retinoic acid

The reason why naturally occurring sources are well tolerated and non-sensitising is because as a whole plant extract, it contains a myriad of other compounds that mitigate skin irritation. For instance, polyphenols with antioxidant, anti-inflammatory and barrier repair effects. In addition, these protect the skin from UV damage, which further reduces the skin-sensitising potential of retinol.

Retinol Face Serum Alternatives
COSMECEUTICAL SCIENCE

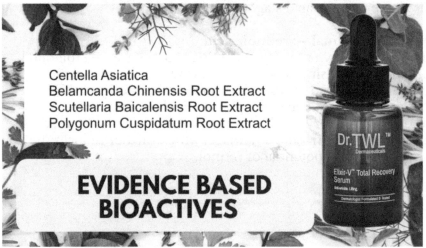

Centella Asiatica
Belamcanda Chinensis Root Extract
Scutellaria Baicalensis Root Extract
Polygonum Cuspidatum Root Extract

EVIDENCE BASED BIOACTIVES

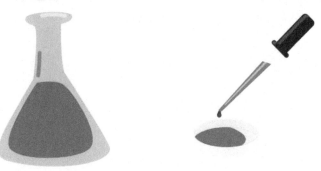

www.twlskin.com

The Elixir-V serum contains brassica extract which is a rich source of natural vitamin A.

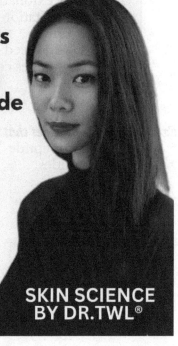

7 Retinol Face Serum Alternatives For Sensitive Skin

Dermatologist Approved

- **Naturally occurring sources of retinol**
- **Retinylpalmitate**
- **Acetylhexapeptide**
- **Oligopeptides**
- **Bakuchiol**
- **Adenosine**

SKIN SCIENCE BY DR.TWL®

2. Retinyl palmitate
Retinol face serums for acne treatment (without skin purging side effects)
Retinyl palmitate undergoes 3 steps of conversion before it becomes retinoic acid, which means it is the least potent of all OTC retinoids. This is my top pick for sensitive skin, especially when it comes to active inflamed acne. Retinoids are helpful in the treatment of comedonal acne but is often blamed as the culprit for acne purging—it induces a pro-inflammatory

response. Retinyl palmitate is the best retinol face serum active for acne prone individuals. Here's why:

- Exfoliates skin cells to reduce pore clogging and comedone formation
- Additional antioxidant effects confer UV protection (minimal photosensitivity)
- Reduces acne scarring by stimulating collagen production and wound healing

The Blemish Spot Cream contains retinyl palmitate which has a triple effect on acne spots

- Gentle skin exfoliation
  - No irritation risk
- Scar prevention
  - UV-induced hyperpigmentation
  - Stimulates collagen production
- Rapid healing
  - Reduces inflammation

Examples of key peptides that can be found in face serums:
- Acetylhexapeptide
- Oligopeptides

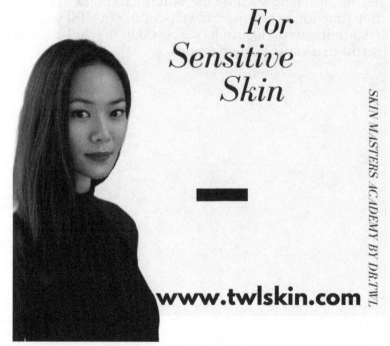

7 RETINOL FACE SERUM ALTERNATIVES

For Sensitive Skin

www.twlskin.com

3. Acetylhexapeptide

Acetylhexapeptide is also known as topical botox— it works directly on the nerve junctions. Specifically, it blocks the release of acetylcholine. This means it reduces the muscle contractions involved in our facial expressions. It also has a remarkable safety profile, as it does not penetrate beyond the uppermost layers of skin. However, acetylhexapeptide containing creams have been shown to improve wrinkles by up to 48% within 4 weeks of twice daily treatment.

4. Oligopeptides
The case for peptide serums: anti wrinkle effects
One major limitation of retinol use is around the eyes and lips. These are what dermatologists refer to as mucosal areas which means the skin is thinner and also more prone to irritation. This is why many who use retinol containing eye creams develop sensitivity with time Peptides are considered well rounded actives which mimic what is naturally found in skin. It's also known as nature's very own anti-wrinkle ingredient—for good reasons too. The best part about peptide serums is that they act holistically. Apart from anti-wrinkle effects, peptides are retinol alternatives that also help stabilise the skin microbiome. This is because they function as anti-microbial peptides (AMPs) which are small, naturally occurring molecules on skin that kill harmful germs that cause skin infections.

Retinol Face Serum Alternatives
FORMULATION SECRETS

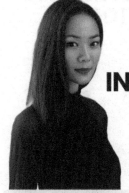

INGREDIENT PAIRING MASTERCLASS

By Dr.TWL®

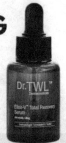

CASE STUDY: ELIXIR-V SERUM

- BASE/VEHICLE
- HUMECTANT/BARRIER REPAIR
- AMINO ACIDS
- BOTANICAL ACTIVES/ADAPTOGENS

www.twlskin.com

5. Bakuchiol
Vegan retinol that's suited for sensitive skin
Bakuchiol is derived from the seeds and leaves of psoralea corylifolia. It's also described as a functional analog of retinol—which means it activates the same nucleic acid receptors as synthetic retinol. This has been validated in studies which show similar gene expression profiles. Remarkably, the side effects associated with traditional retinols are also absent, as it is with other plant sources of retinol. The whole plant extracts include antioxidant and anti-inflammatory properties that

mitigate signs of skin irritation such as redness, stinging and flaking.

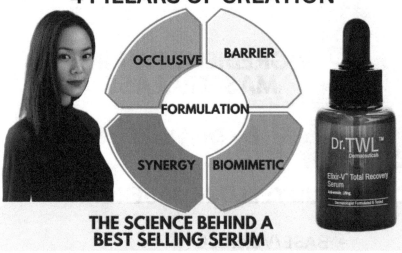

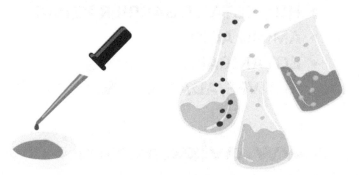

www.twlskin.com

6. Adenosine

Remember adenosine triphosphate (ATP), the molecule you learnt about at school? Adenosine is the amino acid present in ATP itself. When it comes to skincare, adenosine was first observed for its ability to penetrate the human stratum corneum. Later scientists realised that it was also an effective anti wrinkle ingredient in skincare. Specifically, it was tested in clinical studies which showed that it significantly improved frown lines between the brows and also crows feet.

DERM'S PRO TIP: When describing wrinkles on the face, the correct terms would be
- Between the brows : corrugators
- Forehead: glabellar
- Around the eyes: crows feet
- Around the mouth: nasolabial

Retinol Face Serum Alternatives
PLANT-BASED SKINCARE

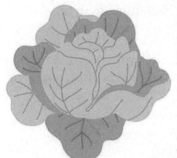

Contains Larecea™ our trademarked extract of Brassica oleracea (a botanical extract from cruciferous family plants) and a super-power Japanese Knotweed plant extract which is a source of trans-resveratrol, a potent anti-oxidant that enhances cellular regeneration at night, without the irritation effects of traditional retinoids.

Integrated humectant formula with polyglutamic acid & hyaluronic acid for intensive hydration and reducing appearance of pores. Polyglutamic acid is 5x more potent than hyaluronic acid in trapping moisture under the skin.

LARECEA + POLYGLUTAMIC ACID
Brassica oleracea

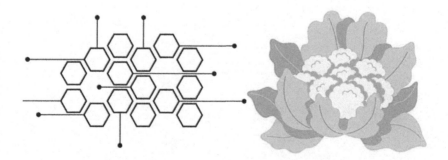

www.twlskin.com

7. Sea buckthorn oil

Fatty acids

Balanced composition of fatty acids which include

- Unsaturated fatty acids
    - palmitooleic acid (omega-7)
    - gamma-linoleic acid (omega-6)
- High linoleic to oleic acid ratio
    - ideal composition for barrier repair

1. Proanthocyanidins

Directly targets oxidative stress related skin aging

- Enhance superoxide dismutase (SOD), glutathione (GSH)
- Remove excess free radicals
- Stimulates collagen 1 synthesis
- Block degradation of collagen 1
- Maintain skin structure (extracellular matrix)

A blend of fatty acids, micronutrients and vitamins with skin regenerative properties that targets all signs of photoaging

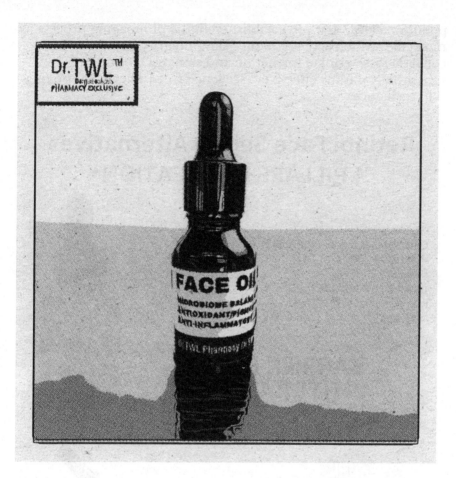

This is a lesser known active that deserves its spot on our list of retinol face serum alternatives. The secret to this anti-aging skincare active is in the balanced composition of fatty acids that mimic the natural lipid ratio of the skin barrier. Specifically, the ratio of linoleic to oleic acids that make up the ideal composition for barrier repair. Sea buckthorn oil has a high linoleic to oleic acid ratio and is particularly rich in unsaturated fatty acids such as omega 6 and omega 7.

The second key feature that makes it an excellent retinol alternative is its proanthocyanidin content. These are highly bioactive compounds which target the key source of aging—free radical damage. Free radicals are highly unstable molecules that are formed by environmental stress such as UV radiation and pollution. They are well established in the photoaging process as molecules which actively reduce skin integrity leading to collagen loss, wrinkle formation and skin discolouration. Proanthocyanidins effectively scavenge free radicals, improving skin resilience.

Retinol Face Serum Alternatives
4 PILLARS OF CREATION

Glycerin
Glyceryl Glucoside, Leaf Water
Panthenol
Betaine
Sodium Hyaluronate
Polyglutamic Acid
Serine, Methionine, Histidine

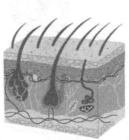

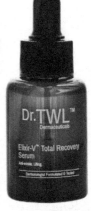

BARRIER REPAIR HYDRATION

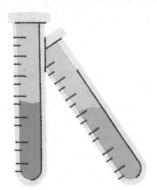

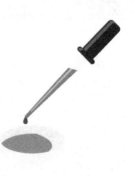

www.twlskin.com

MINI TUTORIAL: THE SCIENCE BEHIND FACE OILS

DR.TWL'S FORMULATION TIPS

- **PURITY MATTERS**

Water-based face serums are assessed for synergistic ingredients that boost overall efficacy. In contrast, face oils are best formulated as pure distillates (without additives) from a whole plant ingredient, carefully selected for its dermatological effects.

- **CAREFUL SELECTION OF PLANT ACTIVE**

Not all plant extracts are suitable actives in face oils. Oils are usually formed from fatty parts of the plant such as the nuts/seeds, rather than leaf/flower parts. This oil itself is a natural carrier of the multiple bioactives innately present in the seed itself, i.e. enhancing absorption. Essential oils used for aromatherapy are not recommended for skin application as these are caustic on skin. Safflower oil, jojoba oil, olive oil and sea buckthorn are the top oils ideally used as whole plant extracts in face oils.

SKIN EXPERT FAQ

What is the best alternative for retinol?
If you have suffered retinol allergies before, you may find yourself searching for alternatives. Here's my list of retinol alternatives:

- Bakuchiol
- Peptides
    - Oligopeptides
    - Acetyl hexapeptide

Also consider actives with retinol-like effects on skin aging such as

- Sea buckthorn oil
- Adenosine (amino acid)

Is there a natural alternative to retinol?
Plants can be a source of natural retinol. For instance the cruciferous vegetables are sources of natural retinol which do not irritate skin because these are whole plant extracts which also have anti-inflammatory effects unlike synthetic derivatives.

Retinol Face Serum Alternatives
HERBAL FORMULA

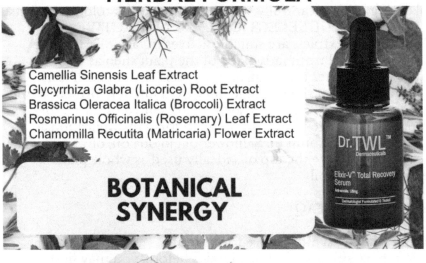

Camellia Sinensis Leaf Extract
Glycyrrhiza Glabra (Licorice) Root Extract
Brassica Oleracea Italica (Broccoli) Extract
Rosmarinus Officinalis (Rosemary) Leaf Extract
Chamomilla Recutita (Matricaria) Flower Extract

**BOTANICAL
SYNERGY**

Dr.TWL™
Dermaceuticals

Elixir-V™ Total Recovery
Serum
Anti-wrinkle. Lifting.
Dermatologist Formulated & Tested

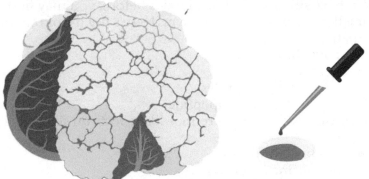

www.twlskin.com

Are retinol alternatives as good as retinol?
The truth is retinol is only as effective as...how well you tolerate
it. It simply isn't true that as long as the dose is low, as long as
you skin cycle—that you won't get side effects. What you can do
instead to to switch out of retinol to other alternatives.
Retinaldehyde for example is well tolerated even by those with
sensitive skin because it requires a 3 step conversion process,
which is gentler on skin.

Which is safer than retinol?
Peptides are recommended especially for those with sensitive skin and or a known history of retinol sensitivity/allergy. For areas such as around the eyes or the mouth area, the skin is thinner and may be more vulnerable to irritation. Look for eye creams that contain natural sources of retinol such as brassica or retinol alternatives such as peptides.

Retinol Face Serum Alternatives
INGREDIENT PAIRING

Centella Asiatica [Acne Scar Lightening]

Larecea™ [Regeneration]

Resveratrol [Anti-oxidant]

Potent Oligopeptides [Lifting] [Repair]

Polyglutamic Acid/Hyaluronic Acid [Humectant] [Pore Reduction]

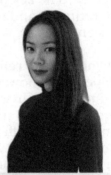

INGREDIENT PAIRING
ANTIOXIDANT + PEPTIDE +HUMECTANT

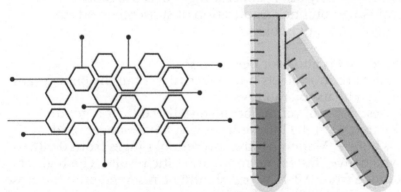

www.twlskin.com

Do retinol alternatives work?
Yes. Studies have shown that oligopeptides have equivalent effects as retinol does, sans skin irritation risks.

Is natural retinol home made?

No. Natural retinol refers to plant-based or botanical sources of retinol. Examples are bakuchiol, rose hip seed oil, carrot seed oil and sea buckthorn oil. Proper distillation processes are essential to ensure purity of the product and efficacy.

What does retinol serum do for the face?

Retinols belong to the family of retinoids which stimulate cell renewal and collagen production. Retinol serums are over-the-counter cosmeceuticals, distinct from prescription retinoids. The key differences are that retinols are less potent than retinoids and require a longer period of use before results are seen.

Is it good to use retinol serum everyday?

It depends on how well you tolerate it. If you are using a retinol product for the first time, it is advisable to start at a lower frequency i.e. 2-3 times a week or as directed by the manufacturer. Different formulations of retinol also confer different tolerability levels, so it is best to do a patch test before you apply to the entire face. For example, under the jawline, left on overnight is good practice. Check for signs of irritation such as redness, flaking, stinging or burning.

Remember to only use retinols at night because of its sunsensitising potential. Application of sunscreen and sun avoidance is also advisable.

Which retinol is good for beginners?

The dose of retinol affects how effective it is but the benefits are also limited by its tolerability.
The lowest doses of retinol begin at 0.01-0.03%. It is good practice to start at the lowest doses if you have never used retinols before. Moderate-strength retinol ranges from 0.03% to 0.3% which gives faster and more dramatic results. The highest doses range from 0.3-1% which should be reserved only for those who have tolerated lower doses.

What are the side effects of retinol serum?

Most commonly, local skin irritation such as redness, burning, stinging and flaking. Some individuals have true retinol allergy which results in a more exaggerated response. Care must be taken not to apply retinol formulations close to the eye area unless specifically formulated for that region.

Should I use retinol or retinoids?
If you already use retinol, prescription retinoids may be an option for highest efficacy. However, bear in mind that sensitisation can still occur. This is why at the pharmacy, our formulations are all retinol-free. Instead, we focus on non-sensitising retinol alternatives such as bakuchiol, sea buckthorn oil and oligopeptides.

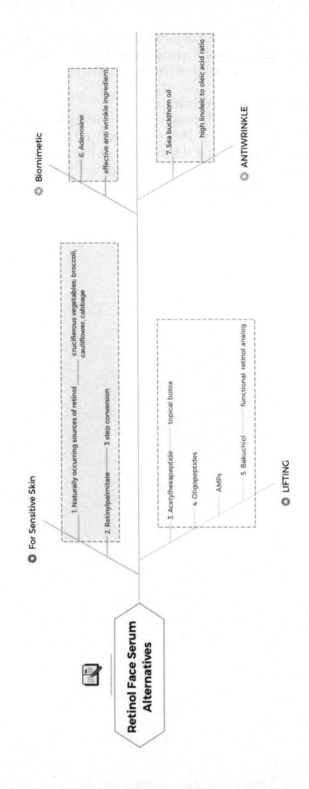

Retinol Face Serum Alternatives

For Sensitive Skin

1. Naturally occurring sources of retinol — cruciferous vegetables: broccoli, cauliflower, cabbage

2. Retinylpalmitate — 3 step conversion

Biomimetic

6. Adenosine — effective anti wrinkle ingredient

ANTIWRINKLE

7. Sea buckthorn oil — high linoleic to oleic acid ratio

LIFTING

3. Acetylhexapeptide — topical botox

4. Oligopeptides

AMPs

5. Bakuchiol — functional retinol analog

SHORT NOTES

- Korean skincare: retinol alternatives
- Best retinoids, retinols for sensitive skin
- Skin cycling techniques for retinol/retinoid use
- Frequency: using retinoids daily vs weekly regimens

Cosmeceutical korean skincare regimens notably exclude retinol/acids as leave on skincare products. Instead, these are incorporated as wash off peels which can be used weekly or as often as tolerated. The whole idea here is you should completely avoid retinoids and retinols if you have sensitive skin—choose peptides and bakuchiol instead. Skin cycling techniques are essential but that also means you limit the effectiveness of the product—the whole idea of a topical in your skincare regimen is that you want to apply it—and in my opinion the profile of retinoid side effects simply screams—do not use! Frankly, that's the gold standard skincare ingredient for skin barrier damage. In 2023, when retinol alternatives like peptides are evidenced-based. They have similar effects on skin, sans irritation.

This is where skin flooding becomes relevant:

The reason why I stopped using retinoids myself was because of a bad bout of retinoid dermatitis, which occured after 10 years of use. In theory, my skin was already hardened to retinoids, so I should not have been particularly at risk. But that also reminded me how these reactions are idiosyncratic. That means we cannot predict when it happens, to whom. Certainly I would avoid retinol use in those who have eczema or sensitive skin, but even those without sensitive skin can develop delayed sensitivity.

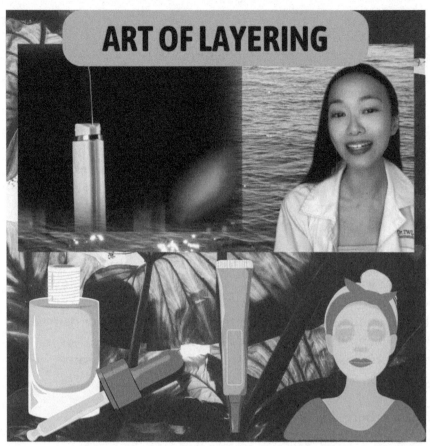

ART OF LAYERING

I adopted instead the korean skincare routine which prioritises healing the skin barrier. The skincare layering steps are really about maximising concentration of active ingredients delivered to skin. By separating the ingredients into serum, lotion, emulsion and cream formulations respectively, the end result is that a higher overall dose is achieved per application.

Skincare layering also creates a moist wound healing environment which essentially enhances the effectiveness of each skincare routine step. The moisture occlusion sandwich works.

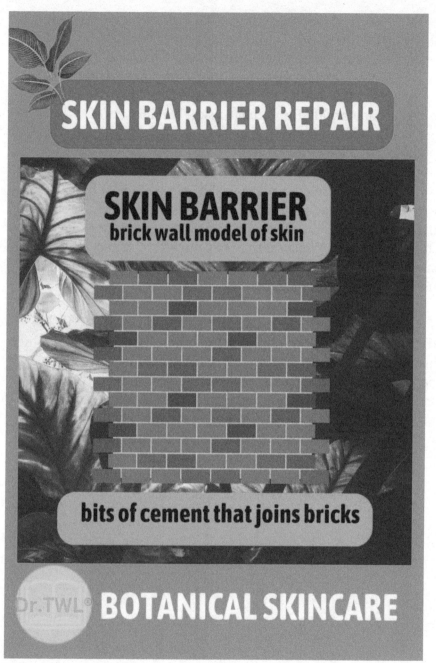

Retinoid & Skin Barrier Damage
- Damaged skin barrier before after how to recognise

- Retinol damaged skin barrier, retinol ruined my skin: truth or scam?
- Can skin barrier be permanently damaged
- How to treat acne with a damaged skin barrier
- How to know if skin barrier is damaged
- Niacinamide for damaged skin barrier
- Oral retinoids

- Retinol and skin barrier damage

Retinol does cause disruption in the skin barrier. What looks to be exfoliation that targets skin renewal also leads to a breakdown in the glue that joins skin cells known as corneocytes together. Is there a solution? Well you may have heard of skin cycling, but in simpler terms that just means not using retinols everyday and using moisturiser. Not genius.

Trouble is even that does not solve the problem of barrier dysfunction. I suspect that immunological reactions occur which also disturbs the microbiome, all of which constitute skin ecology. Immediate barrier damage occurs in the form of irritant contact dermatitis, delayed barrier damage in the form of a hypersensitivity reaction. The latter was what happened to me after 10 years of religiously using prescription retinoids.

- Damaged skin barrier before after how to recognise
- How to know if skin barrier is damaged

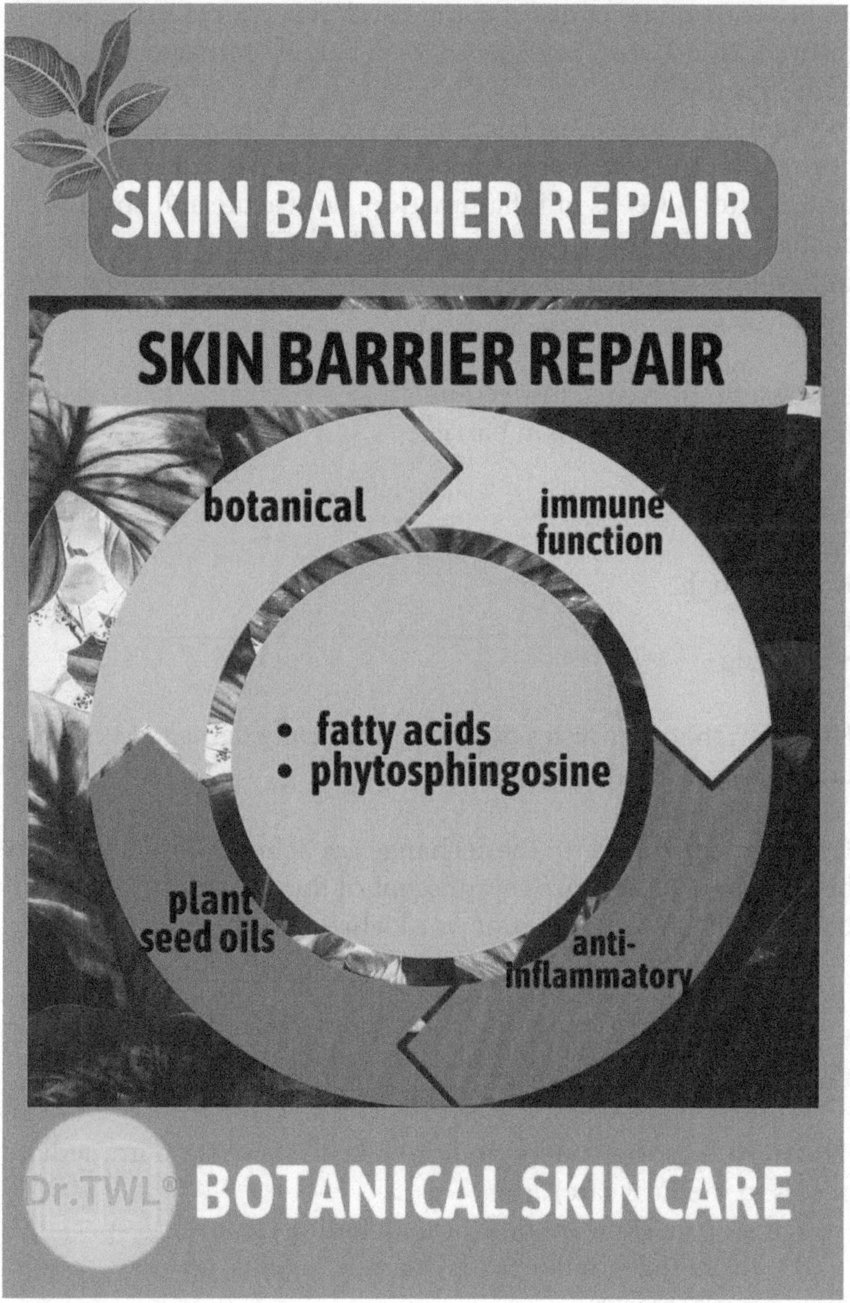

SKIN BARRIER REPAIR

SKIN BARRIER REPAIR

botanical

immune function

- fatty acids
- phytosphingosine

plant seed oils

anti-inflammatory

Dr.TWL® BOTANICAL SKINCARE

So how do you recognise a damaged skin barrier? First up we distinguish between the types of skin barrier damage:
Acute vs chronic
In general anything that has gone on for less than 6 weeks dermatologists consider as acute. Chronic skin barrier damage occurs after 6 weeks of inflammation, both acute and chronic changes can appear simultaneously. The underlying cause is inflammation which causes skin to react with visible changes on the surface.

Here's a tip for visual inspection:
For acutely damaged skin barrier:

F Flaking
A Angry
R Red, rough
P Pain
S Stinging

However, there are also signs of a chronically damaged skin barrier you should not miss:

Dermatologists refer to these changes as lichenification, which is because the changes are reminiscent of the thickening of a tree bark i.e. lichen itself the root word which it refers to.

T Thickening
L Lines
D Dullness

The most important steps you can take (if there is no immediate access to medical care) are:
- Stop all skincare products including cleansers (especially those that contain acids, foaming agents, retinols), toners, peels, masks
- Use only a dermatologist-recommended intensive moisturising cream

Apply 5 times a day on damp skin

Wet occlusion sheet masking (without essence): Use a reusable face mask (polysaccharide material to enhance moisture delivery) or use a soft microfibre towel that is dampened. This increases delivery of moisture to the skin.

How to choose a moisturiser: active ingredients should include Ceramide (phytoceramides like shea butter included, synthetic) Hyaluronic acid

Glycerin

In general I would avoid lanolin (sensitising) and fragrance for damaged skin barrier.

- OTC Hydrocortisone (1% available where I practice)

Use twice a day before applying moisturiser for 3 days strictly. If there is no improvement with the above regimen. A consultation with a dermatologist is necessary. If there is any sign of: Allergy, burn, swelling, fever, should seek medical attention immediately.

*Caution: do not self-medicate with topical steroids. In the medium to long term this can impact effectiveness of medical therapy and can also cause severe irreversible damage to the skin i.e. thinning, ulceration, permanent redness.

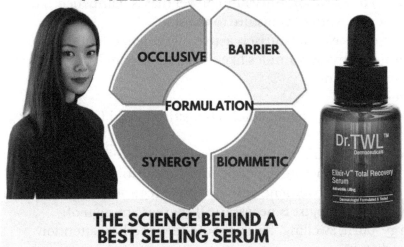

BEST FACE SERUM
4 PILLARS OF CREATION

OCCLUSIVE | BARRIER

FORMULATION

SYNERGY | BIOMIMETIC

Dr.TWL™
Dermaceuticals

Elixir-V™ Total Recovery Serum

THE SCIENCE BEHIND A BEST SELLING SERUM

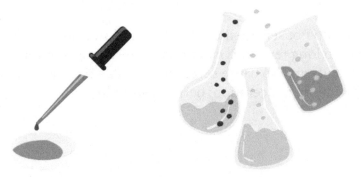

www.twlskin.com

In this tutorial, we go through the core ingredients and formulation of a gold standard antiaging serum for universal skin types.

BEST FACE SERUM
PLANT-BASED SKINCARE

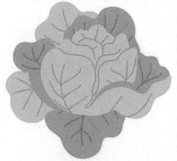

Contains Larecea™ our trademarked extract of Brassica oleracea (a botanical extract from cruciferous family plants) and a super-power Japanese Knotweed plant extract which is a source of trans-resveratrol, a potent anti-oxidant that enhances cellular regeneration at night, without the irritation effects of traditional retinoids.

Integrated humectant formula with polyglutamic acid & hyaluronic acid for intensive hydration and reducing appearance of pores. Polyglutamic acid is 5x more potent than hyaluronic acid in trapping moisture under the skin.

LARECEA + POLYGLUTAMIC ACID
Brassica oleracea

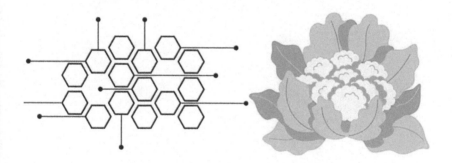

www.twlskin.com

Barrier repair actives and stabilising vehicle
- Glycerin
- Glyceryl Glucoside, Leaf Water
- Panthenol
- Betaine
- Sodium Hyaluronate
- Polyglutamic Acid
- Serine, Methionine, Histidine

The first category of actives we shall discuss are those that work on the superficial layers of skin. Humectants like hyaluronic acid, polyglutamic acid, amino acids and glycerin which trap moisture under the stratum corneum and prevent transepidermal water loss. Soothing actives like panthenol and amino acids also double up as building blocks for the skin's own reserve of natural moisturising factors.

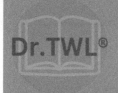

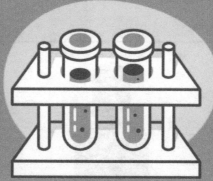

HOW PRODUCTS IMPROVE SKIN RESILIENCE

01 **INCREASE ANTIOXIDANT CAPACITY**

02 **STIMULATES CELL REPAIR**

03 **BUILD HEALTHY SKIN CLIMATE**

04 **IMPROVE PHYSICAL APPEARANCE OF SKIN**

05 **ENCOURAGE CELL TALK**

DERMATOLOGIST RECOMMENDED SKINCARE ROUTINES

CASE STUDY INGREDIENT ANALYSIS

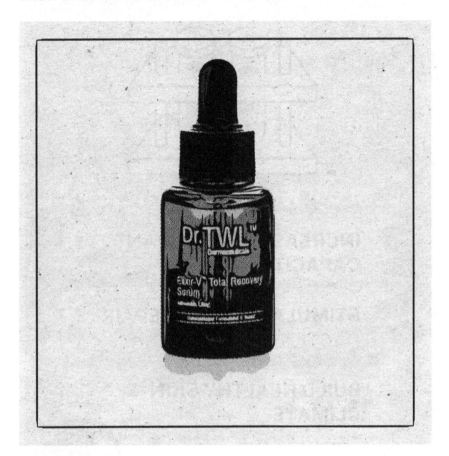

Glycerin
Glyceryl Glucoside, Leaf Water
Panthenol
Betaine
Sodium Hyaluronate
Polyglutamic Acid
Serine, Methionine, Histidine

Centella Asiatica
Belamcanda Chinensis Root Extract
Scutellaria Baicalensis Root Extract
Polygonum Cuspidatum Root Extract

Camellia Sinensis Leaf Extract
Glycyrrhiza Glabra (Licorice) Root Extract
Brassica Oleracea Italica (Broccoli) Extract
Rosmarinus Officinalis (Rosemary) Leaf Extract
Chamomilla Recutita (Matricaria) Flower Extract

Beta-Glucan
Oligopeptide-1

*Ingredients discussed in decreasing order of concentrations.

BASE/VEHICLE: POLYGLUTAMIC ACID VS HYALURONIC ACID

The ideal serum vehicle is water-based which allows for a lightweight texture fit for the skincare layering technique. Polyglutamic acid is my choice for the combination serum base as it enhances the synergistic effects of the other additives. It holds 5X more water than hyaluronic acid but is significantly more expensive. Hence, it is best formulated with other actives rather than as a pure serum for cost-efficiency. Higher concentrations of polyglutamic acid do not necessarily translate into increased efficacy and can increase the stickiness sensation of the product.

HUMECTANT/BARRIER REPAIR: AMINO ACIDS

The serum includes a mixture of amino acids (methionine, serine, histidine) both in synthetic and derivative form. For instance, whole plant extracts contain naturally occurring methionine, also known as Vitamin U, which is essential for wound healing and has additional UV-protective properties. Glycerin is a well-known traditional humectant and is part of ideal serum formulations to enhance effect of actives.

Humectants are not just barrier repair actives, glycerin for instance actually creates a micro-climate within the formulation itself that enhances the activity of other ingredients.

BOTANICAL ACTIVES/ADAPTOGENS

Adaptogens help skin to "adapt" to environmental stressors. When UV damage occurs, free radicals generated cause a form of physiological stress to the skin, known as oxidative stress.

Plant actives are the most effective form of adaptogens as plants are innately selected to adapt to their environment. Different plant parts possess varying properties—the roots, stems, leaves and flowers contain varying actives that can be incorporated to strengthen skin. Skin resilience respects the entire skin eco-system, encouraging beneficial cell talk activity and improving skin immunity. A key function of adaptogens is to enhance skin resilience, which means it is able to repair DNA damage from daily stressors such as UV radiation, carcinogens and airborne pollution. In addition, adaptogens increase the skin's natural reserve of antioxidants that combat the effects of cell inflammaging, caused by biological aging processes.

RESVERATROL
LEARNING OBJECTIVES

- ☐ SOURCES (NATURAL VS SYNTHETIC)
- ☐ MECHANISM OF ACTION/HOW IT WORKS
- ☐ WHAT IS IT USED FOR
- ☐ DR.TWL FORMULATION SECRET: JAPANESE KNOTWEED

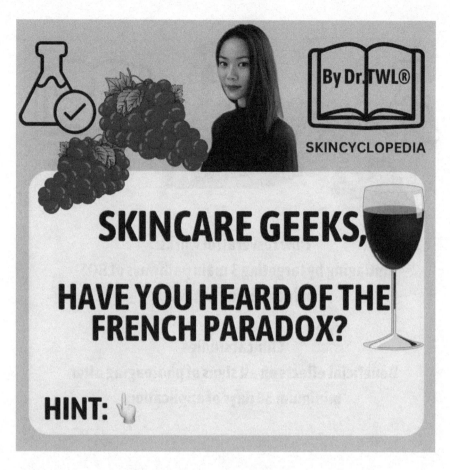

SKINCARE GEEKS,

HAVE YOU HEARD OF THE FRENCH PARADOX?

HINT:

SOURCES (NATURAL VS SYNTHETIC)

Resveratrol was made prominent in 1992 as researchers unraveled the "French Paradox" which associated health benefits with moderate wine consumption. Turns out, grapes contain this key ingredient resveratrol which has potent physiological effects throughout the body. The key actives are known as polyphenols which belong to the stilbenoid group of compounds. Resveratrol exists in 2 forms, as the active trans-isomer and the inactive cis-isomer. Over 70 plant sources of reseveratrol exist, the most prominent of which are grapes (found in the seeds/skin), red wine, peanuts and soy.

- Polyphenols (stilbenoid group)
- Two forms (active *trans*-isomer, inactive *cis*-isomer)
- Natural sources (>70 plant sources)
- Dietary (grape seeds/skin, red wine, peanuts, soy)

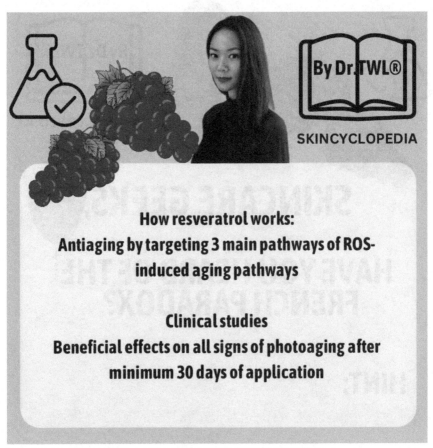

How resveratrol works:
Antiaging by targeting 3 main pathways of ROS-induced aging pathways

Clinical studies
Beneficial effects on all signs of photoaging after minimum 30 days of application

MECHANISM OF ACTION/HOW IT WORKS

- **Antioxidant**

Protect cells against hydrogen peroxide-induced oxidative stress, UV-damage

- Direct: Free radical scavenger
- Indirect: Modulates cell antioxidant pathways

- **Anti-inflammatory**

Helps auto-immune and chronic inflammatory diseases

- NFKB, IL6, eicosanoids
- TLR2, TLR3, TLR4 signalling
- Reduces TLR7, TLR8, TLR9-mediated inflammation (psoriasis)

- Anti-cancer effects
- Regulate metabolism (whole body fat and blood sugar levels)
- Specific skin targets:
  - Wound healing
  - Scarring
  - Photoaging

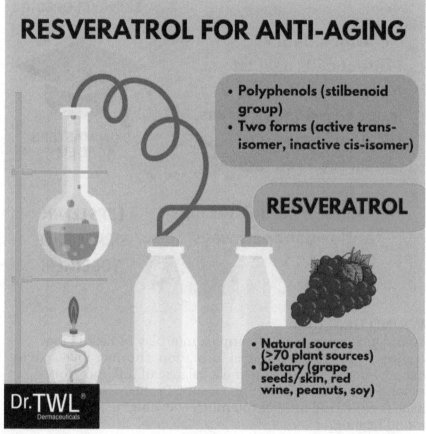

RESVERATROL FOR ANTI-AGING

- Polyphenols (stilbenoid group)
- Two forms (active trans-isomer, inactive cis-isomer)

RESVERATROL

- Natural sources (>70 plant sources)
- Dietary (grape seeds/skin, red wine, peanuts, soy)

Dr.TWL®
Dermaceuticals

Reseveratrol is a well-rounded skincare active that has holistic effects on skin. The "anti" effects are as follows: as an antioxidant which neutralises cell damaging free radicals, an anti-inflammatory agent that reduces inflammation in various skin diseases, and also as an anti-cancer agent which prevents the growth of abnormal mutant skin cells. There are other specific "pro" effects such promoting wound healing (minimising scarring), cell repair which slows down photoaging and also promoting cell metabolism for healthy skin functioning.

MECHANISM OF ACTION HOW IT WORKS

By Dr.TWL®

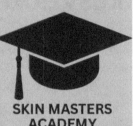

SKINCYCLOPEDIA

SKIN MASTERS
ACADEMY

LET'S LEARN
SKIN SCIENCE
TOGETHER!

- **Antioxidant**
Protect cells against hydrogen peroxide-induced oxidative stress, UV-damage
  - **Direct: Free radical scavenger**
  - **Indirect: Modulates cell antioxidant pathways**

WOUND HEALING

Wound healing involves a complex interplay of factors that requires sufficient blood vessel formation, antimicrobial activity that prevents skin infection and a balance of inflammatory responses that result in wound closure. Problems arise when the tissue is either too little or too much—leading to improper wound healing.

Resveratrol promotes wound healing by exerting the following effects:
The 4 'A's of Resveratrol
- Anti-inflammatory
- Anti-oxidative
- Angiogenesis (blood vessel formation)
- Anti-microbial (fights infections)

MECHANISM OF ACTION HOW IT WORKS

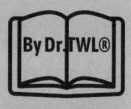

SKINCYCLOPEDIA

- **Anti-inflammatory**
- **Helps auto-immune and chronic inflammatory diseases**
- **Regulate metabolism (whole body fat and blood sugar levels)**

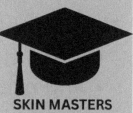

SKIN MASTERS ACADEMY

- **Wound healing**
- **Scarring**
- **Photoaging**

LET'S LEARN SKIN SCIENCE TOGETHER!

How it works
- Protects collagen-producing cells (fibroblasts)
- Stabilise skin structure
- Promote blood vessel formation (VEGF)
- Antibacterial effects (Staph aureus, Pseudomonas aeruginosa, Candida albicans, superior to commercial antimicrobial ointments)
- Special medical applications: treat non-healing wounds i.e. diabetic ulcers

Resveratrol exerts potent effects that contribute towards healthy skin repair and functioning. For instance, it promotes cell stability by protecting collagen, stabilises the deeper structure of skin known as the extracellular matrix and also exerts antibacterial effects superior to topical antibiotic creams when it is used on wounds. Additional skincare benefits include scar lightening, barrier repair and UV-protection.

189

Resveratrol Benefits

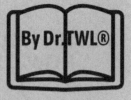

SKINCYCLOPEDIA

The 4 'A's of Resveratrol

- Anti-inflammatory
- Anti-oxidative
- Angiogenesis (blood vessel formation)
- Anti-microbial (fights infections)

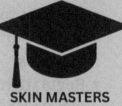

SKIN MASTERS ACADEMY

LET'S LEARN SKIN SCIENCE TOGETHER!

Skincare benefits
- Anti-scarring

Prevents development of abnormal scars in laboratory studies
- Photoprotection
- Barrier function (moisture delivery)

Crucial to a solid grasp of this aspect of how resveratrol works is the understanding of UV-related skin damage. You may have heard of oxidative stress, as well as the term antioxidant. These terms are meaningful only when you understand how UV-damage actually occurs. Here is a step-by-step explanation.

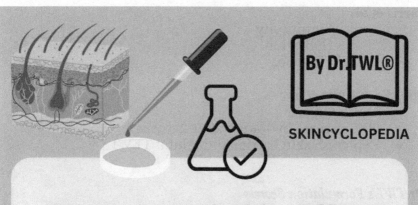

Resveratrol Skin Effects

- **Luminosity**
- **Hydration**
- **Elasticity**
- **Tightening**
- **20% increase hydration after 2 weeks**
- **Replenish skin barrier and inhibit TEWL**

How UV damages skin:
Chronic UV exposure results in activation of 3 major aging cascades known by the acronym MIA

- **Reactive oxygen species (ROS) production**
  - Metalloproteinases MMP-1 mediated
  - Inflammaging IL-6, 8 mediated
  - Apoptosis-induced via NFKB, caspase 3

How resveratrol works:
- Antiaging by targeting 3 main pathways of ROS-induced aging pathways

Clinical studies
- Beneficial effects on all signs of photoaging after minimum 30 days of application

Farris et al
- ○ Luminosity
- ○ Hydration
- ○ Elasticity

Igielska-Kalwat et al
- Tightening
- 20% increase hydration after 2 weeks
- Replenish skin barrier and inhibit TEWL

Dr.TWL's Formulation Secrets

Proanthocyanidins: Nature's Anti-aging Fingerprint

The best-selling Elixir-V Serum contains Japanese Knotweed, also known as polygonum cuspidatum. It is a source of trans-resveratrol which is an active form of the compound. It is lesser known in western pharmacology but is well established in ethnobotanical applications. Biochemical analysis has shown it to be a rich source of proanthocyanidins, a potent antioxidant, specifically found in the roots of the plant.

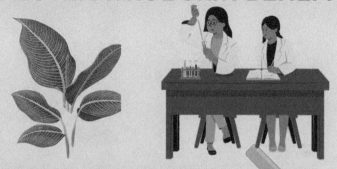

RESVERATROL SKIN BENEFITS

PROANTHOCYANIDIN: BIOACTIVE COMPOUNDS

- **Anthraquinones**
- **Flavanoids (rutin, apigenin, quercetin)**
- **Stilbenes (resveratrol)**
- **Catechin, epicatechin, epicatechin-gallate**
- **Procyanidin B12**

www.twlskin.com

Native to East Asia, it is an invasive plant that also has medicinal properties.

Chromatographic studies have isolated the following

- Anthraquinones
- Flavanoids (rutin, apigenin, quercetin)
- Stilbenes (resveratrol)
- Catechin, epicatechin, epicatechin-gallate
- Procyanidin B12

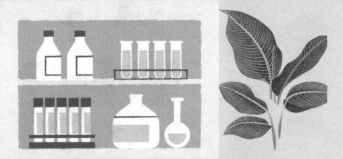

RESVERATROL SKIN BENEFITS

PROANTHOCYANIDINS:
Holistic effects on skin physiology

- Antioxidant
- Antimicrobial (stilbenes, anthraquinones)
- Anti-inflammatory
- Inhibit pigment formation
- Anti-tumor
- Barrier repair

www.twlskin.com

By virtue of it being a whole plant extract rather than a chemically synthesised copy, there are additional benefits such as:

Holistic effects on skin physiology
- Antioxidant
- Antimicrobial (stilbenes, anthraquinones)
- Anti-inflammatory

- Inhibit pigment formation
- Anti-tumor
- Barrier repair

Sirtuin, the youth protein

The sirtuin family of proteins are an important target of antiaging and skin cancer research. Specifically, sirtuin 1 is a NAD+dependant acetylase which regulates multiple biological pathways involved in aging cells. By modifying SIRT1 activity, the lifespan of organisms can be prolonged. This is where the study of botanicals such as resveratrol becomes relevant—several plant compounds have been proven to directly impact SIRT1 expression.

FERULIC ACID

LEARNING OBJECTIVES

☐ SOURCES (NATURAL VS SYNTHETIC)
☐ MECHANISM OF ACTION/HOW IT WORKS
☐ WHAT IS IT USED FOR
☐ DR.TWL FORMULATION SECRETS

SOURCES (NATURAL VS SYNTHETIC)

- Whole grains
- Spinach, parsley, grapes, rhubarb
- Cereal seeds: wheat, oats, rye, barley

MECHANISM OF ACTION/HOW IT WORKS
'ANTI-EFFECTS'

- Super antioxidant
  - Fights free radical damage
    - Direct neutralisation
    - Inhibits free radical catalytic enzymes
    - Enhance scavenger enzymes
- Antioxidant activity
    - Forms stable phenoxyl radicals
    - Radical molecule + antioxidant molecule formation
    - Blocks complex reaction cascade of free radical generation
    - Prevents UV-induced cell/DNA damage

- o Free radical scavenging
- o Bind transition metals i.e. iron, copper
- o Block lipid peroxidation
- Anti-inflammatory
- Antimicrobial
- Anti cancer

'PRO STIMULATORY EFFECTS'
- **Regeneration & wound healing**
  - o Blood vessel formation via VEGF, PDGF, HIF01
  - o Immunomodulatory
  - o Cell repair

☐ **WHAT IS IT USED FOR**
- Stabiliser/pairing
  - o Paired with Vitamin C, Vitamin E as stabiliser, boost UV-protection
  - o Paired with niacinamide as skin brightener
  - o Paired with hyaluronic acid for barrier protection
  - o Paired with lipohydroxycarbones (keratolytic) for enhanced absorption
- Anti-pollution, UV-protective
  - o Boost intracellular antioxidant defense
  - o Protects cell structures
- Depigmenting
  - o Inhibits tyrosinase (melanogenesis)
  - o Inhibits melanocyte growth

☐ **DR.TWL FORMULATION SECRETS:**
- OTC: 0.5-1% concentration
- Cosmeceutical: 12% concentration
- Adjunct: microneedling, chemical peels
  - o Skin aging /photoaging
  - o Hyperpigmentation, melasma
  - o Seborrheic(oily) skin
  - o Acne

GINGKO BILOBA
BIOACTIVES
- Flavanoids (quercetin, kaempferol, isorhamnetin)
- Terpenoids (Gingkolide A, B, C, biloba like)
- 1%-5% cream

- Good skin penetration
- Improves
  - Wound healing
  - Barrier function
  - Anti-wrinkle effects
  - Rosacea treatment
- Ingredient pairing: Green tea extract (EGCG)

CHAPTER SIX

Cosmeceutical Skincare FAQ—Facts, Myths, Retinol Before/After

Fact: prescription creams damage the skin barrier
Myth: prescription creams are superior and are always effective

Retinoids for one are prescription only, for a good reason. It can cause severe damage to healthy skin—like it did to mine. Functional dermatology is the approach I take formulating skincare—choosing retinoid alternatives such as peptides and botanical equivalents that have additional benefits: for instance, they are anti-inflammatory, repair the skin barrier and also restore the skin microbiome...which retinoids and prescription creams don't do. So in this section I'll try to piece everything together for you to understand and formulate an individualised approach for yourself or your client.

We begin with one of the most pressing questions about retinoid related skin barrier damage:
 • Can the skin barrier be permanently damaged?
Nothing is ever impossible when it comes to the human body—the fundamental rule of science is that there will always be exceptions. However, it is quite unlikely, if you follow these principles I've discussed, that you'll end up with permanent skin barrier dysfunction. But for instance if best practices are not followed, one can potentially accelerate and worsen barrier dysfunction to the extent that it becomes a chronic skin condition. I have seen patients who were prescribed retinoids, either oral or topical despite their personal history of sensitive skin or even eczema—and they go on to suffer life long skin

barrier dysfunction which can be quite severe. Even requiring immunosuppressant treatment. But in general, for individuals who develop retinoid allergies, as long as the retinoids are stopped and treatment initiated, most cases will recover. The trouble also is that it's often difficult for those who have used retinoids for many years, like me—over a decade, to give it up. I think it is partly psychological, since access to retinoids usually begins with a medical prescription for a skin concern. Retinoids do work, and when you find that your skin condition improves, even when you develop side effects like irritation, it's easy to enter into denial. So that's one thing to watch out for.

- How to treat acne with a damaged skin barrier

Here's the paradox: acne is associated with oily skin, but oily skin can have a damaged skin barrier too. Why? Pharmaceuticals, most of the time.

It's a chicken and egg situation here. Traditional acne treatment has long advocated use of astringents like toners, salicylic acid, benzoyl peroxide, retinoids—based on an outdated mindset that acne was caused by greasy skin. Period.

That's patently false: here's why.

Acne is now understood to be a multi factorial condition. Sufferers of acne do tend to have oily skin, but primarily have a strong genetic predisposition which increases the activity of a certain gene known as PPAR-y receptor. At puberty, the surge in the hormone testosterone causes an increase in oil production, which stimulates inflammation. I.e. the process of comedone formation.

Yet, actives like toners, salicylic acid, benzoyl peroxide do not target acne holistically—they address only the aspect of oil production.

The trouble also is that oil production is not an outside-in issue. It's inside out. We've mentioned genetics. But the key here is sebum regulation. There is excess oil being produced, partly also because the skin's sebaceous glands are getting the wrong signals. When you apply barrier disrupting skincare to acne prone skin, the signals go further haywire.

199

What do you do instead:
Choose holistic actives—in my research I've identified botanical actives which address acne inflammation. None of the traditional acne creams are anti-inflammatory, which is a problem. To reduce inflammation, dermatologists opt for topical steroids for a short duration —since steroids themselves cause steroid-induced acne. When it's an angry looking cyst, intralesional steroid injections are applied. But none of these are medium to long term solutions...and acne is unfortunately a chronic condition.

For instance, berberine, which was first discovered and used widely amongst practitioners of traditional chinese medicine, targets multiple pathways of acne:
- Inflammation
- Comedogenesis
- Post-inflammation hyperpigmentation (scarring)
- Oxidative stress (anti-oxidant effect)

With this in mind, we carry on with our list of best practices for using retinoids to minimise adverse events, although it must be noted that in spite of all this, sensitisation can still occur.

- How to choose retinoid skincare products, retinol recommendations

Retinols are the form of retinoids available OTC, whereas retinoid compounds like tretinoin and adapalene are strictly via prescription only.
Here are the key principles to abide by when choosing a retinol skincare product. It also applies to skincare that contains glycolic acids, salicylic acids. These are all products that can disrupt the skin barrier, so common principles apply:

- Vehicle: choose a cream formula, not serum or lotion

Leave on products which contain irritating ingredients must ideally be formulated in a moisturising base. The best retinol formula should include ceramides, glycerin and hyaluronic acids. Since retinols are only to be used at night, there is no concern with texture or greasiness. In fact we want the skin to be hydrated and repaired overnight rather than having the skin barrier disrupted.

- Ingredient pairing: avoid retinol with salicylic, glycolic, lactic acids
- The concept of skin cycling can be condensed into this: moisturise and give your skin a break from retinols/acids, which means the product you apply should itself be moisturising to reduce risk of irritation
- Consider alternatives, i.e. vegan retinol is really bakuchiol which targets similar molecular pathways as compounds in the retinoid family. The key advantages of this active are:
  - non-irritating/stimulating
  - repairs the skin barrier instead of disrupting it
  - in-built anti-inflammatory effects (no need for skin cycling)

- Retinoids before and after, what to expect

RETINOIDS BEFORE
First, let's discuss who should never use retinoids on any part of their face:
  - Anyone with a personal or family history of sensitivity, reactivity
  - Dry skin symptoms
  - Broken skin (see a dermatologist to find out the underlying cause)
  - Active inflamed acne bumps (will make the acne worse, not better)
  - Any signs of a damaged skin barrier
  - Pregnant/breastfeeding states
  - Lifestyle considerations (outdoor activities, sun exposure—regardless of sunscreen use)

Such candidates should opt for retinol alternatives like peptides, bakuchiol for antiaging, botanicals like berberine for acne, because of the risk of photosensitivity.

The ideal candidate for retinoids:
- o Oily skin type
- o 20s-early 30s: decline in skin barrier function after may increase risk of skin irritation
- o Predominantly comedonal acne (whiteheads, blackheads)
- o Lifestyle involves low sun exposure, can practice sun avoidance

RETINOIDS AFTER
- Retinoids are no miracle workers. To see results, one must consider the following
  - o Consistency of use (for ideal effects, nightly use which may not be possible on sensitive skin)
  - o Duration of use minimum 2-4 weeks to see results

- Retinoid rosy glow

The retinoid glow, also referred to as retinoid facies in dermatology is the characteristic complexion of one who uses retinoids. It's slightly pink which in 2023 is not a good marker of skin health —refers to inflammation caused by a disrupted skin barrier. But in the past has been lauded as a rosy glow, when dermatology research was less about the skin barrier function and the role it plays in the skin ecological system.

Retinoids can cause a lifted, tightened skin appearance, because it stimulates collagen and elastin production. This is one of the key benefits of retinoid therapy.

- Retinol vs retinoids: a dermatologist's take

Retinoids are prescription only, so it may limit access. If you are dead set on including retinoids, you may find it more worthwhile to get your hands on retinoids instead of retinols, which are weaker and in my experience carry similar risks of sensitisation.

- Retinoid side effects
  - Retinoid dermatitis
  - Photosensitivity

Both these conditions overlap. Here are some guidelines to diagnosing retinoid dermatitis (for medical professionals only)

  - History of retinol or retinoid use (duration does not matter because delayed reactions can occur)
  - Signs of damaged skin barrier
  - Location of retinoid use also does not matter that much—when retinoids are absorbed they can be distributed to an area locally. For instance affecting the cheeks even when the product has been applied on the nose only.
    - Retinol purging

Described as an acne flare after using retinoids. This has been attributed to the phenomenon of comedogenesis i.e. before pimples appear on the surface of skin, they start by forming mini whiteheads and blackheads under the skin.

  - ***Retinol purging, retinoid purging (they are one and the same thing)***

The theory is that while retinols and retinoids work by targeting comedone formation, it also triggers off inflammation. This is why dermatologists don't recommend applying retinoids or retinols when you have active inflamed acne bumps. Ditto for acne cysts. What happens if you do so? Well your angry pimple gets even angrier. I.e redder, bigger, more painful...and may even develop into a cyst.

ADDITIONAL NOTES
- Oral retinoids

Isotretinoin is best known for treatment of acne vulgaris. It is prescription only and works by stopping sebum production. Skin becomes dry, and retinoid dermatitis is also a common side effect. Additionally, cheilitis (lip eczema) and peri-orofacial dermatitis can occur, due to disrupted skin barrier function and change in skin microbiome.

CHAPTER SEVEN

Other Core Cosmeceuticals

GLYCOSAMINOGLYCANS

By the end of this section you should be able to answer these FAQ

- What are glycosaminoglycans
- Where are glycosaminoglycans found in skin
- Glycosaminoglycans the same as hyaluronic acid?
- What is the main function of glycosaminoglycans
- What are glycosaminoglycans used for in cosmetics

PROTEOGLYCAN FAMILY

Hyaluronic acid & Natural Moisturising Factors

We begin by unravelling the significance of proteoglycans in aging skin.

First, what is aging skin?

Aging skin is associated with a decline in skin quality and consists of 2 broader categories of what is separately considered *intrinsic and extrinsic aging*. There are specific histological features such as a thinned epidermis and loss of volume in the second layer of skin (dermis). These correlate with the development of surface changes such as fine lines and wrinkles. The extrinsic factors are the external environmental aggressors which include UV light, airborne pollution, cigarette smoke exposure which result in physical signs of skin aging collectively known as photoaging i.e. coarse wrinkles, loss of skin elasticity, roughened skin texture etc,

Aging skin= decline in skin quality

- Intrinsic aging

Due to biological, chronological aging, internal factors

- Fine lines

- Thinned epidermis
- Dermal atrophy (gradual process)

- Extrinsic aging (photoaging)

Sum of external aggressors i.e. UV light, airborne pollution, cigarette smoke exposure
- Coarse wrinkles
- Loss of elasticity
- Rough texture

Physiologic CELL changes in aged skin (intrinsic vs extrinsic)
Fully appreciating the role of hyaluronic acid in antiaging skincare requires one to grasp the minute physiological changes in the deeper layers skin. Firstly, intrinsic or biological aging reduces the amount of hyaluronic acid and other proteins in the dermis, collectively referred to as glycosaminoglycans.
Apart from hyaluronic acid, other important molecules identified as anti-aging cell targets are: perlecan, decorin—the latter has been shown to cause skin fragility.

Intrinsic aging
- Reduced GAG
- Reduced HA

Extrinsic aging (photoaging)
- Increased GAG
- GAG distribution: papillary dermis vs between collagen/elastin fibres (normal skin)
- Reduced HA but increased LMW HA (inflammation)

Additional notes for Proteoglycans in Aged Skin :
Reduced Perlecan (Proteoglycan)
*identified as target for anti-aging treatments
Reduced Decorin
*causes skin fragility

What really happens visually is this:
- Improved skin quality
- Increased radiance due to enhanced skin cell renewal
- Tight, lifted facial skin due to increased collagen synthesis and glycosaminoglycans deposition

Glycosaminoglycans form an integral part of skin. As skin ages, GAG and proteoglycans change in the following ways:
- Structure
- Function

Alteration of both GAG and PG occurs in both intrinsic and extrinsic aging processes, with differences. Hyaluronic acid is a well-known example of direct topical GAG application. However, other approaches exist, such as molecules like C-xyloside that promote GAG release within the skin itself.

Glycosaminoglycans
- AKA Mucopolysaccharides
- Moisturising: water-binding molecules (1000 times its own weight, draws moisture to skin)
- Supports skin structure
- Strong biological activity: Involved in collagen, elastin growth for skin elasticity
- Improves skin quality
- Unsulfated (HA), sulfated (chondroitin sulfate CS, dermatan sulfate DS, heparan sulfate HS, keratan sulfate KS)

Both Glycosaminoglycans & Proteoglycans
- Participate in cell talk
- Regulate growth factor activity
- Promote wound healing: re-epitheliasation, blood vessel growth (angiogenesis), collagen growth (fibroblast proliferation), cell survival (vs cell death)

Hence, these are important targets for cosmetic interventions in skincare to improve quality of aged skin, targeting both intrinsic and extrinsic aging.

Topical Skincare Applications
Topical HA is best known.
Issues to consider
- Acts directly but also need to consider
- How well penetrates skin
- How stable it is in the formula

Hyaluronic acid
- The most important unsulfated GAG
- Structural component of ECM (extra-cellular matrix)
- Scaffold in bottlebrush formation
- Participates in cell talk (cell-cell signaling)

High molecular weight (HMW)
- Suppress inflammation
- Promote angiogenesis (blood vessel formation)

Low molecular weight (LMW)
- Promote inflammation
- Promote wound healing process
- Stimulate collagen
- Increase blood vessel growth for scar formation
- Antioxidant scavenger (wound healing)
- Assist Langerhans cells (LC) for skin immune function

Skin benefits of Hyaluronic acid
Beneficial effects on skin are visible to the naked eye! Especially, OTC formulations with high levels of HA show
- Reduction in wrinkle depth
- Improvement in skin laxity
- Hydrates skin
- Repairs skin barrier
- Minimal adverse effects

Module summary
- What are glycosaminoglycans?

Glycosaminoglycans are mucopolysaccharides best known for their moisturising properties. Commonly incorporated in topical skincare formulations like hyaluronic acid and polyglutamic acid, GAGs bind water molecules effectively. For e.g. it can hold 1000 times its own weight in water and draws moisture to skin. It also acts as a humectant, meaning it prevents water loss to the environment. This is a phenomenon known as transepidermal water loss. Glycosaminoglycans supports skin structure—it is responsible for elastic, plump and healthy looking skin. Glycosaminoglycans are effective in skincare because of its strong biological activity. It stimulates collagen growth and elastin production, increasing skin elasticity. These are markers for a healthy skin appearance. As a result, there is an improvement in skin quality. There are 2 major types of glycosaminoglycans, the unsulfated and the sulfated. Hyaluronic acid is an example of an unsulfated glycosaminoglycan. Sulfated glycosaminoglycans include chondroitin sulfate, dermatan sulfate, heparan sulfate and keratan sulfate.

- **Where are glycosaminoglycans found in skin?**

They are found in the second layer of skin, known as the dermis, where they form the bulk of the extra cellular matrix.

Choosing Products with glycosaminoglycans
- **Are glycosaminoglycans the same as hyaluronic acid?**

Hyaluronic acid is a form of glycosaminoglycan. Hyaluronic acid is best known amongst the glycosaminoglycans because it is readily incorporated into topical skincare formulations. It has all the beneficial effects of naturally occurring glycosaminoglycans in skin, i.e. regulating immune cell activity, stimulating growth factors, collagen production and improving overall skin quality.

- **What are glycosaminoglycans used for in cosmetics?**
- **What is the main function of glycosaminoglycans?**

Glycosaminoglycans provide structural support to skin. When skin ages, skin quality deteoriates because of loss of glycosaminoglycan function and quantity. This affects the immune as well as barrier function of skin. Application of glycosaminoglycans in cosmetics helps to restore visual characteristics of healthy, youthful looking skin. Glycosaminoglycans work by targeting skin cells from the inside, resulting in beneficial effects such as increased skin elasticity, plumpness and a lifted appearance. These are all markers of healthy, resilient skin and good skin barrier function.

<u>Must-know cosmeceuticals</u>
VITAMIN C

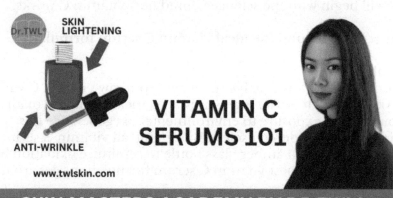

SKIN LIGHTENING

ANTI-WRINKLE

www.twlskin.com

VITAMIN C SERUMS 101

SKIN MASTERS ACADEMY BY DR.TWL®

FORMULATION SECRETS

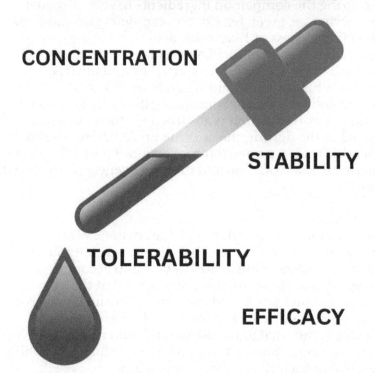

CONCENTRATION

STABILITY

TOLERABILITY

EFFICACY

Which vitamin C serum do dermatologists recommend? The ideal formulation follows certain criteria which we will go through in this chapter..

We will begin with the science behind how vitamin C works.

The science behind the ideal vitamin C serum formulation:

1. Stability

L-ascorbic acid is the active molecule from raw vitamin C which works on skin. It is also highly unstable, meaning it gets oxidised rapidly upon exposure to environmental oxygen. Once it is oxidised, it is rendered useless. By default, all vitamin C serums are packaged in an amber glass bottle to minimise oxidation by light as well. The best vitamin C serum formulations get around this problem by:

- Increasing the concentration of L-ascorbic acid to ensure there is still a sufficient amount that works on skin taking into account the oxidation process
- Ensuring the companion ingredients have anti-oxidant properties i.e. green tea extracts can synergise and boost the effectiveness of L-ascorbic acid
- Instead of L-ascorbic acid, vitamin C can be formulated as a salt known as sodium ascorbyl phosphate (SAP) which is highly stable and resistant to oxidation

In the case of sodium ascorbyl phosphate (SAP), its functional form is still L-ascorbic acid. It is absorbed via the epidermis and when it reaches the dermis, the enzyme phosphatase transforms it to L-ascorbic acid in a one-step conversion. There is hence no atmospheric related oxidation and the effectiveness is preserved. Clever, isn't it?

2. Concentration

The concentration of L-ascorbic acid does matter. When L-ascorbic acid is chosen as the active vitamin C compound, concentrations generally are at 20% to take into account environmental loss. However, this also means that the formulation becomes acidic and can irritate sensitive skin. For SAP on the other hand, concentrations at 4-5% are sufficient because there is minimal to no risk of oxidation as it is a stable salt. In fact concentrations of just 1% have been shown to inhibit the acne-causing bacteria, cutibacterium acnes.

Acne purging can be a nightmare—it's also a myth that acne treatments cause purging. It occurs mainly with retinoid treatment.
Microcomedones form under the surface of skin 2-4 weeks before they

appear, and retinoid therapy drives the comedones to the surface. The beneficial effects occur when it increases skin cell turnover, so there is less follicular plugging. But here's the problem. Retinoids are also pro-inflammatory. Which means it causes acne flare-ups. Before it even gets to work, we see the side effects first. But here's a secret—certain botanicals can treat acne without the purging side effect. Berberine for example treats acne by suppressing inflammation and comedone formation. It also regulates sebum production and reduces post-inflammation hyperpigmentation which means your scars heal faster.

3. Tolerability
This refers to the sensitising potential of vitamin C. As an acidic compound, it can irritate skin when concentrations are too high especially when applied to sensitive skin types. This is why vitamin C serums should not be applied to areas of active eczema, raw or broken skin. The exception is with acne bumps and cysts, as vitamin C itself creates a beneficial antioxidant environment that prevents acne bacteria from proliferating. It also prevents the oxidation of sebum, which contributes to comedone formation. However, when sodium ascorbyl phosphate is used, there is minimal to no risk of irritation. This is because it is a stable salt and the concentrations used are lower. Unlike L-ascorbic acid, there is no need to take into account environmental oxidation.

4. Efficacy
What's in the ideal vitamin C serum?
It is important to include synergistic actives such as
  • Botanicals
Certain botanical extracts have an anti-inflammatory effect on skin. For instance our pharmacy's formulation contains camellia sinensis, sage extract, brassica and belamcanda chinensis root extracts which also create a profound antioxidant environment to enhance the efficacy of the product.

We know the importance of an intact skin barrier—a damaged skin barrier leads to conditions like eczema and dermatitis. But did you know the skin barrier is also a barrier to absorption? This is why dermatologists are concerned with enhancing transdermal absorption, which refers to the ability of cosmeceuticals to cross the skin barrier into the deeper layers of skin such as the dermis where it exerts its effects on target cells.

- Humectants i.e. sodium hyaluronate
- Occlusives i.e. castor oil

Hyaluronic acid is a well known humectant, which means it traps water under the skin. It is a hygroscopic molecule which means it attracts water and in fact is known to hold 1000 times its own weight in moisture levels. The ideal vitamin C serum formula should contain a humectant which can also be polyglutamic acid or glycerin as this enhances the effects of vitamin C on skin—by creating a moist environment it increases epidermal permeability. This enhances absorption of vitamin C via the skin barrier. Plant-derived oils like castor also facilitate transdermal absorption by increasing the overall occlusivity of the product.

You may have heard of wet wrap therapy which refers to using layers of wet fabric on top of moisturisers to enhance absorption of skincare. Sheet masking is a concept based on this technique as well. But did you know that when formulating skincare, ingredients can also be paired in order to boost its effectiveness? For instance, vitamin C paired with humectants and occlusives can be better absorbed via the epidermis. When paired with botanicals, it can enhance the overall anti-oxidant and anti-inflammatory effects on skin. For acne prone skin ingredient pairing can also help regulate sebum production.

- Natural moisturising factors i.e. amino acids methionine
- Peptides

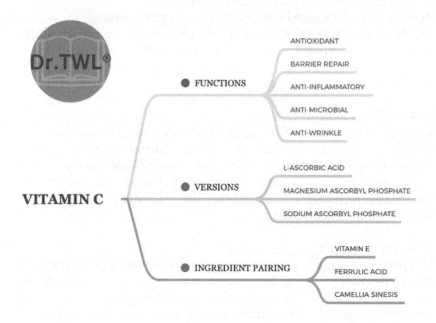

VITAMIN C

- **FUNCTIONS**
  - ANTIOXIDANT
  - BARRIER REPAIR
  - ANTI-INFLAMMATORY
  - ANTI-MICROBIAL
  - ANTI-WRINKLE

- **VERSIONS**
  - L-ASCORBIC ACID
  - MAGNESIUM ASCORBYL PHOSPHATE
  - SODIUM ASCORBYL PHOSPHATE

- **INGREDIENT PAIRING**
  - VITAMIN E
  - FERRULIC ACID
  - CAMELLIA SINESIS

Notes

How vitamin C can be used to treat acne purging

Vitamin C serums are underrated, especially when it comes to treatment of acne. I generally don't recommend application of vitamin C serums on areas of raw or broken skin—but the exception really is with inflamed acne bumps and cysts. Here are the reasons why.

1. Inflammation related to sebum oxidation
Firstly, the type of inflammation in acne is slightly different from what occurs in eczema or areas of injury. It's inflammation that's driven by an oxidative process, namely from oxidation of sebum. Acne prone skin tends to produce excess oil, and this isn't just uncomfortable. It's actually driving the inflammation which makes acne flare-ups worse.

2. Infection/Colonisation with C Acnes

Acne is also associated with bacteria—in particular Cutibacterium acnes. Vitamin C serums create an anti-oxidant environment which inhibits the growth of this bacteria. This means vitamin C serums can be used for acne prevention and long term maintenance treatment as well.

3. Speeds up wound healing

Vitamin C is essential for collagen production and wound healing. Acne scars develop as a result of inflammation. The commonest type of scar is known as post-inflammatory hyperpigmentation and fades with time. Using a vitamin C serum can reduce melanin production and this also has a brightening effect on skin.

4. Reduces scarring

Deeper acne scars known as ice pick or box car type of scars are due to dermal scarring, for eg due to an acne cyst or an infected acne papule. Since vitamin C stimulates collagen production, it can encourage proper wound healing and reduce the risk of developing acne scars

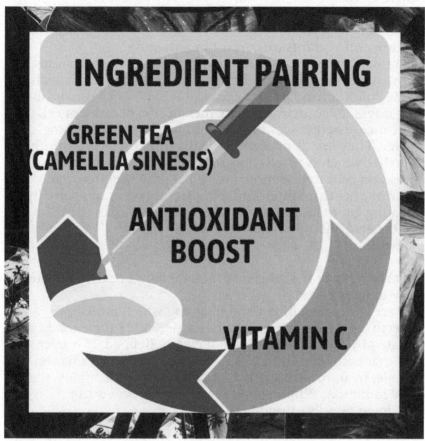

Vitamin C paired with EGCG results in a complementary effect via the following mechanisms.

Focus on Epigallocatechin Gallate (EGCG)

EGCG is a well known polyphenol found in green tea. It is primarily regarded as an anti-oxidant ingredient, but it also enhances skin barrier repair. Specifically, by the following mechanisms:

- Enhancing the expression of natural moisturising factor-related genes filaggrin (FLG), transglutaminase 1, HAS-1 and HAS-2
- Antioxidant effect
- Prevents free-radical damage associated cell death by downregulating caspases

A study by Eunji Kim in 2018 found that EGCG exerted a positive effect on skin moisture levels, wrinkles and hyperpigmentation via the above.

Why are antioxidants important in antiaging?
First understand how and why aging occurs. External causes also known as extrinsic aging refer to environmental factors such as UV, air pollution and particulate matter like PM2.5. Intrinsic aging refers to biological aging which occurs because of cell senescence, essentially, when cells grow older they become sleepier. They lose functions gradually until they stop working altogether which is when cancerous cells develop. Aging also causes skin cells to lose moisture, which is why actives like hyaluronic acid are important. HA increases skin moisture by regulating genes known as hyaluronic acid synthase (HAS). Retinoic acid (vitamin A) also effectively regulate HA in the epidermis

What are natural moisturising factors? How are they affected by UV damage?
NMF are composed of HA and filaggrin, which directly or indirectly affect the skin moisture barrier. NMF themselves are regulated by factors which are not clearly defined. However we know that components of NMF are affected by UV radiation. For example, hyaluronidase which breaks down HA is highly altered by UV radiation. When EGCG is added, it prevents the breakdown of cells caused by UV-damage.

How does pairing vitamin C with EGCG improve overall efficacy?
One of the key ways vitamin C works is by engulfing free radicals generated by UV-damage. It is an antioxidant, which means it fights the oxidative stress. However, L-ascorbic acid itself is also susceptible to UV-damage and when it undergoes oxidation, it will become ineffective. Pairing vitamin C with EGCG preserves the integrity of L-ascorbic acid or SAP formulations as it stabilises the vitamin C extract itself.

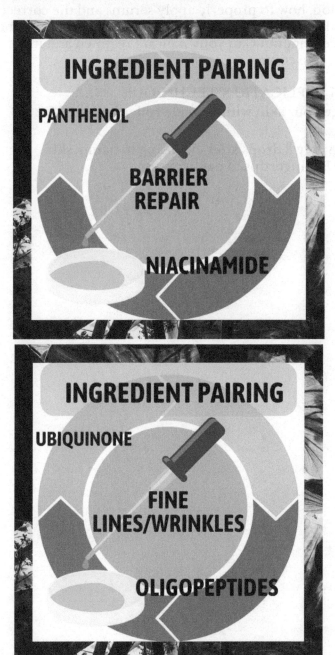

In the next section, you'll learn about enhancing serum absorption, how to properly apply serums and the correct steps to include in your skincare routine. Learn to maximise the benefits of vitamin C in your skincare regimen and make every skincare step count.

SERUM APPLICATION TECHNIQUE
Massage your skin with the jade roller included for 1-2 minutes.
- Apply 3 drops after cleansing to damp skin
- Use fingertips to pat in excess

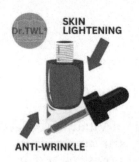

SKIN LIGHTENING

ANTI-WRINKLE

VITAMIN C SERUMS 101

SKIN MASTERS ACADEMY BY DR.TWL®

FORMULATION SECRETS

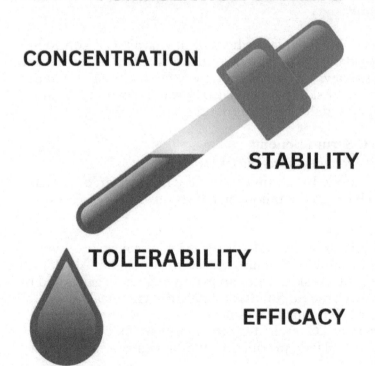

CONCENTRATION

STABILITY

TOLERABILITY

EFFICACY

Formulation Secrets Revealed
Let's lay the foundation first by defining what Vitamin C really is.

L-Ascorbic Acid
- chemically active form of Vitamin C
- essential nutrient
- antioxidant fights free radical cell damage
- facilitate cellular repair
- topical L-ascorbic acid for targeted skin efficacy

Essentially, it is the chemically active form of Vitamin C that is used by the body as an essential nutrient. As an antioxidant, it also fights free radical cell damage and promotes cell repair. When one ages, cell repair slows down and that's when damaged cells persist, leading to textural skin irregularities like spots. Skin dullness is usually because of reduced skin cell turnover in aging skin, due to a lengthened skin cycle. Dead skin cells then accumulate on the skin surface, resulting in perceived dullness of skin tone.

In this section, I'll explain why topical vitamin C is considered a key antioxidant in skincare formulations as well as benefits on skin physiology. You will learn how to choose the best vitamin C serum for your skin type and also how to incorporate it into your day and night skincare routine.

Vitamin C Serum Benefits
What does Vitamin C serum do for your face?
Topically applied Vitamin C is usually in the form of L-ascorbic acid which exerts the following effects on skin:

1. Anti-wrinkle
Vitamin C is required in the production of collagen, which is depleted in aging skin. It also acts as an antioxidant shield, which means it protects skin from environmental damage caused by UV rays, airborne pollutants and harmful chemicals. As an antioxidant it engulfs free radicals that are generated by oxidative stress. Overall, it exerts an anti-wrinkle effect by stimulating collagen production and blocking breakdown of collagen.

Anti Wrinkle Effect
- required to produce collagen
- anti-ageing shield prevents future damage

- cofactors of enzymes that augment the stability of collagen fibers
- increases expression of collagen
- block collagen breakdown

2. Skin-lightening

Vitamin C is known as a tyrosinase inhibitor which means it blocks the enzyme tyrosinase which in turn prevents conversion to melanin. When there is less melanin produced, a skin lightening effect is achieved. This is how vitamin C can address hyperpigmentation.

Skin-Lightening Effect
- inhibits tyrosinase
- blocks tyrosine to melanin conversion
- produce less melanin

3. Anti-Inflammatory Effect
- combats oxidation (sebum)
- reduces comedogenesis

VITAMIN C SERUM BENEFITS

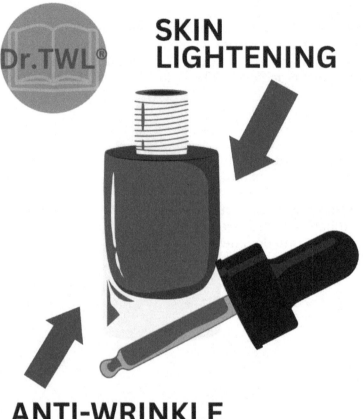

SKIN LIGHTENING

Dr.TWL®

ANTI-WRINKLE

www.twlskin.com

The best vitamin C serum formulations target various skin concerns by acting on specific cell targets in the dermis. In the case of oily, acne prone skin, it also works as an antioxidant. This also helps reduce inflammation that leads to comedone formation. Excess sebum on acne skin types leads to inflammation when the sebum itself undergoes oxidation, leading to stress that triggers off comedone formation. As a result, using a vitamin C serum can reduce formation of comedones also known as blackheads and whiteheads.

UV protective

As the best known antioxidant, vitamin C essentially boosts the skin's natural reserve of cells that fight damaging free radicals. Essentially, antioxidants "eat up" or engulf the damaging free radicals generated at the surface of skin as a result of environmental damage.

Dr.TWL's Tips

What are the pros and cons of L-Ascorbic Acid?
L-Ascorbic Acid based Vitamin C serums

- highly unstable under atmospheric conditions
- react almost instantly with oxygen in the air and degraded
- formulated with higher concentrations 20% L-Ascorbic Acid in order to survive the degradation & reasonable efficacy
- increases acidity
- sensitive or eczema-prone skin (irritation and flare ups)

L-Ascorbic Acid or raw Vitamin C, whilst fundamentally important as an antioxidant and driver of cellular repair in the human body, may not confer the most benefit when applied topically as it is, in its raw form, to the skin.

Chemically, L-Ascorbic acid is highly unstable in solution under atmospheric conditions, being the potent antioxidant that it is which inadvertently causes the molecule to react almost instantly with oxygen in the air and be degraded of its functional form.

VITAMIN C SERUM BENEFITS

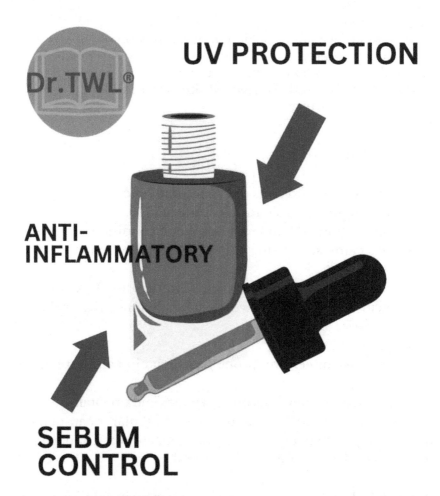

UV PROTECTION

Dr.TWL®

ANTI-INFLAMMATORY

SEBUM CONTROL

www.twlskin.com

The best vitamin C serum is formulated according to the following key principles
- Readily absorbed

- Does not degrade rapidly when exposed to the environment
- Effective and gentle on all skin types

This often results in L-Ascorbic Acid based Vitamin C serums having to be formulated with higher concentrations - for instance 20% L-Ascorbic Acid formulations may quite frequently be marketed, in order to survive the degradation in some manner and have any reasonable efficacy by the time the molecule is absorbed by the epidermis and dermis.

A consequence of high concentrations of L-Ascorbic Acid however is that, as may be suggested by its chemical nomenclature, it increases acidity on the skin.

For individuals with sensitive or eczema-prone skin, it is not uncommon to experience irritation and flare ups following the use of such highly concentrated L-Ascorbic Acid formulations.

Which vitamin C derivatives would you recommend, and why? Are there any derivatives that you particularly like?
Sodium Ascorbyl Phosphate (SAP)
- stable precursor of L-Ascorbic Acid
- adjunctive treatment to and pigmentation conditions
- salt of ascorbic acid
- stable in solution under atmospheric conditions
- intact on exposure to environmental oxygen up till absorption
- in dermis, the enzyme phosphatase cleaves off the phosphate group attached
- converted back to functionally active L-Ascorbic form
- deliver the efficacy of the vitamin without the same losses
- lower 5 percent concentration of SAP, avoiding potential irritation from high concentrations
- 1 percent concentration of SAP shows strong antimicrobial efficacy against Cutibacterium acnes

In my practice, I use Sodium Ascorbyl Phosphate (SAP), a stable precursor of L-Ascorbic Acid, in the formulation of a stabilized Vitamin C serum - the Vita C GOLD Serum, which is a cosmeceutical often opted for by patients as adjunctive treatment for hyperpigmentation. The SAP is a salt of ascorbic acid and is stable in solution under atmospheric conditions. This allows the molecule to be kept intact mostly on exposure to environmental oxygen up till absorption through the epidermis and dermis, where the enzyme phosphatase is abundant to cleave off the phosphate group attached to the Ascorbic Acid molecule. From here, the SAP is converted back to its functionally active L-Ascorbic form, to deliver the efficacy of the vitamin optimally right into the skin without the same losses that may be experienced by conventional Vitamin C serums, due to intermediary exposure to environmental oxygen. What this means is that a much lower 5 percent concentration of SAP (which is the amount present in the Vita C GOLD) for example, could have sufficient potency for similar if not stronger efficacy than more concentrated raw L-Ascorbic formulations, whilst avoiding the pitfalls of potential irritation from high concentrations.

In fact, studies have shown that a mere 1 percent concentration of SAP has strong antimicrobial efficacy against Cutibacterium acnes. Also, one added benefit of the SAP is that skin cells are understood to continuously take up the SAP and convert it into ascorbic acid by the process of dephosphorylation. This continuous process allows elevated levels of ascorbic acid to be maintained in the skin for considerable lengths of time after the initial introduction of SAP, to deliver more sustained benefits to the skin.

VITAMIN C SERUMS

L-ascorbic acid

- highly unstable under atmospheric conditions
- react almost instantly with oxygen in the air and degraded
- formulated with higher concentrations 20% L-Ascorbic Acid in order to survive the degradation & reasonable efficacy
- increases acidity
- sensitive or eczema-prone skin (irritation and flare ups)

www.twlskin.com

SAP

- stable precursor of L-Ascorbic Acid
- adjunctive treatment to and pigmentation conditions
- salt of ascorbic acid
- stable in solution under atmospheric conditions
- intact on exposure to environmental oxygen up till absorption
- in dermis, the enzyme phosphatase cleaves off the phosphate group attached
- converted back to functionally active L-Ascorbic form
- deliver the efficacy of the vitamin without the same losses
- lower 5 percent concentration of SAP, avoiding potential irritation from high concentrations

FAQ
How to use vitamin C serum
Serums are regarded as leave-on skincare products (as opposed to wash-off i.e. facial cleansers or gel masks), so they can be applied directly and left on skin. For optimal absorption, applying on clean skin is recommended.

Here is Dr.TWL's recommended method to optimise absorption:
- Massage your skin with a Jade roller for 1-2 minutes.
- Apply 3 drops after cleansing to damp skin
- Use fingertips to pat in excess

When to use vitamin C serum
Incorporate serums as the step right after cleansing. Vitamin C and hyaluronic acid are the two essential serums recommended by dermatologists in your skincare routine. It is important to apply it on clean, slightly damp skin. Right after cleansing as damp skin increases absorption of skincare actives. Unlike actives like retinol, you can use vitamin C both in your day and night skincare routine as it generally does not increase sun sensitivity. Follow with your facial essence and moisturiser right after application of serums and finish with sunscreen for your day skincare routine.

Is it okay to use vitamin C serum everyday?
Yes. In fact it is recommended as an essential step both in the day and night skincare routine to improve the antioxidant reserve of skin. This directly enhances skin resilience, which means skin is better able to handle stressors and repair damaged skin cells.

Which is the best vitamin C serum?
The ideal vitamin C serum should fulfil the following criteria
- Non-sensitising (reduced acidity)
- Balanced with barrier repair actives like glycerin and other humectants
- Highly stable and resistant to environmental oxidation
- Readily penetrates the epidermis and dermis where it converts to active form L-ascorbic acid for antioxidant effects

- Non-sticky residue
- Ideally paired with camellia sinensis (green tea) which is synergistic and increases antioxidant capacity

Who should not use vitamin C serum?
Everyone can benefit from a well-formulated vitamin C serum. The point really should be that no one should use a poorly formulated vitamin C serum—one that is unstable, too acidic or one that frankly has already oxidised and will not work at all. However, if you are having an active flare-up of eczema/any sensitive skin condition, it is advisable to hold off vitamin C until your condition has stabilised and to use a dermatologist-recommended formulation suitable for your skin type. Vitamin C serums should also not be applied directly on areas of raw, broken skin. It however, can be applied to inflamed acne bumps and cysts as it has an anti-inflammatory effect.

How to choose the best vitamin C serum for oily skin
Oily skin generally tolerates all types of vitamin C well. Use of a vitamin C active calms oxidative stress caused by excess sebum production. The ideal vitamin C formulation should also include companion ingredients that synergise with the active.
The Vita C Gold Serum contains Camellia Sinensis (green tea extract) which specifically boosts the antioxidant properties and improves stability of the vitamin C active delivered to the skin.

How to choose the best vitamin C serum for hyperpigmentation
The Vita C Gold serum contains a combination of botanicals that synergise to inhibit melanin production. The active form of vitamin C in our formulation is sodium ascorbyl phosphate, the environmentally most stable form of vitamin C. It is absorbed via the epidermis and via the enzyme phosphatase, it is converted into L-ascorbic acid which then exerts its effects in the deeper layers of skin.

How to choose the best vitamin C serum for over 50
The over 50s must focus on correction and reversal of photoageing. If skin aging has already progressed and sun spots, textural irregularities have already appeared, the key may be to use prescription or laser therapy to achieve reversal in conjunction with a topical regimen. Home options for laser

therapy-like results may include microcurrent, microdermabrasion, hydrodermabrasion and LED light therapy. The Vita C Gold serum contains a botox-alternative known as oligopeptides which directly act on muscle junctions to relax fine lines and wrinkles.

How to choose the best vitamin C serum for dry skin
Dry skin is characterised by impaired skin barrier function. This means that L-ascorbic acid based vitamin C serums can irritate skin, due to its acidity. The Vita C Gold serum is based on a neutral salt compound of vitamin C known as sodium ascorbyl phosphate, which firstly is highly stable in the atmosphere. When L-ascorbic acid is exposed to environmental oxygen, it degrades rapidly. Not so with SAP, which is the key benefit of Dr.TWL's pharmacy formula. SAP is also gentle on sensitive, dry skin, as it does not have the acidity associated with L-ascorbic acid. Furthermore, it requires a much lower concentration as there is no wastage via environmental oxidation. Higher concentrations are used in L-ascorbic acid formulations due to expectations of compound instability when exposed to oxygen in the air. Since SAP penetrates the epidermis first before it is converted to L-ascorbic acid which is the active form, there is minimal to no risk of loss of concentration or efficacy unlike pure L-ascorbic acid formulations.

How to choose the best vitamin C serum for sensitive skin
Sensitive skin may be different from dry skin—not all sensitive skin types are dry. For instance, those with reactive skin i.e. rosacea or even severe cystic acne may react to environmental changes. However, the skin barrier may not actually be impaired in these conditions. Sensitive skin may experience stinging and pain when L-ascorbic acid is applied on skin, due to its acidic nature. It is best to opt for SAP or MAP formula (magnesium ascorbyl phosphate).

Ideal Vitamin C serum for sensitive skin
- stabilized
- dermatologist-tested
- formulated at concentrations no more than 5%

Safety considerations

- type and concentration of Vitamin C in topical formulations
- do not concoct your own Vitamin C ie citrus juice causes phytophotodermatitis

Which derivative is best suited for sensitive and sensitised skin, as well as those who are new to using actives?
I would recommend the use of stabilized Vitamin C, dermatologist-tested and formulated at concentrations no more than 5% to avoid potential irritation to sensitive skin individuals.

In your opinion, who should use vitamin C in their skincare routine, and who should avoid it? How should we incorporate vitamin C into our routines, for maximum efficacy and safety?
In general, Vitamin C, being a powerful antioxidant and essential nutrient that helps drive cellular repair and wound healing in the human body, is suitable in any skincare routine, much like a healthy diet being suitable for anyone. However, for sensitive skin individuals especially, it is important to discern the type and concentration of Vitamin C used in topical formulations, and do also look out for dermatologist-tested and formulated labels for added assurance. Avoid concocting your own Vitamin C, as it may lead to phytophotodermatitis - inflammation of the skin from contact with light sensitizing botanicals followed by sunlight exposure, which is somewhat common with patients who DIY using lemon, lime or oranges etc.

On top of the use of stabilized Vitamin C, my patients also often opt for a lightweight moisturising emulsion (oil-in-water for a comfortable texture in humid climates) - the Radiance Fluide Hydrating Emulation, which is imbued with an added mix of antioxidants and plant extracts that help to augment the anti-aging effects of Vitamin C, via hydration to the skin and a boost to collagen production. Above all, however, I can't stress enough the importance of a healthy balanced diet (which includes consumption of dietary Vitamin C) and regular exercise to maintain healthy youthful skin.

SUMMARY
In this tutorial, we've covered the following:
- How to choose the best vitamin C serum for different skin types
- How vitamin C can suppress inflammation, improve acne and oily skin
- The advantages of sodium ascorbyl phosphate over L-ascorbic acid formulations

INGREDIENT SPOTLIGHT
L-Ascorbic Acid or Vitamin C is required by our bodies to produce collagen, making this vitamin crucial for anti-ageing. Think of it as an anti-ageing shield your skin needs to reduce the damage your skin suffered, and also to prevent future damage. The vitamin forms cofactors of enzymes that augment the stability of collagen fibers. It also increases expression of collagen and synthesizes inhibitors to block enzymes from degrading collagen, thereby contributing to the treatment of wrinkles - which are frequently caused by the loss of collagen and skin elasticity with age.

In addition, Vitamin C plays an important role in skin-lightening as it inhibits an enzyme called tyrosinase which participates in the metabolism of melanin that causes pigmentation on skin. This enzyme works by converting tyrosine into melanin, so by reducing the activity of tyrosinase, our skin cells inadvertently produce less melanin. Furthermore, topical Vitamin C can help improve conditions by combating oxidation of sebum and comedogenesis (also commonly referred to as the clogging of pores), by its sheer potent antioxidative strength to neutralise free radicals and reduce oxidative stress. This neutralisation of free radicals also protects the individual from UV light exposure, which may lead to photodamage such as via sunburn cell formation and DNA fragmentation.

NIACINAMIDE
5 Things to Know
1. Form of Vitamin B3
2. forms in cosmeceuticals: niacinamide (nicotinamide) & nicotinic acid (interchangeable terms usually)
3. Difference between **niacinamide** (nicotinamide) & nicotinic acid. Worthwhile to note that nicotinic acid may be more beneficial because of increased NAD (niacinamide adenosine dinucleotide) effects on skin, by interacting with nicotinic receptors on skin. But nicotinic acid causes skin flushing (vasodilation), changes in body temperature, blood pressure, pulse. Niacinamide is generally preferred
4. Precursor of NAD, NADP cofactors which are involved in more than 40 cellular biochemical reactions
5. Star anti-aging ingredient: exerts multiple effects on skin via different cellular targets

COSMECEUTICAL FRAMEWORK

1. ABSORPTION
Evidence of absorption

2. MECHANISM OF ACTION/EFFECTS ON SKIN

What does niacinamide do to your skin?
Niacinamide=NADP coenzymes precursor = >40 biological effects
- Improve skin barrier function
- Improve skin elasticity
- Reduce hyperpigmentation
- Reduce fine lines & wrinkles
- Reduce redness, uneven skin tone
- Decrease sallowness, dullness
- Antioxidant
  - Niacinamide works by increasing antioxidant capacity of skin, via reduced form NADPH* best known anti-aging effect

- Improve skin barrier function

Enhances skin's ceramide levels

Encourages cell differentiation, skin cell renewal

- Reduce redness, uneven skin tone

Improved barrier function, reduced sensitivity

- Exfoliant

Speeds up skin cell renewal

- Improve skin elasticity
- Reduce fine lines & wrinkles
- Why wrinkles appear: reduced collagen & protein production
    - Importance of proteins in anti-aging skincare
    - Reduced proteins in aging skin leads to wrinkle formation & deficient barrier function
    - Proteins are natural moisturising factors i.e. fillagrin, involucrin which stabilise the stratum corneum
    - Niacinamide increases collagen & protein production

- Reduce hyperpigmentation

5% niacinamide moisturiser reduces melanosome transfer from melanocytes

- Decrease sallowness, dullness

Why does skin yellow with age?

We know that collagen decreases with age, but something else increases, these are known as Amadori products, which essentially are collagen oxidation products.

From age 20-80, there is a 5 fold increase in these COP in human skin.

Maillard reaction: glycation of proteins in skin

Protein + sugar in an oxidative reaction, resulting in a adore products which are yellow-brown in color and fluorescent.

3. CLINICAL STUDIES

5% niacinamide cream: improvement in hyperpigmentation
2% niacinamide cream
2.5% niacinamide: exfoliant, smoothens skin roughness
2%, 5% niacinamide 12 weeks: dose dependent effects

4. COMMON FAQ

Niacinamide for damaged skin barrier?
Yes. Although it would depend on the formulation.The best way
to repair a damaged skin barrier is by moisture sandwiching,
essentially an occlusion effect achieved by layering. This is why a
1 size fits all product, prescription or not that's standalone does
not work. The predominant active should not be a single
ingredient, rather a synergy of actives that work on every single
layer of the skin and targets specific cell layers.

Should I use niacinamide everyday
You can. It is a non-irritating ingredient, provided the rest of the
formulation does not contain AHAs, salicylic, lactic acids or
retinols.

Which is better vitamin C or niacinamide
Vitamin C works differently. It is an antioxidant which helps to
combat free radical stress. It is best to include both in your
skincare routine.

What not to mix with niacinamide
Nothing in particular. However with any product I advise the
following:
Do a patch test on the underside of your jawline, leave on
overnight and observe for any reaction. If irritation occurs at
any point of time, even months or years after using a product,
stop and visit a dermatologist. Delayed reactions are possible.

GREEN TEA (CAMILLIA SINENSIS)

- Types
  - Green (highest EGCG content)
  - White (least processed)
  - Black (fermented)
- Active: Polyphenols aka catechins (epicatechin, epicatechin-3-gallate ECG, epigallocatechin-3-gallate EGCG*
- *EGCG largest catechin, most active antioxidant, highest concentration in green tea

Active polyphenol content: 30-35% dry weight

Green tea extract is another key cosmeceutical ingredient to know. There are 3 types, green, white and black which all contain polyphenols the most bioactive antioxidant of all—EGCG which has been found to exist in the highest concentrations in green tea specifically.

1. ABSORPTION

Evidence of absorption:
3 key challenges exist when it comes to formulations:

I. Unstable compound

- Green tea polyphenols highly unstable
- Easily oxidised
- Best paired in vitamin C serum formulation (for synergistic antioxidant capacity)

II. Limited penetration of epidermis

- Hydrophilic i.e. water loving, difficulty penetrating the lipid-rich stratum corneum
- Key is the formulation for maximum effectiveness

III. Polyphenol content vs Green Tea Content

- E.g. of why cosmeceutical manufacturing standards differ: evidence-based formulation methods: 90% polyphenol content vs green tea extract concentration i.e. 5% which causes product to appear brown.

2. MECHANISM OF ACTION/EFFECTS ON SKIN
What does green tea do to your skin?
- Antioxidant
  - Polyphenols quench ROS (Reactive Oxygen Species)
  - Prevent/limit UV-damage (lipid peroxidation process)
- Anti-inflammatory

EGCG suppresses free radical damage

RECAP: FREE RADICALS ARE HARMFUL Free radicals are generated by UV-damage, pollution, stress and biological aging. These cause skin cells to age, losing their ability to repair damaged DNA.
  - Increase collagen breakdown (via enzymes known as collagenases)—> skin wrinkles!
  - Increase inflammation (PRO-INFLAMMATORY)
- **Promotes collagen synthesis**

Green tea polyphenols are FREE RADICAL SCAVENGERS
  - Suppress collagenase, stops collagen breakdown
  - Increase collagen growth via fibroblast cells
- **Photoprotective (EGCG, ECG components)**
  - Suppress UV-induced erythema (redness)
  - Reduce DNA damage
  - Reduce sunburn effect (lowers number of sunburn cells)

3. CLINICAL STUDIES
Chiu et al: 40 women with moderate photoaging given green tea supplements & green tea cream. At 8 weeks, no visible changes but significantly improved elastic tissue content under microscopic examination. This means it's likely a longer duration is required for effects visible to the naked eye to be observed. Bottom line: weighting evidence, these are definitely safe, beneficial for human health and preferred over potentially skin irritating actives.

4. SUMMARY SECTION & COMMON FAQ:

Green tea extract is a cosmeceutical active that is safe for sensitive skin and also has been shown to have beneficial effects on skin.

Green tea extract benefits:

The list of skincare benefits of green tea include its anti-inflammatory, antioxidant properties. Anti-inflammatory skincare is a buzzword because it can reverse a key process in aging known as inflammaging.

The *skin exposome concept* refers to internal and external factors that affect skin aging, with one thing in common. Lifestyle factors, biological factors and the skincare you apply —all these ultimately affect the inflammaging process. And this is the role skincare ingredients like green tea extract plays.

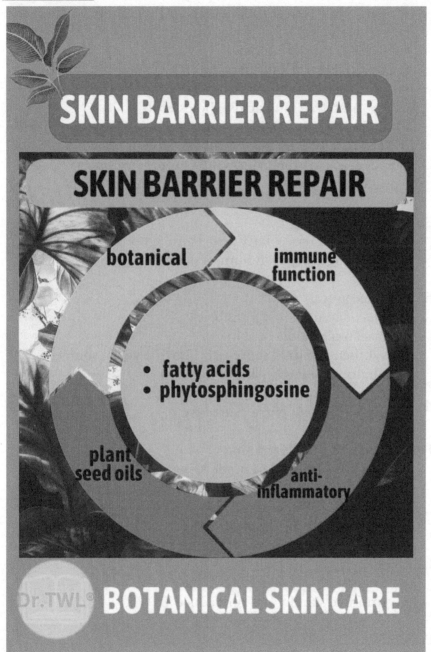

Role in skin homeostasis i.e. harmony & balance
- Part of stratum corneum (barrier function from allergens, reduce TEWL)
- Brick & mortar model:
- Bricks: keratin + fillagrin
- Mortar: fats between skin cells i.e. lipids (ceramides 50% by mass, free fatty acids, cholesterol)
- Disruption of barrier: environmental damage, increased TEWL

Deficiency leads to atopic dermatitis i.e. eczema due to Filaggrin gene mutations

Structure:
- Spinghoid base + fatty acid + amide bond
- 12 different types in human skin

As a cosmeceutical
- bits of cement that joins bricks
- brick wall model of skin
- synthetic, animal sources, i.e. bovine vegan source: phytoceramides (plant ceramides)
- botanical, plant seed oils, shea butter.
- repair the skin barrier effectively

Hydroxypalmitoyl sphinganine
- When added to skin models, increase Cer 1, 2, 3
- Improve skin hydration, reduce TEWL, increase stratum corneum CER in patients with eczema or on tretinoin therapy

CER 1, 3
- Synergistic
- Improve skin hydration, reduce TEWL

Pseudo-CER
Pseudoacyl CER
- Asian skincare

- Treats essential fatty acid deficiency
- Similar behaviour to true CERs

Phytoceramides
- botanical, plant seed oils, shea butter.
- repair the skin barrier effectively
- fatty acids, phytosphingosine

Examples:
- Shea butter, sunflower oil, moringa and meadowfoam seed oil
- Improve the recovery rate of damaged stratum corneum
- Enhance hydration better than synthetic ceramide
- Improved immunity
- Anti-inflammatory

Dr.TWL's notes
Skin Intelligence: Barrier & Beyond

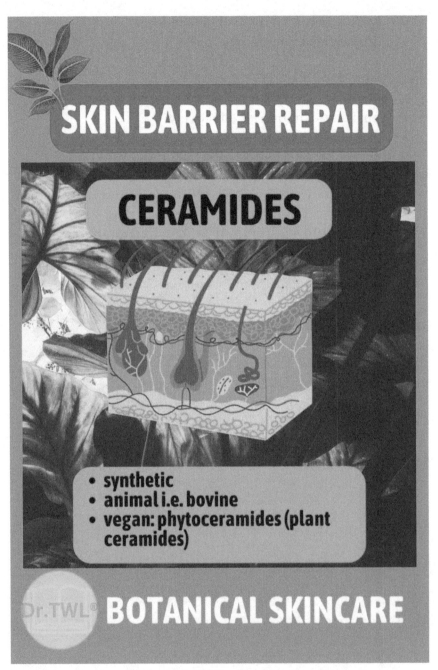

SKIN BARRIER REPAIR

CERAMIDES

- synthetic
- animal i.e. bovine
- vegan: phytoceramides (plant ceramides)

Dr.TWL® **BOTANICAL SKINCARE**

As a complete ecosystem, the skin plays host to diverse microorganisms collectively known as the microbiome. Barrier function is a critical component of skin health that ensures the survival of good germs. effective cell communication and self-regulation.

Sensitive skin isn't really all that allergic, it all boils down to an impaired skin barrier

Decades ago, atopic dermatitis was interpreted as a predominantly allergic type skin condition—it's true. Sufferers tend to be allergic to house dust mite, pollen and VOCs. They also have associated conditions under the umbrella term of the "atopic triad"—asthma, allergic rhinitis/hay fever.

Then, studies emerged which showed that eczema was really due to a deficiency in filaggrin gene expression—a fact already established in conditions such as icthyosis vulgaris. This led to impaired ceramide production, which meant that the epidermis became "leaky". Out of this emerged the brick and mortar model of the skin barrier— the bricks are superficial skin cells known as corneocytes, and the fatty lipids which join the corneocytes together, the cement. This lipids known as ceramides could be replenished with ceramide-dominant moisturisers which fill the "gaps" between the bricks.

When sensitive skin is treated with barrier repairing moisturisers, it becomes less reactive to environmental triggers.

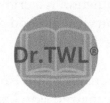

BARRIER REPAIR
SKIN MASKING
HACKS

POLYSACCHARIDE MASK DRY MASKS

NORMAL SHEET MASK MATERIAL

WWW.TWLSKIN.COM

The art of replacing like for like

Over 340 types of ceramides exist within the human stratum corneum alone. The composition of which is varied. From the 12 classes identified researchers conclude the following:

The basic ceramide structure is composed of:

- Sphingoid base joined to a fatty acid via an amide bond

YOUR SKIN'S CERAMIDE FACTORY

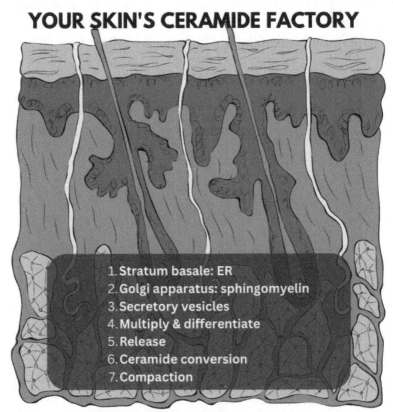

1. Stratum basale: ER
2. Golgi apparatus: sphingomyelin
3. Secretory vesicles
4. Multiply & differentiate
5. Release
6. Ceramide conversion
7. Compaction

www.twlskin.com

Notes

Healthy skin—your ceramide factory:

- Beginning at the bottom most layer of the epidermis, the stratum basale. Ceramides are made within the endoplasmic reticulum

- Converted to sphingomyelin in the Golgi apparatus
- Packed into secretory vesicles (bubble-like)
- These vesicles multiply as skin cells (keratinocytes) differentiate and move towards the surface of skin
- The bubbles burst and release sphingomyelins
- Sphingomyelins converted back to ceramides
- Ceramides, free fatty acids & cholesterol are compacted into layers in the stratum corneum to form the skin barrier

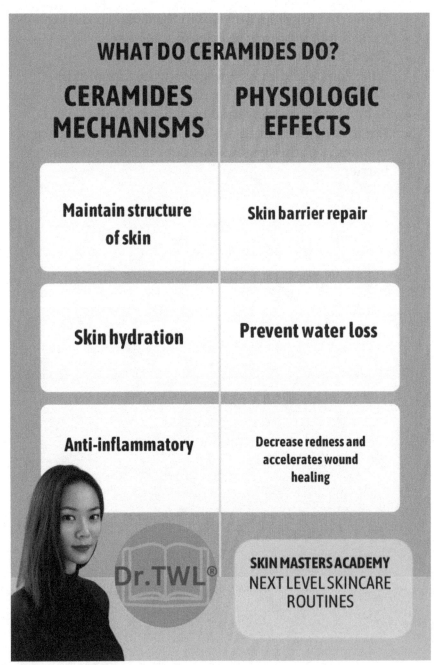

WHAT DO CERAMIDES DO?

CERAMIDES MECHANISMS	PHYSIOLOGIC EFFECTS
Maintain structure of skin	Skin barrier repair
Skin hydration	Prevent water loss
Anti-inflammatory	Decrease redness and accelerates wound healing

Dr.TWL®

SKIN MASTERS ACADEMY
NEXT LEVEL SKINCARE ROUTINES

The skin on our body is sometimes neglected—and that's a mistake because skin ages uniformly. Meaning, that you would expect a similar characteristics in aged skin whether it's on the face or on the body. This undermines the importance of overall good health, doctors consider that organ systems like your heart, lung, brain, liver, kidney and gut must function well for your entire body to be in an optimal state of health—that is true for the skin too. In fact many of these internal organ conditions manifest as skin symptoms first—this is the case for instance in a condition we term pruritus.

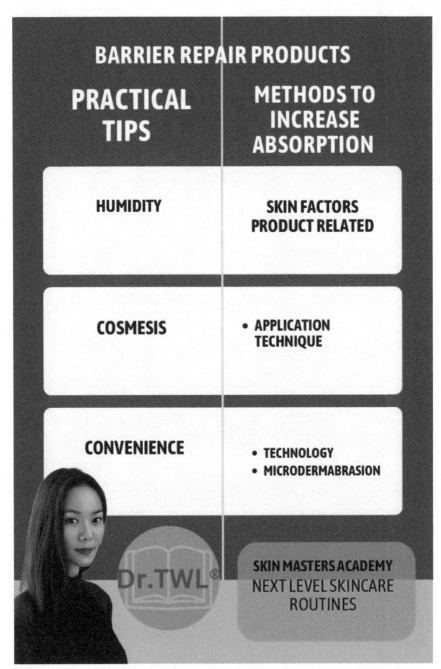

BARRIER REPAIR PRODUCTS

PRACTICAL TIPS	METHODS TO INCREASE ABSORPTION
HUMIDITY	SKIN FACTORS PRODUCT RELATED
COSMESIS	• APPLICATION TECHNIQUE
CONVENIENCE	• TECHNOLOGY • MICRODERMABRASION

Dr.TWL®

SKIN MASTERS ACADEMY
NEXT LEVEL SKINCARE ROUTINES

Ceramide containing cosmeceuticals can be considered the foundation of skincare routines. It is the one ingredient upon which we can build a fuss-free skincare routine not just for facial skin but for the rest of our skin. We must bear in mind that it is an important constituent that forms the bulk of the surface area of the largest organ of the body— skin itself.

I want to draw your attention to phytoceramides. You may have heard about ceramides for skin barrier—essentially these are the bits of cement that joins the bricks together in the well-known brick wall model of skin. Most ceramides beauty brands refer to are synthetic or animal sources, i.e. bovine in origin—which is also a concern for those preferring a vegan lifestyle. My top pick for ceramides is actually a lesser known subtype known as phytoceramides. These are botanically derived from plant seed oils and the most prominent phytoceramide of all is shea butter. Derived from the shea tree, shea butter provides a rich source of natural origin plant-based ceramides that can repair the skin barrier effectively. Most importantly, scientific studies in recent years have actually shown the benefits of using phytoceramides in skincare formulations. Specifically, natural oils are sources of fatty acids and a compound known as phytosphingosine which directly repair the skin barrier. Shea butter, sunflower oil, moringa and meadowfoam seed oil were observed to improve the recovery rate of damaged stratum corneum and enhance hydration even better than synthetic ceramide versions. Benefits include increased hydration as well as improved immunological function, partly because of anti-inflammatory properties inherent in botanical actives.

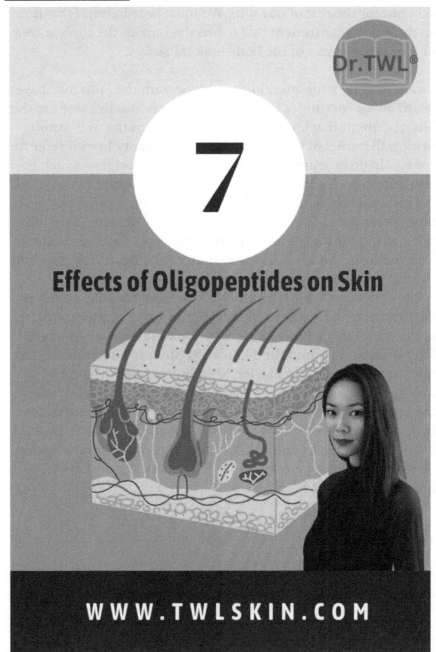

7

Effects of Oligopeptides on Skin

WWW.TWLSKIN.COM

Oligopeptides are nature's own topical botox with extra anti-microbial benefits. These are biomimetic molecules which are synthesised to mimic the naturally occurring peptides produced by healthy skin. When incorporated into cosmeceuticals, oligopeptides are effective retinol/retinoid alternatives that are suited for sensitive skin types. It can also be used as an adjunct to retinoid treatment as part of a holistic antiaging skincare regimen.

We will discuss the key applications of oligopeptides for anti wrinkle treatment here:

Botox-like effects
Oligopeptides AMPs for wrinkles
- Botox-like effect
- Affect neurotransmitter release
- Wrinkle formation, expression lines due to: repetitive facial muscular contractions
- Botulinum toxin works by blocking acetylcholine release at neuromuscular junction, relaxes facial muscles and soothes lines
- Oligopeptides are topical mimetic
- Targets proteins (SNARE) at neuromuscular junction, less neurotoxic, safer, effective in reducing facial lines, wrinkles

WHAT DO PEPTIDES DO?

PEPTIDE MECHANISMS

PHYSIOLOGIC EFFECTS

- Oligopeptides (Antimicrobial peptides i.e. AMPs)
- Bioactive peptides
- Regulate & modulate biochemical reactions
- Physiological processes:
  - Cell proliferation & migration
  - Inflammation
  - Angiogenesis (blood vessel formation)
  - Melanogenesis (pigment formation)
  - Immune system (innate immunity)
- Latest dermatological applications:
  - Antimicrobial
  - Neurotransmitter

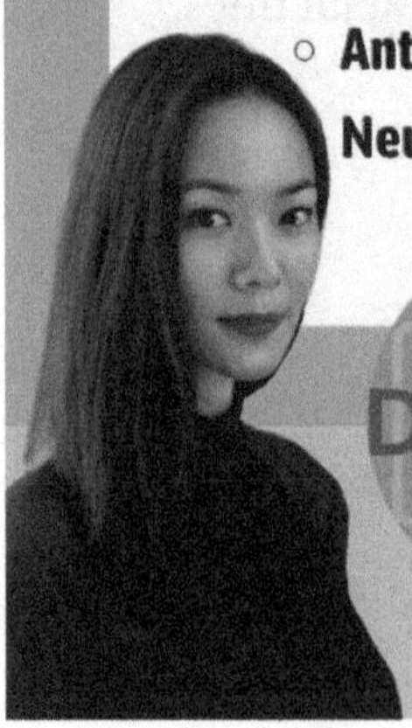

Dr.TWL®

SKIN MASTERS ACADEMY
NEXT LEVEL SKINCARE
ROUTINES

Important oligopeptides for anti-wrinkle effects

- Acetyl-hexapeptide aka argireline i.e. 5% similar potency as BoNT , reduce depth of wrinkles up to 17% after 15 days, 27% after 30 days
  - Well tolerated, no primary irritation at high doses
- Pentapeptide 3
  - 0.05% concentration
  - 49% decrease in wrinkle size, 47% decrease in skin roughness after 28 days
  - Effective for smoothening periorbital, forehead, nasolabial fold wrinkles
  - Immediate skin tightening effect
- Leuphasyl
  - Synergistic with argireline
- Tripeptide
  - Reversible reduction in muscle contraction
  - 4% concentration, 52% reduction of wrinkle size after 28 days

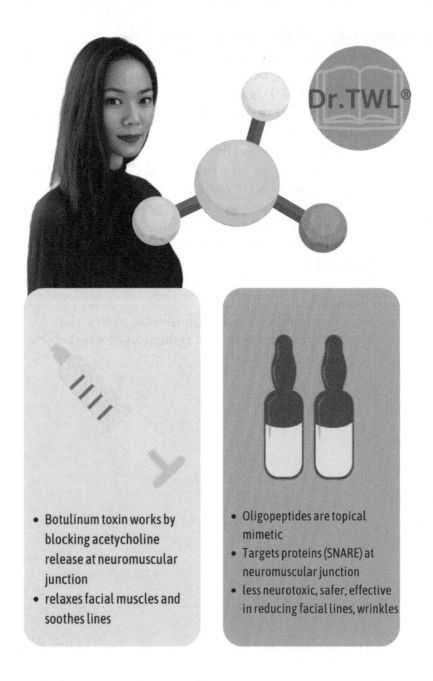

- Botulinum toxin works by blocking acetycholine release at neuromuscular junction
- relaxes facial muscles and soothes lines

- Oligopeptides are topical mimetic
- Targets proteins (SNARE) at neuromuscular junction
- less neurotoxic, safer, effective in reducing facial lines, wrinkles

Oligopeptides (Antimicrobial peptides i.e. AMPs)
- Bioactive peptides

- Regulate & modulate biochemical reactions
- Physiological processes:
    - Cell proliferation & migration
    - Inflammation
    - Angiogenesis (blood vessel formation)
    - Melanogenesis (pigment formation)
    - Immune system (innate immunity)
- Latest dermatological applications:
    - Antimicrobial
    - Neurotransmitter

Another important function that oligopeptides play is in terms of regulating the skin microbiome. They are also known as AMPS (anti-microbial peptides).

AMPs for skin microbiome & immunity
- Skin barrier protects against pathogenic germs
- Nature designed skin defense mechanism minimise problems of antibiotic resistance
- AMPs (antibiotic-like antimicrobial peptides) are small molecules on skin that kill germs i.e. dermicidin, cathelicidin, defensin
- Disrupt bacterial cell walls
- Trigger immune response to kill germs
- AMPs especially important in atopic dermatitis, i.e. staphylococcus aureus colonisation due to decreased AMPs defensins, dermicidins

One of the key challenges of peptide delivery is enhancing transdermal absorption. The limiting factor of topically applied cosmeceuticals is that the stratum corneum is a physical barrier that naturally inhibits absorption of topicals, which is part of its protective defense mechanisms. However, enhancing the effects of cosmeceuticals require methods of increasing epidermal permeability. This can be achieved through the various technologies available which include sonic waves, low level electric current, ultrasound and microdermabrasion.

Transdermal delivery techniques
How to increase skin absorption of oligopeptides
- Electroporation
- Sonophoresis
- Microdermabrasion/dermal infusion

Good-to-know cosmeceuticals

Adenosine :
- nucleoside associated with the body's energy-transferring processes
- present in adenosine triphosphate (ATP)
- occurs naturally in the body
- good penetration
- effective anti-wrinkle ingredient
- periorbital, glabellar frowns, crows feet
- skin smoothness

Acetyl Hexapeptide:
- 10% concentration of acetyl hexapeptide-8
- topical botox mimetic
- inhibits acetylcholine release
- reduces repetitive facial muscle contraction
- effective in reducing wrinkles
  - efficacies up to 48% upon 4 weeks of twice daily treatment

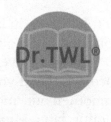

**ANTIAGING
SKINCARE ROUTINES
FOR SENSITIVE SKIN**

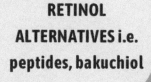

RETINOL
ALTERNATIVES i.e.
peptides, bakuchiol

Retinols,
retinoids

W W W . T W L S K I N . C O M

Retinol alternatives like peptides have significant anti-wrinkle properties sans irritation.

Botulinum toxin is touted as a wrinkle cure, but is it? Well if you consider a cure one that lasts 6 months, paralyses your muscles so you can't move them—whatever that looks like to you. The theory is that if you stop using those expressions, the lines will smoothen out, and it does. Until you begin to use them again 6 months later. Mini-botox is another fad—inject a small amount. So it's less obvious.

All that is true. Except that wrinkles aren't the only sign of aging, and more importantly aging isn't defined by wrinkles. The latest evidence points towards addressing inflammaging as the key process in cellular death and decay in all our organs, which applies to skin as well. Botulinum toxin does not intervene in this process and hence should not be regarded as a therapeutic.

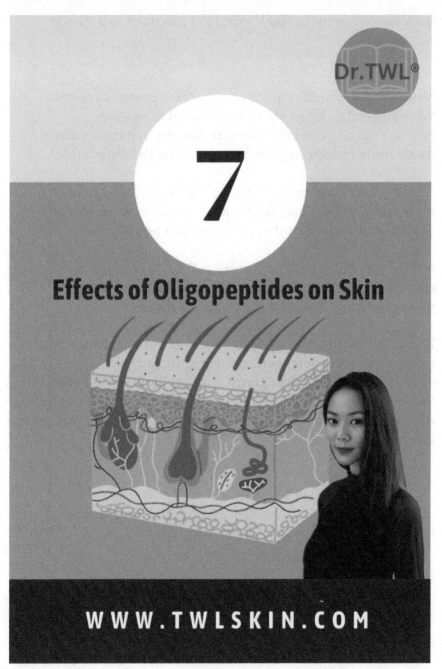

7

Effects of Oligopeptides on Skin

WWW.TWLSKIN.COM

Dr.TWL®

Oligopeptides target skin via multiple cellular pathways. Peptide skincare benefits include stimulation of collagen production, relaxing facial muscles for anti wrinkle effects and also stabilising the skin microbiome.

Nature's anti-wrinkle cure is one that also protects your skin. Women need to know about botox alternatives like cosmeceuticals. The evidence is mounting that these offer a much more holistic approach to antiaging than injectables.

Oligopeptides are topical skincare ingredients that treat skin holistically, rather than just paralyse muscles, these are biomimetic molecules that promote skin health

Nature's way of skincare is brilliant. Peptides known as anti-microbial peptides AKA AMPs are our body's natural defences against harmful germs and pathogens.

Unlike antibiotics, these AMPs help to restore a balanced skin microclimate via defensins, cathelicidins and dermicidins—killing bad germs without harming the good guys. What we call the skin flora refers to the host of beneficial germs that help protect against harmful invasions by germs that cause disease.

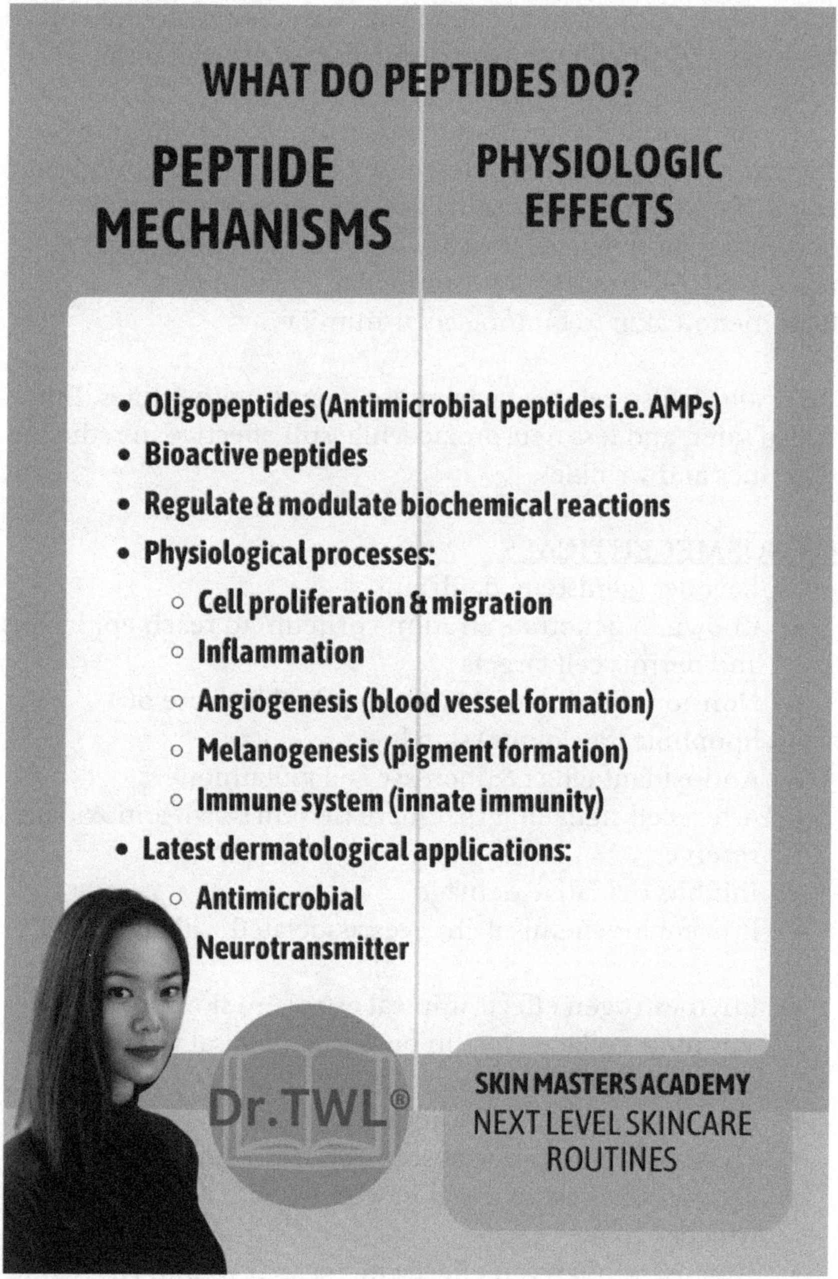

WHAT DO PEPTIDES DO?

PEPTIDE MECHANISMS

PHYSIOLOGIC EFFECTS

- **Oligopeptides (Antimicrobial peptides i.e. AMPs)**
- **Bioactive peptides**
- **Regulate & modulate biochemical reactions**
- **Physiological processes:**
  - **Cell proliferation & migration**
  - **Inflammation**
  - **Angiogenesis (blood vessel formation)**
  - **Melanogenesis (pigment formation)**
  - **Immune system (innate immunity)**
- **Latest dermatological applications:**
  - **Antimicrobial**

  Neurotransmitter

Dr.TWL®

SKIN MASTERS ACADEMY
NEXT LEVEL SKINCARE
ROUTINES

Antibiotics kill all germs, good and bad, leading to an imbalance in the flora. There's also the issue of antibiotic resistance, which causes the development of super-bugs that creep into the entire ecosystem. Eventually causing more disease via mutations.

Turns out, peptides also target the neuromuscular junction by affecting neurotransmitter release. But not in the way botulinum toxin does, which is by blocking acetylcholine release at neuromuscular junction. Instead, synthetic peptides target proteins (SNARE) at the neuromuscular junction in a phenomenon akin to biomolecular mimicry.

The result? It also relaxes facial muscles and soothes lines. But it's also safer, and less neurotoxic while still effective in reducing facial lines and wrinkles.

SOY COSMECEUTICALS
Soy isoflavones (genistein, daidzein)
- Known to penetrate stratum corneum to reach epidermis and dermis cell targets
- Non-ionised version better absorbed because of lipophilic (fat-loving) skin layer
- Antioxidant effect & increase cell glutathione
- Affect cell signalling that increase skin's own antioxidant reserve,
- Inhibits oxidative damage
- Prevent biochemical changes associated with aging cells

- Phytoestrogen effects (topical estrogen) slow down skin thinning, collagen loss in post-menopausal women via estrogen receptors in skin
- Stimulate collagen synthesis
- *Low risk of systemic absorption from application of creams, but best to avoid in women with active breast cancer
- Glucosaminoglycan effects: increase GAG and HA (tissue repair, skin hydration) in aging skin

SOY FOR PIGMENTATION
- Soy protease inhibitors
  - Treats hyperpigmentation
  - Soy trypsin, protease inhibitor with depigmentation activity, prevents UV-induced pigmentation

However, the use of soy products in melasma patients must be carefully considered as whole soy potential ca worsen the condition due to its estrogenic properties. In research settings, isolated soy protease/trypsin constituents are used instead.

PLANT HORMONES
Kinetin
- Plant growth hormone
- Regulates growth and cell differentiation
- Reduces leaf yellowing/cell senescence
- Slows fruit ripening/rotting process
- Uncertain skin absorption profile
- Stable, easily incorporated
- Studies on human fibroblasts in cell culture: delay age related changes
- Uncertain mechanism
- Antioxidant
- Improved skin texture
- Decreased hyperpigmentation
- Decrease TEWL (water loss to environment)
- Improves fine lines, hyperpigmentation
- Barrier repair

Studies:
- 0.1% kinetin lotion McCullough et al: improve photoaging signs
- Restore barrier function 12-24 weeks application
- 0.03% kinetin paired with niacinamide 4%combination improved pigmentation, blotchiness, hydration

Good-to-know cosmeceuticals

Hydroxyacetophenone:
- phenolic antioxidant
- synthetic antioxidant
- free radical scavenging
- anti-inflammatory

N-acetylglucosamine:
- inhibits conversion of protyrosinase to tyrosinase
- inhibit pigmentation
- 2% NAG reduced the appearance of facial hyperpigmentation
- ingredient pairing: 4% niacinamide

CHAPTER EIGHT

Cosmeceuticals for Functional Dermatology and the Art of Acne Skincare Routines

Cosmeceuticals for inflammaging & the skin exposome

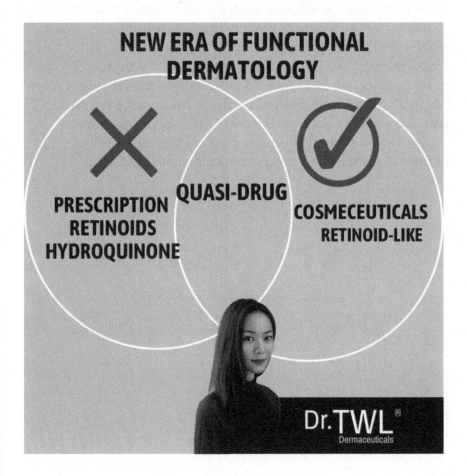

Why a **cosmeceutical skincare routine** matters more than traditional prescription actives in the light of new research on inflammaging and the skin exposome. Traditional actives like retinoids and hydroquinone have a targeted effect and were designed to be used under medical supervision. The effects were quite quickly observed, but there were side effect effects such as skin barrier dysfunction and immunological reactions. For instance, courses of topical hydroquinone were limited to 3-6 months in order to avoid paradoxical rebound phenomena. Retinoids were recommended to be used in the context of regular moisturiser therapy, tailing doses, a gradual escalation of concentrations as tolerated—under medical supervision. Both are associated with barrier dysfunction, sensitisation (indicative of immunological pathway being involved), photosensitive side effects and very likely, also a disruption of the skin microbiome (more targeted studies required to investigate this phenomena. The increasing recognition of cosmetic intolerance syndrome may also serve an impetus for dermatologists to examine approaches to over-the-counter skincare actives as well as traditional prescription cosmeceuticals such as retinoids.

DR.TWL®
PRESCRIPTIVE APPROACH

RETINOL/RETINOID FREE	PRESCRIPTION RETINOIDS
COSMECEUTICALS WITH RETINOID-LIKE EFFECTS	SKIN IRRITATION
ENCOURAGES CELL TALK	DISRUPTS SKIN MICROCLIMATE
RESTORES MICROBIOME	DISRUPTS MICROBIOME
HEALS THE SKIN BARRIER	SUN SENSITIVITY DAMAGES SKIN BARRIER
PREGNANCY SAFE	NOT SAFE FOR PREGNANCY

With cosmeceuticals we are looking at mainly botanicals or synthetics that mimic natural cell components, they are characterised by

- Low irritation potential, gradual mode of action
- Multi-modal effects vs single cell target
- Need for longer duration of treatment and increased frequency of use because of mechanism of action (requiring holistic approach to multiple cell pathways, i.e. green tea extracts showed histological improvements in skin tissue quality after 8 weeks but this was not apparent by clinical observation alone.
- Prescribed method of application: korean dermatologists created the skincare layering method with serums, emulsions/lotions, moisturising creams, masks and facial

mists. This method achieves the following: modification of wet occlusion therapy to enhance dermal absorption, creation of an artificial skin microclimate mimicking the moist wound healing environment and flooding of skin cells with hygroscopic molecules like sodium hyaluronate and amino acids with humectant effects for skin barrier repair.

- Pairing botanicals with biomimetic synthetic molecules to enhance stability and efficacy. I.e. antioxidant Vitamin C paired with Camilla sinensis extracts (green tea polyphenols) ensure stability of the latter.
- Variety of actives vs single active i.e. multiple botanicals at low concentrations observed to have synergistic interactions
- Focus on vehicles to address issues of dose delivery, compliance to ensure consistent and frequent use to achieve desired results: i.e. serum formulations concentrate water-soluble actives, facial mists allow frequent reapplication without discomfort or cosmetic issues
- Use of novel sheet mask materials such as polysaccharides which further enhance the wet occlusion effect with innate humectant properties
- Pairing with home-user friendly technologies such as hand-held sonic cleansing, electroporation, radiofrequency and hydrodermabrasion devices to increase epidermal penetration and cosmeceutical absorption.

Aestheticians, skin experts and dermatologists need to be updated on advancements in cosmeceutical research in order to better prescribe skincare routines. The korean cosmeceutical industry works closely with dermatologists, who are well positioned to feedback on clinical aspects such as topical treatment of rosacea, acne and sensitivity.

Functional dermatology: an advanced approach to skincare

Functional dermatology is a holistic approach to skin health. It involves using botanical actives as cosmeceuticals to harmonise the skin microenvironment. What exactly are cosmeceuticals? Well, these are what dermatologists consider bioactive skincare ingredients that fulfil 3 criteria:

- Acts by a known mechanism on a cellular target
- Can penetrate the skin barrier and exert the intended effect
- High quality clinical studies exist to support skin benefits i.e. double blind, randomised clinical trials

There are traditional cosmeceuticals such as hydroquinone and retinol/retinoids which have sensitising potential and can disrupt the skin barrier. These are not the focus of our research at the pharmacy. Instead we are examining plant-based alternatives which besides being gentler on skin, provide an added benefit of stabilising the microbiome, repairing the skin barrier and also additional anti-inflammatory benefits that protect aging skin. By targeting inflammation, these cosmeceuticals are also beneficial for adjuvant treatment of conditions such as acne, rosacea, pigmentation and eczema.

Here are some ways cosmeceuticals can help skin conditions without the need for prescription medications.

Skincare cocktails are both an art and a science: Understanding ingredients also includes how pairings can boost synergistic effects of cosmeceuticals.

<u>**Dr.TWL's Must-Know Ingredient Pairings**</u>

1. Niacinamide + Panthenol for barrier repair & anti-inflammatory effects
2. Ubiquinone (AKA Vitamin U) + Oligopeptides for anti-aging
3. Camellia sinensis + Vitamin C for enhanced stability and efficacy.

Beginning with advanced skincare routines that specifically target acne:

The ideal acne skincare routine recommended by dermatologists is one that treats the skin environment.

In a nutshell, when it comes to acne skincare routines, here's what I'd recommend. I'll also explain how newer acne skincare ingredients differ from traditional skincare actives.

Daily treatment:
- A gentle, hydrating and oil balancing cleanser
- Serum: antioxidant and sebum regulation
- Non-irritating pimple cream with anti-inflammatory ingredients
- Hydrocolloid patch
- Moisturising mist, emulsion

This discussion also applies to those with acne-prone sensitive skin. If your condition is moderate-severe, topical skincare alone may not be sufficient. You will need adjunct medical therapy. However, an acne skincare routine is still essential for long term maintenance and prevention of flare-ups.

You may already be aware of subtypes of acne such as hormonal acne and fungal acne. We will now learn the key features and how we should address these problems with skincare.

Hormonal acne skincare routine

Hormonal acne is mostly associated with adult women diagnosed with polycystic ovarian disease. However, all acne is actually hormonal in nature. Except in teenage acne, we consider that physiological. The surge in testosterone in both males and females triggers the production of sebum. In those who are genetically prone, acne develops. The dermatologist recommended acne skincare routine for all subtypes of acne is standard. The key principles are:
- Stabilise the microbiome with a good balance of bacteria

- Regulate oil production instead of drying skin out
- Reduce inflammation to prevent new formation of pimples
- Encourage quick healing of pimples to reduce scarring i.e. post-inflammatory hyperpigmentation and deeper dermal scars like ice pick, box car type scars

Fungal acne skincare routine

Fungal acne is a misnomer. Fungal acne is actually not acne at all. It's folliculitis, which is inflammation of the hair follicles. It can be associated with infection, but most of the time it is an immune reaction that occurs. Pityosporum folliculitis is the accurate scientific name for fungal acne. The fungus in this case is a yeast known as malessezia furfur, which is a commensal on healthy skin. This means that it lives on human skin without causing any problems. However, in those who have too much of this yeast, a condition caused by genetics, environmental factors such as excess heat and humidity, the fungus causes this acne-like condition. It can occur on the forehead, near the hairline and also the jawline. It can look quite similar to comedonal acne. When around the jawline, it is sometimes mistaken as hormonal acne. Treatment is with anti-dandruff shampoos applied on the scalp to reduce the population of yeast on the scalp. Prescription anti-dandruff shampoos include ketoconazole also known as Nizoral. However, these can be quite drying and sensitising when used long term. Non-prescription anti-dandruff shampoos are helpful for long term treatment and maintenance. These contain zinc pyrithone, salicylic acid which helps to inhibit the growth of the yeast. When the dandruff symptoms improve, fungal acne around the face will also resolve. In more severe cases or when there is an overlap with true acne conditions, oral medications may be necessary. Oral erythromycin, doxycycline prescribed exert an anti-inflammatory effect which works well for both fungal acne and acne vulgaris itself. For severe cases, oral isotretinoin which stops all sebum production may be prescribed. However it is important to note that oral isotretinoin itself can disrupt the balance of skin bacteria. The disturbances in the skin microbiome can cause folliculitis as well. Seek medical advice if you think you have been affected.

SKIN EXPERT MASTERY
ACNE SKINCARE ROUTINES
As a skin expert, one of the commonest concerns you will be addressing is acne. This section equips you to become competent in the teaching of advanced skincare steps for acne sufferers.

Acne Treatment

The 3 pillars of spot acne treatment

1. Targeted Treatment: Anti-Inflammatory
2. Acne Scar Removal
3. Resolve pigmentation

Step #1
- A gentle, hydrating and oil balancing cleanser

The goal of an acne skincare routine is to harmonise the skin microenvironment. Acne is genetic and driven by inflammation as well as excess sebum production. Addressing the latter 2 factors is the goal of an ideal acne skincare regimen.
Options: botanical emulsifiers and amino acid surfactants are gentler options of acne face washes compared to SLS-laden cleansers.

CLEANSING
Acne itself is caused by genetics, bacteria and oil production triggered by hormones all of which lead to inflammation and formation of comedones, papules and cysts.
The ideal acne skincare routine treats the skin microbiome, regulates the skin microenvironment, oil production and also reduces inflammation and flare-ups.

Cleansing plays a huge role, as do spot acne treatments. The Honey Cleanser is suitable for universal skin types, aids in skin barrier repair and also is anti-inflammatory. It is boosted with botanicals such as Arnica Montana flower which reduces skin flaking, hydrolysed collagen which improves skin resilience and also CICA for radiance and treating pigmentation.

THE SLS-CLEANSING MYTH
Are all foaming cleansers harsh for the skin?

No. The key is understanding the constituents of what makes the product foam.

On the topic of gentle skin cleansers that actually make your skin look and feel clean:

- Laureth-sulfates can be gentle, in ultra low concentrations but these cleansers end up feeling sticky
- Pure botanicals like soy and honey are mixed with laureth or amino sulfates to enhance the cleansing effect
- Added benefit: leaves a moisturising layer on skin to prevent trans-epidermal water loss (humectant effect)

Step #2

- Serum: antioxidant and sebum regulation

The 2 essential serums for acne prone individuals are vitamin C and hyaluronic acid serums.

Antioxidants like vitamin C change the skin microenvironment. Lipid peroxidation is due to increased sebum on skin of acne-prone patients. This process worsens skin inflammation and formation of whiteheads/blackheads. When comedones get infected, red bumps like papules emerge. Acne cysts are when the papules get infected at a deeper level, causing the skin cells to form a wall around the infection. This requires injections with intralesional steroids like triamcinolone. But in serious cases when the cyst recurs over many months, surgery may necessary.

How Vitamin C serums work for acne treatment

- Reduce inflammation i.e. purging due to retinols/retinoids
- Decrease bacteria count
- Reduce scarring, post-inflammatory hyperpigmentation

The bacteria Cutibacterium causes acne. Reducing growth improves acne flare-ups.

How hyaluronic acid serums work for sebum regulation
Hyaluronic acid is a humectant molecule that attracts moisture from the environment and traps it under the skin. Moisturising oily acne-prone skin is important because it sends a signal to skin to regulate oil production. Oily skin occurs when there is excess stimulation of the oil glands known as sebaceous glands. When oily skin is stripped of moisture with strong lathering agents, the skin barrier is also damaged. This triggers sebaceous glands to produce even more oil, a condition known as reactive seborrhea. It is a paradoxical condition whereby oily skin feels dehydrated and tries to compensate.

Step #3
- Non-irritating pimple cream with anti-inflammatory ingredients

ACNE SPOT TREATMENT:
Inflamed acne papules cause significant scarring, post inflammatory hyperpigmentation and may become infected cysts. Early spot treatment must be non irritating and create a moist wound healing environment for rapid healing. The Blemish spot cream based on the latest dermatological research on the skin microenvironment, it contains botanical extracts like chlorella vulgaris, argan oil and synthetic mimics of amino acids such as methionine. Chlorella has an anti-inflammatory effect, argan oil extract helps with treating pigmentation and methionine boosts wound healing. The formulation ensures that it is suited for all skin types including sensitive skin as it treats acne while healing the skin barrier.

Traditional acne treatments involved creams that dried up the skin barrier. The idea that oily skin is the cause of acne is outdated. In fact, dermatologists know acne is caused by a combination of genetics, excess oil triggered by hormones at puberty, bacteria and inflammation. Benzoyl peroxide, tea tree oil and salicylic acid all dry up the skin. However it worsens inflammation. This may be the reason why you find your acne bump redder, more inflamed after applying your acne cream.

Retinoids are usually prescribed for comedonal acne. However, retinoids worsen inflammation and should not be applied on actively inflamed acne bumps like papules and cysts. This is one reason why individuals experience acne purging.

Topical antibiotics should be avoided, i.e. erythromycin, clindamycin. These quickly breed resistance and lose effectiveness. Combinations with benzoyl peroxide, also known by trade names Epiduo commonly cause irritation. A side effect known as irritant contact dermatitis is actually due to skin barrier damage. Antibiotic resistance can also be a serious problem

Choose botanical actives that treat inflammation. Berberine, chlorella and argan oil are the actives used in our pharmacy recommended acne spot creams. Berberine in particular acts on multiple pathways. It is naturally antibacterial without the same risks of antibiotic resistance common to topical antibiotics. There are additional benefits which include antioxidant properties, this makes the acne bacteria less likely to thrive. In addition, anti-inflammatory effects help the pimples resolve faster. There is also an effect on comedogenesis. This means that blackheads and whiteheads are less likely to form. The key advantage is the absence of irritating side effects which are associated with traditional acne creams.

EXERCISE: Dr.TWL's PIMPLE CREAM FORMULATION

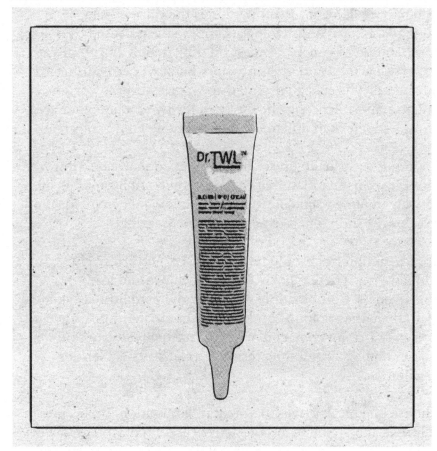

The ideal pimple cream formula should possess the following functions:

- Treat pimple quickly and effectively
- Promote rapid healing (glycerin, niacinamide)
- Repair skin barrier
- Peptides, amino acids (copper tripeptide, methylmethionine, arginine)
- Minimise scarring by inhibiting pigment formation (centella asiatica CICA)
- Anti-inflammatory (more than 16 different botanicals)
    - Argania spinosa
    - Sesamum indicum

- o Chlorella vulgaris
- o Serena serrulata
- o CICA
- o Sophora augustifolia root
- o Sambucus nigra flower
- o Polygonum cuspidatum root
- o Scutellaria baicalensis
- o Camellia sinensis
- o Soy isoflavones
- o Licorice root
- o Chamomile recutita
- o Rosemary
- o Artemisia vulgaris
- o Gentiana lutea root
- o Archillea millefolium
- o Arnica Montana flower
- Prevent new pimples from forming
- Target inflammation & comedone formation
  - o Retinyl palmitate (gentlest retinol)
- Encourage cell turnover
- Antimicrobial effect (chlorella vulgaris)
- Microbiome friendly ferment tetrad
  - o lactobacillus +soybean
  - o lactobacillus + punica gunatum
  - o lactobacillus +pear juice ferment

SUMMARY: Botanicals can restore a healthy balance, regulate the skin microenvironment, sebum production in acne.

Why do you need an effective pimple cream?
When the pimple has already formed, you want the pimple cream to rapidly heal the bump. An effective pimple cream does so by exerting anti-inflammatory effects. However, active pimples are also areas where skin barrier damage has occured. So it should repair the skin barrier to prevent secondary infections and scarring. Scarring first begins with redness, known as post-inflammatory erythema. This progresses to

pigmentation, when skin turns reddish-brown. Dermatologists call that post-inflammatory hyperpigmentation. When inflammation is severe, for example, with an acne cyst, a deep scar occurs. Ice pick and box car scars are examples of dermal scarring. Skin responds to inflammation and injury by sending chemical signals to other skin cells. The cells then coordinate with each other in a process known as cell talk to begin repairing skin tissues. There is collagen being produced, which helps to heal the injured skin. When inflammation goes deep like in an acne cyst, this process can be impaired. Eventually resulting in an indented scar.

Step #4
- Hydrocolloid patch

I recommend pimple patches as spot treatment. First of all it helps to reduce picking and squeezing. There are many other benefits:
  - Reduces inflammation with antibacterial effect
  - Encourages healing with the ideal skin microenvironment
  - Rapid healing means a lower risk of scarring

Hydrocolloid patches that come with infused medicated oils or essences can irritate skin, avoid these. Choose plain hydrocolloid patches or ideally, one that is formulated with skin barrier repairing ingredients like glycerin. The hydrocolloid patch from our pharmacy contains glycerin and urea. Urea is a keratolytic which means it breaks down dead skin cells. In acne, there is retention of keratinocytes which are dead skin cells—this leads to comedone formation via a process known as follicular plugging.

EXERCISE: THE IDEAL HYDROCOLLOID PATCH:

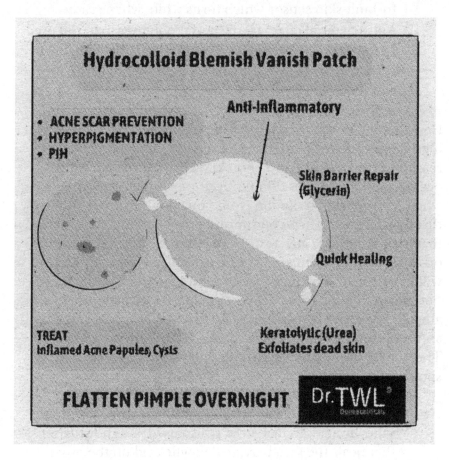

An essential part of acne spot treatment is the use of hydrocolloid patches. There are different types of hydrocolloid patches and not all are created equal. For instance the hydrocolloid patch we designed has additional built-in anti-inflammatory and skin healing properties such as glycerin that helps to repair damaged and broken skin, urea which is a gentle keratolytic, meaning it exfoliates dead skin cells. It can treat inflamed acne papules and cysts and also prevent acne scars such as post-inflammatory hyperpigmentation (PIH). Additional benefits include

☐ Prevents squeezing and picking

- [ ] Repairs skin barrier (infused with hydrating glycerin)
- [ ] In-built skin sensor which turns white when ready
- [ ] Anti-bacterial effect from special polymer material used
- [ ] Exfoliates dead skin cells with urea —gentle and effective for sensitive skin
- [ ] NO ESSENTIAL OILS*

Here's why you should not use pimple patches that have active ingredients infused in them, essential oils, salicylic acid etc. The reason for this is a phenomenon known as occlusion. Under occlusion, skin behaves differently, for example, remember when you got skin irritation from your pimple cream? Multiply that by 10 times. When you suffocate the skin under any sort of material, skin magically absorbs much more of what is applied on skin. So unless you are using a moisturiser, everything else will irritate skin. The point about pimple patches is that they are not meant to treat acne per se—too late. The acne bump has already formed. The point here is to help skin heal. Essential oils and acids only serve to irritate broken skin rather than heal it. There are 2 important features in the patch that treats acne spots:

- Repairing the skin barrier
- Exfoliating dead skin with a keratolytic, urea vs using salicylic acid. In fact, urea is also used as a moisturiser that heals the skin barrier. Salicylic acid on the other hand can burn through skin causing irritant contact dermatitis.

Most skin irritation occurs under occlusion, because absorption is enhanced. So non-irritating acne treatment ingredients when used with the hydrocolloid patch instead enhance skin healing and repair.

Step #5
- Moisturising mist, emulsion

A moisturising mist or emulsion is the best moisturiser for oily, acne prone skin types. Cream formulations or ointments are too heavy on oily skin to be comfortable. Definitely avoid paraffin, common in skincare trends known as slugging. That occludes skin and increases flare ups of acne.

Look for these ingredients in your facial mist:
- Hyaluronic acid
- Polyglutamic acid
- Botanical extracts like rice bran
- UV protective antioxidants i.e. portulaca oleracea

Layer your emulsion or face lotion with facial mists
- Use your facial mist before, after or anytime in between your skincare steps
- When used before and after facial lotions, it increases absorption of moisturising skincare actives

The ideal face moisturiser for acne prone skin should contain
- Panthenol
- Niacinamide
- Glycerin
- Hyaluronic acid & polyglutamic acid

These synergise to repair the damaged skin barrier.

Step #6 Sunscreen
If you are using prescription retinoids, it may not be enough to just use sunscreen. It is wiser to also practice sun avoidance. However here are some important things to bear in mind when choosing a sunscreen for acne-prone skin:
- Lightweight texture
- Easily absorbed, does not leave a sticky residue
- Non-comedogenicity

In general, sunscreen is quite a tricky skincare product for those who suffer from acne. It is true that some sunscreens can worsen acne. This is because of the oil vehicle as well as chemical sunscreen components which sometimes irritate areas of broken skin. My best advice is to sample sunscreens if you are not sure. The sunscreen formulation at our pharmacy has been tested on those with acne prone skin with good clinical outcome.

Am and pm skincare routine for acne prone skin
Apart from sunscreen use in the daytime only, there are no differences in the am and pm skincare routine for acne prone skin according to the regimen prescribed here.

An acne skincare routine is an essential component of acne treatment. If your acne is moderate-severe, or you have co-existing, overlapping skin conditions such as sensitive skin, rosacea or perioral dermatitis, you may wish to consult a dermatologist for a clinical examination and diagnosis.

If you wear makeup, double cleansing is necessary. Choose a milk or emulsion makeup remover cleanser for the first step. Milk cleansers are preferred over micellar face washes for acne prone skin because of the following:
- Gentler and leaves moisturising layer
- Easier to remove without friction on skin

Makeup wipes are detrimental for acne prone skin. The harsh surfactants damage the skin barrier.

IN SUMMARY
The ideal acne skincare routine is one that addresses the following
1. Skin hydration levels to repair skin barrier damage
2. Treats the acne microbiome to reduce growth of bad bacteria
3. Regulates oil production to prevent excess oil on skin
4. Anti-inflammatory to reduce comedone formation, post inflammatory hyperpigmentation and scarring

All these strategies are important for long term treatment and prevention of acne. Medical treatment must be used in conjunction with an acne skincare routine as maintenance therapy.

Good to know cosmeceutical for acne:
Zinc:
- essential cofactor for enzymes
- anti-inflammatory
- bactericidal
- oil control
- treat acne

Anti-inflammatory
The proposed anti-inflammatory mechanism of zinc on acne pathogenesis is through inhibition of leukocyte chemotaxis. Chemotaxis is the attraction and movement of molecules to a chemical signal. This process uses signalling proteins such as cytokines and chemokines to attract immune cells such as leukocytes to the site of infection, ensuring that pathogens in the area will be destroyed. This leads to inflammation.

Antimicrobial
Zinc is also antimicrobial and bactericidal. The proposed mechanism of its antimicrobial activity by either interacting with the bacterial surface, or entering inside the bacterial cells. This leads to a disruption in the bacteria's enzyme systems, subsequently killing the bacteria/

Sebum control
Additionally, overproduction of sebum is typically caused by circulating hormones in the body, namely, dihydrotestosterone (DHT). Zinc acts as a DHT blocker, helping to regulate the amount of sebum the skin produces. This regulation helps to prevent acne.

Weekly (up to thrice weekly)
1. Exfoliation
Exfoliation addresses the build up of dead skin cells. Physical exfoliation with abrasive beads damage the skin barrier and are especially bad for those with active acne. Instead choose chemical exfoliation or enzymatic exfoliation. Acids such as

glycolic, lactic and salicylic acids target cell renewal and inflammation. However in sunny climates depending on where you live can cause photosensitivity. Using sunscreen is essential. However, a newer form of exfoliation exists—which is my preference. Enzyme peels based on papain and bromelain, these are derived from papaya and pineapple respectively. Besides breaking down and exfoliating dead skin cells for skin radiance, enzyme peels for acne also have additional benefits of reducing inflammation, scars and have minimal side effects.

2. Masking

Masking in acne prone individuals is mainly to improve skin barrier function. This can help to regulate oil production. However there are added functions when certain active ingredients are included:

- High doses of Vitamin C

This is possible in a wash off gel mask, as leave on formulations like vitamin C serums tend to have lower concentrations. Overall, an antioxidant rich skin treatment can help reduce growth of acne causing bacteria

- Anti-inflammatory

Botanicals in face masks can synergise to improve the skin microbiome and reduce inflammation.

I developed the mask peel range to address both exfoliation and masking in 1 step. There are no abrasives and natural botanical extracts are selected to maintain optimal skin health by strengthening the skin's immune system—a concept known as skin resilience.

ADDITIONAL OTC OPTIONS FOR ACNE TREATMENT
Use of textiles

- Face masks (if applicable)
- Pillowcases

Textiles are a new advancement in skincare. I discussed this in my paper*—as a good therapeutic option for those with acne-prone skin. Biofunctional textiles help to reduce the growth of bacteria without causing antibiotic resistance.

Additionally the release of ions such as copper nanoparticles from materials embedded in pillowcases can also improve scars and reducing formation of acne marks.

Teo WL. Diagnostic and management considerations for "maskne" in the era of COVID-19. J Am Acad Dermatol. 2021 Feb;84(2):520-521. doi: 10.1016/j.jaad.2020.09.063. Epub 2020 Oct 1. PMID: 33011321; PMCID: PMC7528820.

Incorporating blue light LED therapy
Blue light for acne is one of the most underrated treatments. The reason being, it is traditionally offered in dermatologist's offices and the costs per treatment could really add up. Let me go into how blue light works. Essentially research shows that twice a week, 30 minute durations of blue light therapy in-office for a month confers antibacterial effects similar to traditional oral medication therapy for acne.

Hand-held devices do not produce sufficient energy for treatment and LED face masks without eye protection could be dangerous for the eyes. Consider latest designs which are modelled after in-clinic machines but created for home users. An example is the AURORA light therapy machine for acne which has a small footprint and includes options for treatment of body acne and acne scarring.

FAQ
Skincare routine for acne-prone sensitive skin
Acne-prone sensitive skin needs to be understood this way. There are 3 potential problems going on:
1. Acne vulgaris
2. Eczema/dermatitis caused by a damaged skin barrier
3. Misdiagnosis

- Acne vulgaris

We understand this to be a multi-factorial condition which is affected by genetics, bacteria, excess oil producing and hormonal factors.

- Eczema/dermatitis caused by a damaged skin barrier

Those with both acne-prone and sensitive skin may be suffering from side effects of acne treatments. Topical retinoids and retinols commonly prescribed for acne also damage the skin barrier. This can result in sensitive skin reactions such as burning, stinging, pain, flaking and redness.

- Misdiagnosis

Sometimes it is not acne. Rosacea and perioral dermatitis can look similar—this is why visiting a dermatologist is important. Medical treatments are slightly different. If your acne-prone sensitive skin does not seem to get better—get a specialist diagnosis.

THE ACNE SENSITIVE SKIN PARADOX

There are 5 considerations here which we will go through. I'll also include a discussion on what to look out for in specific product formulations tailored to remedy such imbalances.

1. Breakdown of lipid joints i.e. the "cement" in the brick-mortar model of sensitive skin

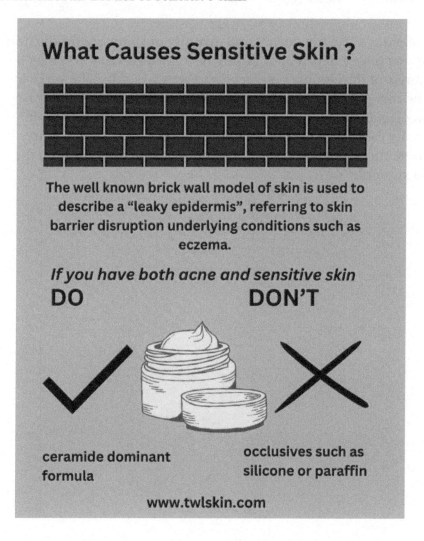

What Causes Sensitive Skin ?

The well known brick wall model of skin is used to describe a "leaky epidermis", referring to skin barrier disruption underlying conditions such as eczema.

If you have both acne and sensitive skin

DO   DON'T

ceramide dominant formula

occlusives such as silicone or paraffin

www.twlskin.com

The well known brick wall model of skin is used to describe a "leaky epidermis", referring to skin barrier disruption underlying conditions such as <u>eczema</u>. The joints of the bricks are sealed by lipids, which is produced by healthy skin. While oil production tends to be beneficial for dry skin types, it does not necessarily translate into a healthy skin barrier. The key is a molecule known as ceramide, produced by the endoplasmic reticulum of healthy skin cells.

Genetics affect the quality and quantity of ceramide production. If you have a personal or family history of eczema, you may be at risk of developing both acne and sensitive skin. The surge in the male hormone testosterone at puberty leads to an increase in oil gland activity—this can compensate for skin dryness in many cases. However, if acne sensitive skin care products are used, this can trigger barrier disruption, which brings us to the next point.

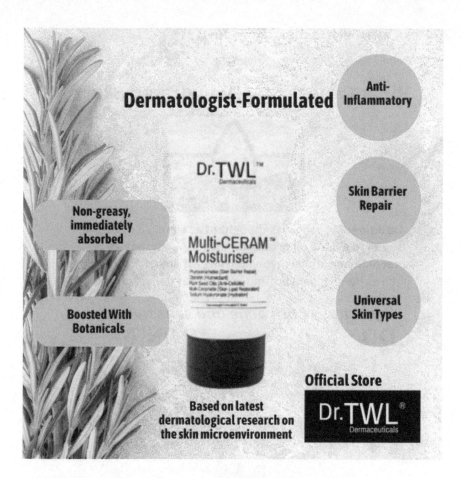

Acne sensitive skin product recommendation tips:

Do use a moisturiser even if you have oily skin. Choose a ceramide dominant formula instead of occlusives such as silicone or paraffin if you are acne prone—the latter can increase comedogenesis.

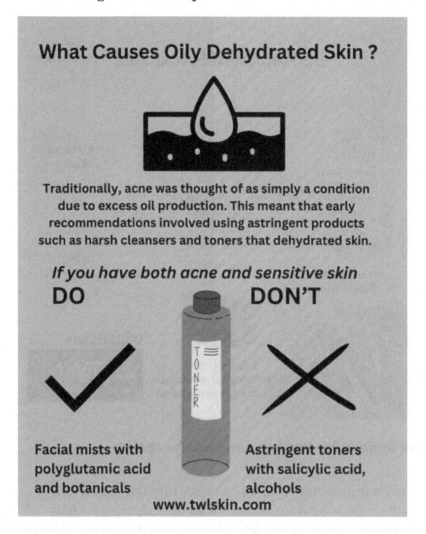

Traditionally, acne was thought of as simply a condition due to excess oil production. This meant that early recommendations involved using astringent products such as harsh cleansers and toners that dehydrated skin. While the effects are quite instantaneous i.e. the shine does disappear, the problem is more complex than that.

The physical removal of grease does nothing to regulate underlying oil production. In fact, what dermatologists have observed is an increase in oil production—a phenomenon described as paradoxical reactive <u>hyperseborrhea</u>. The same problem arises when astringent toners containing salicylic acid, alcohols are used.

Acne sensitive skin product recommendation tips:

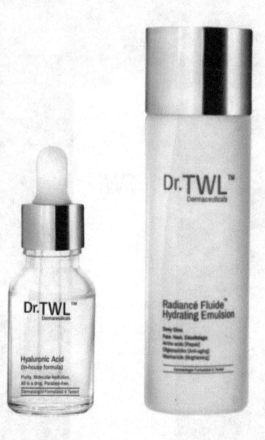

Ceramide moisturisers can be used at night if you are acne prone and live in a humid climate. In the day, a skincare layering method with <u>hyaluronic acid serums</u> and a lightweight

<u>moisturising emulsion</u> can help to keep skin hydrated without triggering off acne flare ups.

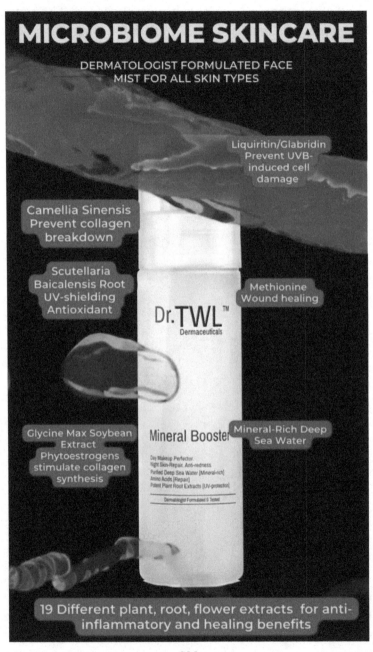

Instead of toners, choose facial mists with polyglutamic acid and botanicals that helps to boost the skin's reserve of antioxidants. Research has shown that oxidative stress caused by excess oil production and environmental stressors worsens comedone formation.

3. Inappropriate use of exfoliation methods to treat acne

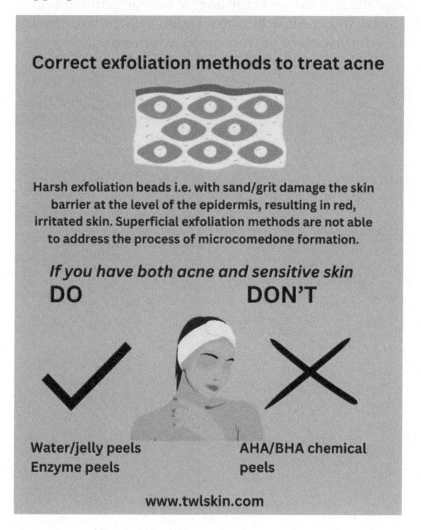

Another common misconception about acne sensitive skin care routines is that physical exfoliation helps to get rid of comedones. Pesky whiteheads and blackheads are merely a symptom of what's going on in the deeper layers. Microcomedones begin forming at least 2 weeks before actual comedones surface—so the key is addressing the root cause of inflammation. Harsh exfoliation beads i.e. with sand/grit damage the skin barrier at the level of the epidermis, resulting in red, irritated skin. Superficial exfoliation methods are not able to address the process of microcomedone formation.

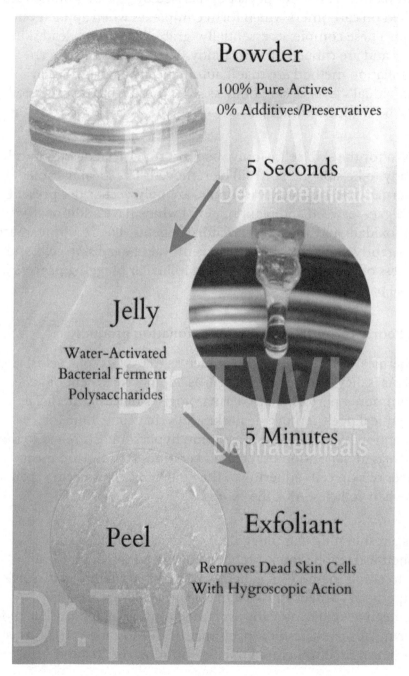

Powder

100% Pure Actives
0% Additives/Preservatives

5 Seconds

Jelly

Water-Activated
Bacterial Ferment
Polysaccharides

5 Minutes

Peel

Exfoliant

Removes Dead Skin Cells
With Hygroscopic Action

Instead of abrasive beads, adopt the J-beauty method of water exfoliation. The water peels popularised by J-beauty brands are based on carbomers which form complexes when applied on skin. These complexes essentially "grab" dirt oil and dead skin cells and are rubbed off skin gently. The benefits of such an exfoliation method are that it automatically adjusts to each individual's level of skin oiliness. This means that no excess oil will be stripped off skin.

Ditto for the skin cells—only the most superficial dead skin cells ready to be sloughed off will be removed. The ideal natural alternative to synthetic carbomers are polysaccharides present in algae, seaweed and plant material which have additional antioxidant and anti-inflammatory benefits. The resulting effect is a gently exfoliated epidermis, removal of dead skin cells and excess oil—factors that worsen the follicular plugging process in acne pathogenesis.

4. Poorly formulated chemical exfoliation products

Chemical exfoliation methods such as AHAs (glycolic acids) and BHAs (salicylic acids) are helpful as adjunct treatment of acne. Commonly performed in dermatologist's offices, superficial chemical peels remove dead skin cells that contribute to retention hyperkeratosis. Retention hyperkeratosis refers to the increased deposition of retained keratinocytes, the top most layer of skin cells adhering to the epidermis. This occurs around the hair follicles, AKA the "pores".

As a result, follicular plugging i.e. pore clogging occurs. Chemical exfoliation is preferred over traditional physical exfoliation methods in general because of its ability to dissolve superficial corneocytes selectively without breaching the protective epidermis. However, the duration of application and formulation of chemical peels matter. For instance, AHAs must be neutralised when used in concentrations of 20% and above—care must also be taken not to leave on the application beyond the prescribed application time.

The challenge is when AHA and BHA containing products are used in home skincare. OTC skincare products are strictly regulated for its acid content, however, this does not always mean that users are reaction-free. Let me explain. Glycolic and salicylic acids do interact with skin immediately and also in the medium to long term. The latter is what is referred to as a cummulative effect. The types of adverse reactions have been described as irritant contact dermatitis and allergic contact dermatitis—the former is much more likely to occur with prolonged use in an acne sensitive skin care routine.

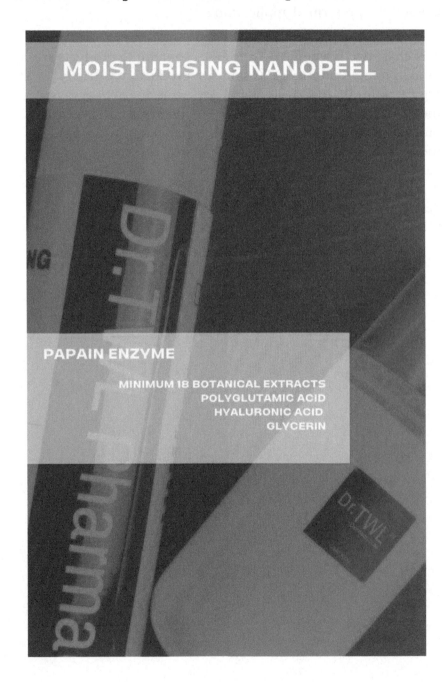

Do choose enzyme peels based on papain or bromelain for home chemical peels. These perform the same functions of microscopic exfoliation, as do traditional AHA/BHA based chemical peels. Additionally, enzyme peels are well suited for sensitive skin types—these whole plant extracts possess anti-inflammatory and anti-microbial benefits while moisturising the skin.

5. Disruption of the microbiome with certain acne medications

Prescription acne medications are required for moderate to severe forms of acne. These include topical and oral forms of retinoids that are really Vitamin A derivatives. Topical retinoid therapy is well-known for disrupting the skin barrier, a side effect due to its rather aggressive exfoliation of superficial skin cells. Oral isotretinoin therapy is reserved for the most severe and/or persistent forms of acne. It remains the most effective form of oral medication for acne as it completely stops sebum production. This however, is not without rather serious adverse events. Cheilitis is a severe form of lip eczema that can lead to bleeding, cracking and infections—it is also a well-known side effect of oral isotretinoin treatment.

What is not spoken about often also is the ability of isotretinoin to disrupt the skin microbiome—the balance of good and bad bacteria on skin. Many of these bacteria are required to maintain healthy skin cell function, cell signaling i.e. cell talk processes that help to regulate sebum production, cell turnover and anti-microbial activity against bad bacteria. Acne sensitive skin conditions such as eczema have been linked to microbiome imbalances as well—microbiome dysbiosis perpetuates the inflammatory cycle that is responsible for persistent flare-ups.

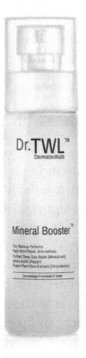

Lactobacillus plus fruit extracts

Rebalancing facial mists are preferred over toners because these are infused with botanical actives that help to encourage a healthy microbiome. The use of bacterial ferments such as lactobacillus plus fruit extracts are a fairly recent development in skincare formulations. These are highly beneficial for stabilising the skin ecosytem—addressing hydration, inflammation and microbial stability.

Dr.TWL's Tutorial Summary

How to treat acne sensitive skin types

The traditional skin typing methods of oily/combination/dry skin does not address the more complex subtypes of oily-dehydrated skin. We have discussed how this arises from the interaction of certain astringent skincare products with acne prone skin. The best intervention would be in the form of carefully selected acne sensitive skin care products that have dual functions—addressing both issues simultaneously.

The Sensitive Skin Hormonal Acne Complex

Hormonal acne is one of the commonest dermatological conditions afflicting adults—one that is perhaps most distressing as well. While its regarded as treatable, the persistence throughout adulthood also means that a sustainable, long-term approach must be in place. Apart from dermatological care and prescription oral medications in the acute phase, acne sensitive skin care routines that target the various pathways we have described in this tutorial can play a critical role in long term maintenance and prevention.

PIGMENTATION TREATMENT:
Hyperpigmentation is due to the following
- Oxidative stress
- UV damage that activates pigment cells (melanocytes)
- Other forms of environmental stress
- Biological aging known as inflammaging

Using an effective vitamin C serum is key to treating and preventing hyperpigmentation. But not all Vitamin C serums are created equal, here are the key features of a vitamin C serum that is precisely formulated as an effective cosmeceutical:

- CONCENTRATION:

Depending on the compound, effective concentrations vary. For instance L ascorbic acid is at 15% and up. But for sodium ascorbyl phosphate 4.5% is the optimal concentration based on studies that can treat acne. Essentially it creates an antioxidant environment that prevents the growth of pathogenic acne bacteria like P.acnes.

- MINIMAL IRRITATION TO SENSITIVE SKIN

The key problem with vitamin C is skin irritation. The problem is mostly with L-ascorbic acid which is acidic and formulated in higher concentrations. Neutral vitamin C compounds like sodium and magnesium ascorbyl phosphate are less irritating and especially when formulated with synergistic extracts like green tea, actually provide a boost in skin benefits.

ECZEMA/DRY/SENSITIVE SKIN:

The key with treating eczema and sensitive skin is by focusing on skin barrier repair. Think of your skin barrier as a brick wall—the bricks are joined together by cement. When you have sensitive skin or eczema, it is the cement that is missing. So when you apply moisturiser what you really want is to replenish like for like. In this case we are referring to ceramides. But there are other criteria for an ideal moisturiser, which is termed in dermatology as a Prescription Emollient Device, which also refers to a moisturiser with steroid-like anti-inflammatory benefits.

- Ceramides repair skin barrier
- Anti-inflammatory botanicals reduce the reliance on steroids without side effects.

Ferment filtrates in skincare

- Inflammaging: low grade chronic inflammation is the process responsible for photoaging
- To counteract inflammation, antioxidants fight oxidative stress generated by UV damage, pollution and biological aging processes
- Inhibit tyrosinase activity & melanogenesis

What is fermentation:
- Metabolic process
- Sugars converted to acids, gases, alcohol
- In skincare: fermented products block melanin production & treat hyperpigmentation

Functional fermented broth components in Dr.TWL skincare:
Natural melanogenesis inhibitors
- Lactic acid (increase epidermal thickness, reduce melanin, increase collagen, increase cell renewal, reduce tyrosinase)
- Flavonoids (fermented rice brain derived kaempferol blocks tyrosinase
- Antioxidants (increased intracellular glutathione blocks melanin)
- Novel melanogenesis inhibitors (albocycline K3 from seed ferments)

Barrier function
Stratum corneum is the outermost layer of the epidermis.

Life cycle of keratinocytes & function of dead skin cells
Keratinocytes start life in the basal layer, moving through spinous & granular layers before they die. But these dead skin cells remain useful at the surface of the epidermis. Corneocytes perform an important skin barrier function, protecting skin against the external environment and regulating moisture levels.

Complete ecosystem at the skin barrier
Goal: maintain healthy skin-water balance with functional ingredients
1. Corneocytes
Form the bulk of the epidermis
2. Lipids (extra cellular lamellar)
Ceramides, cholesterol
3. Natural moisturising factors (NMFs)
Free amino acids, pyrrolidone carboxylic acids, lactates

Glucose, urea, hyaluronic acid, electrolytes

What happens in dry skin:
- Decreased skin hydration
- Increased transepidermal water loss (TEWL)

Effects of a moisturiser:
- Enhances skin hydration
- Decreased transepidermal water loss (TEWL)

Importance of skin hydration
- Dry skin conditions i.e. atopic dermatitis
- Photoaging

Moisturisers with antioxidants
- Reduce facial redness
- Pore size *(Miyamoto 2021)*

Ingredients in your moisturiser: what's really inside?
- Occlusives: petroleum, lanolin are hydrophobic i.e. water repellant reduces water loss through epidermis by 90%
- Humectants: urea, glycerin, AHAs: draw water from deeper layers of dermis and epidermis
- Ceramides
- NMF

Overall effect: increase skin hydration, reduce TEWL, up regulate skin barrier function

Good to know cosmeceutical active

Panthenol: also known as provitamin B5, skin moisturizing, produced significant decreases in TEWL, protects integrity of skin barrier. Works as both a humectant and emollient. Is well tolerated by most skin types.

What is panthenol?
- moisturizing ingredient
- humectant

- emollient
- prevent transpeidermal water loss
  - trap water

- provitamin precursor to vitamin B (pantothenic acid)
- makeup, haircare, skincare
- effect: dewy skin, shiny hair
- AKA provitamin B5, butanimide, depantothenyl alcohol

Panthenol is a popular skincare ingredient found in many skin and hair products, touted for its moisturizing abilities. It has the unique ability to function as both a humectant to draw water, binding it to the skin, as well as an emollient to prevent transpeidermal water loss, trapping water to smooth and hydrate the skin. Hydrated skin helps to improve the overall appearance as well as plumpness and elasticity of the skin.

Panthenol is the provitamin precursor that the body uses to convert to vitamin B, also known as pantothenic acid. It is an ingredient that has been increasingly incorporated in makeup, haircare products as well as skincare products for its ability to give the skin its dewiness, as well as impart shine in hair. In ingredient labels, it is also known as provitamin B5, butanimide and depantothenyl alcohol.

How does panthenol benefit the skin?

- humectant
- bind water molecules
- protect from environmental changes/damage
- transpidermal water loss
  - loss of water from our skin to the environment by evaporation
- wound healing
- anti-inflammatory
  - reduce UV-induced redness/irritation
- relieve itch

Acting as a humectant, it is able to bind to water molecules, holding them in the skin. This makes this ingredient suitable for skin that has to endure harsher climates, exposure to air conditioning or heaters, as it is able to compensate for and prevent the transpeidermal water loss that occurs. Transpidermal water loss is the loss of water from our skin to the environment.

Not only does it retain moisture in the skin, it also acts as an emollient that helps to stimulate cells that promote skin barrier function, maintaining a healthy skin barrier. The skin barrier is the outermost layer of the skin that plays an important role in protection from environmental stressors, irritation and inflammation. Benefits of a strong skin barrier include being able to lock in moisture and keep it from escaping.

As the same cells responsible for skin barrier function are also important for wound healing, panthenol may help to protect the skin while it is healing.

Studies also suggest that panthenol was able to help reduce UV-induced redness and irritation through its anti-inflammatory effect. Furthermore, it could also help relieve itching associated with eczema or dermatitis.

Is panthenol safe for skin?
- well-tolerated
- irritation/sensitivity rare

DERM'S PRO TIP
Skincare products contain several different ingredients and true allergy can only be diagnosed by a dermatologist using specialised patch tests. A good rule when using any new skincare product for the first time is to perform a mini "patch test" by applying the product over a small area of skin for at least 4 hours and watch for reactions. Do not apply any skincare product on

areas of raw, broken skin unless specifically directed by a dermatologist.

Panthenol is considered safe for its intended uses. It is generally well-tolerated by most skin types, rarely causing irritation or sensitivity. However, with any ingredient, an allergy is always possible, even though the chances are low. Therefore, it is always beneficial to perform a patch test before using any new ingredient or skincare and makeup product.

ADVANCED INGREDIENTS TARGETING BARRIER REPAIR & SENSITIVE SKIN
Galactomyces, Lactobacillus ferment filtrates
- Elderly Sake brewers had wrinkle-free youthful skin on their hands which were in constant contact with the sake fermentation process while their faces were wrinkled
- Clinical studies:
    - Improves fluctuations in redness, roughness & pore size
    - Alleviates mask-induced skin irritation (frictional dermatoses)
- Mechanism of action:
  1. Upregulate ceramide production via fillagrin gene expression
    - Tapinarof TAMA-like: therapeutic AHR modulating agents used for inflammatory skin diseases like psoriasis and eczema
    - Via AHR, upregulate fillagrin gene expression (missing in genetic disorders like eczema)
    - Ferment filtrates are Nature's TAMAs
  2. Antioxidant capacity
    - Additional antioxidant effect: neutralises damaging free radicals
  3. Blocks key inflammaging mechanisms i.e. cell senescence
    - Downregulate senescence: cells falling asleep
    - Reduce stress on skin, increase cell repair

4. Increased Caspase-14 *also activated by phytochemicals
5. Increased tight junction molecules
- Cell connections made by proteins
- Affects permeability of skin barrier
1. Increased anti-inflammatory chemical signals (cytokines) i.e. IL-37

CASE STUDY: The ideal cosmeceutical regimen for eczema/dry sensitive skin

☐ Formulated based on latest research in skin barrier function

☐ Ingredients tested on damaged skin models

☐ Botanicals, phytochemicals extracts that target multiple pathways of skin inflammation and reactivity

☐ Ceramide, NMF- dominant skincare

☐ Retinol/retinoid & irritation-free

☐ Advanced cosmeceutical research focus on functional actives

SKIN EXPERT FAQ

Why does sensitive skin develop?
- State of hyperreactivity
- **Barrier function* key**
- Neurological factors
- Inflammatory response

Once skin barrier is damaged, associated proteins change. This stimulates inflammation leading to tissue damage.

Associated with
- High reactivity
- Poor tolerance
- Susceptibility to allergy

Cosmeceuticals investigated with sensitive skin model which mimicked skin barrier damage included:

- Oat extract
- Olive leaf extract
- Brown algae (Phaeophycease extract)
- Stephanie tetranda
- Stachyose
- Erythritol

Chosen for ability:
- Scavenge free-radicals
- Inhibit hyaluronidase

Advanced cosmeceuticals target barrier-related proteins
- Aquaporins
- Fillagrin
- Caspase
- Kallikrein
- IL
- VEGF: *AQP3, FLG, CASP14, KLK7, Cytokines (IL6, 8), VEGF*
- Repair barrier
- Skin soothing effect

Aquaporins (elasticity & hydration)
- Located in cell walls (membranes)
- Transport water, glycerol, urea
- AQP3 role
- Maintain skin hydration
- Regulating keratinocyte growth, proliferation, migration, differentiation
- Absent AQP3: impaired hydration, elasticity, barrier repair

THE IDEAL EYE CREAM FORMULA

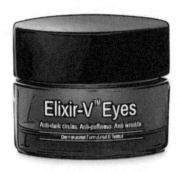

Science of a well-formulated eye cream
- Repair skin barrier
- Lighten pigmentation (dark-eye circles)
- Anti-wrinkle effect (botox alternatives adenosine, acetyl hexapeptide)

- Non-irritating/sensitising (retinol-free, alternatives like oligopeptides)

The eyes are a delicate area and deserve special consideration:
- Formation of expression lines (crows feet, undereye creases)
- Darkening around eyes (racial pigmentation, post-inflammation due to rubbing/sensitivity, fatigue)
- Thinner skin (near mucosa, easily irritated), prone to skin barrier damage
- Increased sagging/laxity with age
- Ocular/dermal absorption can occur (toxicity!)

KEY INGREDIENTS
   1. Skin barrier repair
- Ceramides (phytoceramides)
- Glycerin
- Panthenol
- Sodium hyaluronate

   2. Anti-wrinkle, reduce sagging/laxity
- Adenosine
- Oligopeptide
- Brassica (natural source of ubiquinone, stimulates collagen)

   3. Lightening dark circles, pigmentation
- Niacinamide
- Vitamin E

THE SECRETS TO CREATING THE BEST ANTI-AGING SERUM

1. Vehicle (serum texture)

Serums are excellent for the delivery of high dose skincare actives. Anti-aging serums are skincare products you should not skip. The vehicle refers to the bulk texture of the product. Creams and ointments are oil based and hence feel "creamy" and the texture feels stickier the more oil there is. These are excellent for moisturising skin, healing the skin barrier and preventing water loss. But that also means the bulk of the formula will be an oil and this reduces the dose of the antioxidant actives which are essential to target aging cells.

2. Actives

Before using creams, serums are the ideal skincare step that includes actives that have targeted effects. In the earlier section we've covered the core vitamin C and hyaluronic acid serums essential to a foundational skincare regimen. We are now discussing the third serum which is a must-have for advanced night repair regimens.

When we sleep, our skin cells work hard to repair damaged DNA—-which is responsible for the signs of photoaging. That is why applying the correct night repair serum is crucial. Actives synergise with active skin cells to reboot cell energy, optimising cell function to boost overall DNA repair capacity.

The following is the full list of synergistic active ingredients incorporated in what I consider to be the ideal retinol-free anti-aging face serum that's well tolerated by all skin types including sensitive skin in the long term.

Dr.TWL's Anti-Aging Pot Pourri

This is the specific set of actives which when incorporated in a serum is an ideal retinol/retinoid alternative with additional skin harmonising, microbiome balancing effects. These actives have been lab tested for optimal synergistic effects when applied as a all-in-1 serum on human skin.

- Resveratrol
- Beta-glucan
- Ethnobotanical extracts with bioactive properties
  - Licorice
  - Camellia sinensis
  - Broccoli

- Rosemary
- CICA
- Chamomile
- Scutellaria
- Polygonum cuspidatum
- Belamcanda chinensis
- Peptides (oligopeptides)
- Amino acids (methionine, serine, histidine)

Fragrances in cosmeceutical skincare
Are fragrances in skincare really bad?

First of all, consider this. Would you apply a foul-smelling product to yourself, on your body or even your face?

Dermatologists used to prescribe tar and sulfur-based shampoos a lot—because it had anti-fungal effects and also reduced scalp flaking. But in my experience, patients hated it. By the way, tar is also a carcinogen. Anyway you know what we should say, it's the dose that makes the poison, right? Well. Turns out that our noses can detect things which are potentially harmful to us...

Moving on. 10 years ago, I used to preach that skincare and haircare should be fragrance-free. After all, it is true that many synthetic fragrances trigger allergies and can cause sensitisation. Meaning that even if you aren't allergic, you can become allergic with repeated use. Privately though, I always hated using the generic dermatologist-recommended gentle cleansers which I used to tell my patients to use. They smelt at best, neutral. But the annoying thing was, these gentle cleansers always left my skin feeling sticky. (By the way, SLS-free is a myth.) Many dermatologist-recommended gentle cleansers do contain SLS, but in low concentrations so it does not irritate your skin.

So what I'm trying to say is that I've changed my mind:
- Fragrance-free does not equal good

317

- Fragranced skincare can be bad for skin
- Pleasant aromas are important for a soothing, relaxing skincare & self-care experience

The sweet spot is this:

Hypoallergenic fragrances AKA low allergenicity fragrance, which is what we use in our skincare.

Skincare Advice Section: Use of Skincare to Treat Skin Conditions

This section contains counselling pearls that can be applied in a standard non-medical skin consultation, helpful for skincare coaches.

- Sensitive skin/eczema
- Rosacea
- Acne
- Aging Skin

How Skincare Can Treat Sensitive Skin

Sensitive skin is more than just a problem with the skin barrier. Skin barrier damage presents as redness, flaking, stinging and sensitivity—but what goes on under the skin is a concerted series of interactions between cells that involve the immune cells and neurological system. Ultimately, it's also driven by the itch-scratch cycle which further weakens the skin barrier. If your condition is persistent >2 weeks or if you have a personal or family history of atopic dermatitis, you should seek a medical examination for accurate diagnosis and treatment.

Skincare is an underrated aspect of sensitive skin treatment. Many think that it is just about avoiding harsh ingredients, but over the counter skincare can be used to treat sensitive skin. Here are 5 important steps you can take to manage your sensitive skin problem:

1. Choose retinol/retinoid-free products
Many over the counter antiaging remedies contain a derivative of retinol—and even when it claims to be "gentle", if your skin is sensitive, it will very likely develop a reaction. This is especially so in tropical climates where there is high UV exposure.

2. Moisturise strategically

It's not enough to just moisturise as and when. There is a technique used by dermatologists which you should follow, known as wet wrap therapy:

- Dampen your skin or apply immediately after shower with minimal drying
- Apply a palm-sized amount to your face, or per area on the limb (most people use too little moisturiser)
- Wear a set of wet pajamas for the body. For the face, apply a moist cotton towel or use a polysaccharide material that will retain moisture by trapping it under the skin.

3. Shower with cool or tepid water

Warm or hot water increases transepidermal water loss which significantly worsens dry skin.

4. Get diagnosed by a dermatologist

Not all sensitive skin is eczema, it could be rosacea for example, a condition whereby skin also appears red and reacts to environmental triggers like heat.

5. Choose moisturisers formulated as PEDs

In pediatric dermatology, the ideal moisturiser type is known as a Prescription Emollient Device. This type of moisturiser contains specific ingredients such as ceramides, anti-inflammatory actives that have steroid-like activity and also antioxidants that reduce skin damage.

SECTION 3

Customised Compounding

download textbook resources and printables*

CHAPTER NINE

Ethnobotanical Dictionary

SECTION OVERVIEW

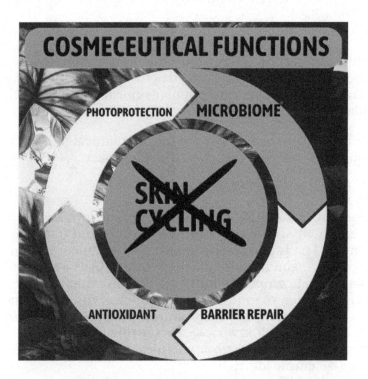

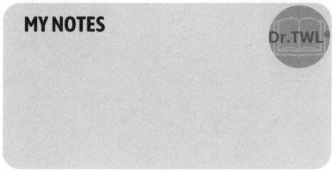

Did you know that the bestselling skincare products have more in common than not? Here's a secret—good cosmetic formulations are universal. This means that they fulfil the criteria set described by Albert Kligman, the father of cosmeceuticals.

- Ability to cross the epidermal barrier i.e. the stratum corneum
- Well-defined mechanisms of action i.e. the cell targets are identified
- Clinical studies back up the efficacy of the ingredient

The following section is a review of the most common ethnobotanical and nature-derived active ingredients compiled from an **analysis of over 300 popular skincare brands/product formulations.**

I conclude with an analysis of the rarest botanical ingredients used our own formulations from the pharmacy.

PRINCIPLES OF ETHNOBOTANY

Ethnobotany is the study of the direct interactions between plants and man, within the context of culture and tradition. A little known fact is that most modern medicines come from plant sources—and it's not difficult to understand why pharmaceutical companies fought to disguise their products with fancy names, manufacturing synthetics which they claim to be their own. In many eastern cultures, traditional medicine is still practiced—which is why we are starting to see the emergence of studies on ethnobotanical actives in peer reviewed, scientific journals.

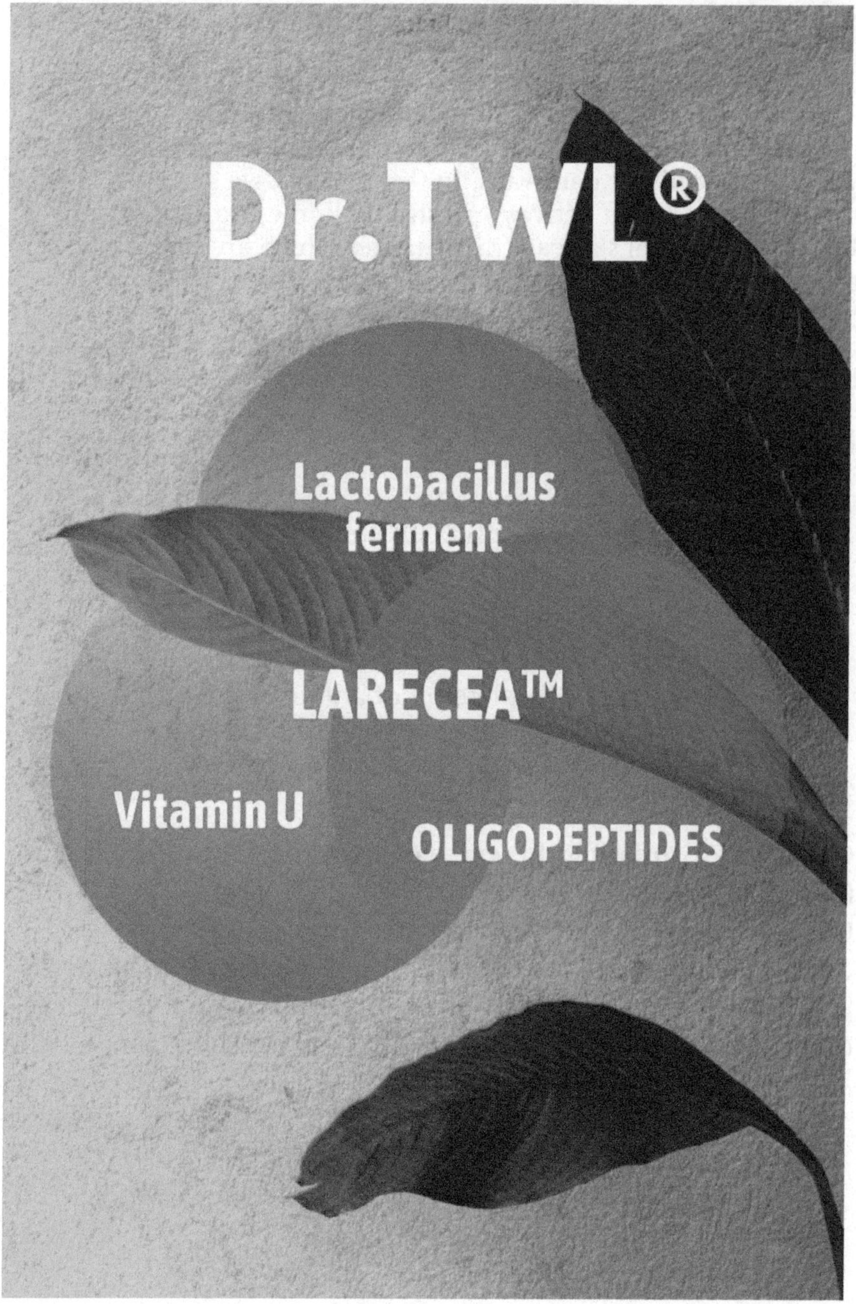

Dr.TWL®
Lactobacillus ferment
LARECEA™
Vitamin U
OLIGOPEPTIDES

Application to modern cosmetic formulation

Tradition isn't dead. Neither is it obsolete. Modern dermatological literature references many of these ancient botanicals which are now shown to intervene in skin conditions via defined cellular pathways. In this section, we shall go through the most important actives you should know as a skin expert. Unlike traditional skincare dictionaries which are listed in alphabetical order, you will find the actives categorised under plant parts i.e. leaves, seeds, flowers, roots. I also go through how the process of bacterial fermentation affects bioactives and can be highly beneficial when incorporated into skincare products.

How to navigate this section

- Register for an account at https://www.twlskin.com/dictionary/ (include a screenshot or photo of book purchase receipt number under comments)
- Receive your verified account within 24 hours
- What you will get:
    - Access complete set of audio lectures that accompany the ingredient dictionary
    - Download your set of study flashcards

Guide to formulating skincare cocktails: how customised formulas work

Custom skincare first originated in a dermatologist's office. Traditionally, topicals would be compounded for skin ailments in the pharmacy—with the dose, concentrations and frequency of application determining the strength of the medicine.

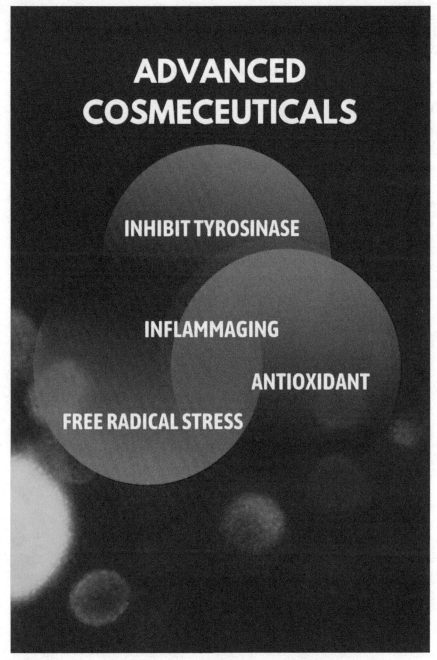

ADVANCED COSMECEUTICALS

INHIBIT TYROSINASE

INFLAMMAGING

ANTIOXIDANT

FREE RADICAL STRESS

When it comes to commercial beauty formulas, there are two ways to create a custom skincare business model:

1. "DIY" consumer customisation model "mix your own"
Most suited for serum formulations. This was popularised in
Japan and involves the creation of a range of serums with an
individually focused active. The requirements of formulation
are as follows:

- Water-based vehicle that water-soluble actives readily
  dissolve in
- The vehicle must be stable and uniformly used
  throughout the entire range
- Care taken not to mix skin irritating actives such as
  salicylic, glycolic acids, retinol within the same
  formula/range
- All actives OTC, cosmeceutical actives with potential
  allergenic or skin irritating side effects excluded
- Focus on skin hydrating actives
- Specific subsets within the range created to ensure when
  consumers "mix and match" their own formulations
  there is no increase in risks of skin irritation/ingredient
  incompatibility that reduces efficacy
- Practical aspects:
  - Instructions provided to consumer
    - Guided use within the subsets
    - Gives sense of personalisation and
      autonomy

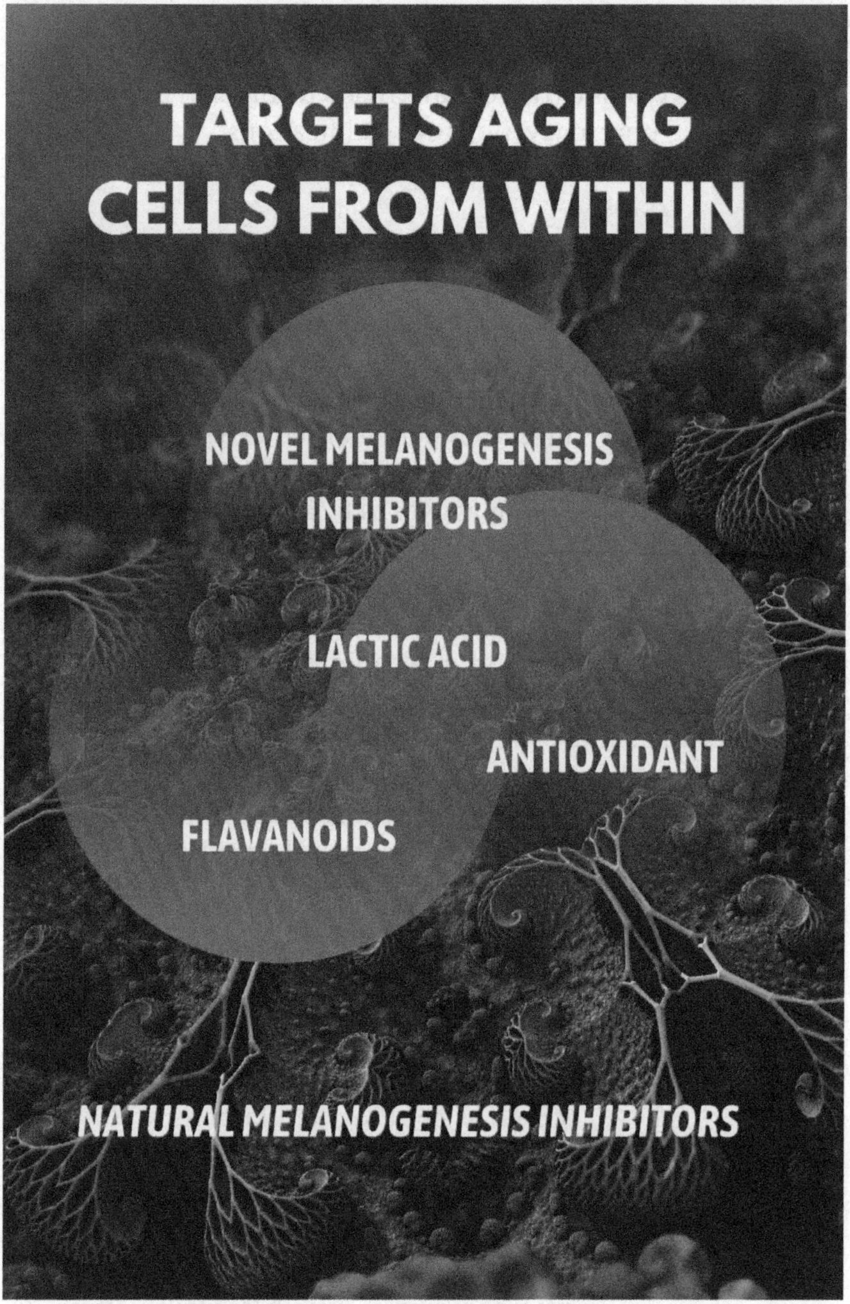

TARGETS AGING CELLS FROM WITHIN

NOVEL MELANOGENESIS INHIBITORS

LACTIC ACID

ANTIOXIDANT

FLAVANOIDS

NATURAL MELANOGENESIS INHIBITORS

2. Traditional pharmacy style customisation model "ready to use"

- On-site trained pharmacy technician present (pharmacy, nursing qualifications)
- Beauty brand expert (without specialised technical skills)
  - Suited for formulations created under 1.
- Product is fully premixed and compounded when consumer receives it
- Advantages:
  - Ease of use
  - Preserves personalised experience without the hassle of DIY
  - Potent actives like chemical peels and retinols can be delivered
  - Doses/concentrations titrated according to skin response
- Best practices for compounding

Unlike cosmeceutical manufacturing which takes place in bulk and should follow the gold standard EUROISO 22716 guidelines, this pharmacy style compounding model is best executed according to the following principles for cost-effectiveness and practicalities:

- Bulk base manufacturing
  - oil or an oil-in-water emulsion base
  - increases effectiveness of ingredients
  - more potent
  - higher concentrations
  - stored as per the manufacturer's instructions
  - shelf-life of 2-3 years as per general cosmetic product
  - necessary preservatives to prevent microorganism growth/contamination

The ideal base differs from the DIY model—instead of a water vehicle, an oil or an oil-in-water emulsion base is preferred. This increases the effectiveness of ingredients being delivered, which are more potent and higher in concentrations than those manufactured under the DIY model. This base should be stored as per the manufacturer's instructions and should contain the necessary preservatives to prevent microorganism growth/contamination and ensure stability.

- Custom ingredients
    - minimum GMP standards
    - organic when available

Whether synthetic or natural, the actives used should be extracted and produced according to minimum GMP (Good Manufacturing Process) standards. Ideally, find a manufacturer with EUROISO22716 certifications. Choose organic raw materials if available—pesticide-free is good news for skin. This means that ingredients generally retain the maximum bioactivity as intended by nature. While there are currently no studies which demonstrate how pesticide residue affects the skin microbiome, it has been established that these chemical residues have the potential to induce allergenicity (allergic type reactions). Lanolin from sheep wool for instance, has been found to be contaminated with pesticide residue accumulated from environmental exposure. This significantly increases the risk of allergenicity. It is also of concern when used as a topical active on the nipples of breastfeeding women.

- Compounding

For prescription level actives i.e. retinoids, hydroquinone, the actual compounding process is best done by a pharmacy technician trained in the calculation of doses/concentrations.

However, there are many non-prescription actives with equivalent potential which I have listed in the directory. In particular, these are all regarded as non-irritating and can be used in high concentrations without adverse effects. In general, the higher the concentration, the greater the efficacy when it comes to these ingredients. However, the concentration used will also greatly depend on costs of labor and raw material.

The actives used in our pharmacy are:

1. Cream based formulations for
  a. spot treatment
  b. leave-on mask treatment with polysaccharide mask

The formulation of our peptide-infused cream base for spot treatment was designed to meet the following criteria:

- Cream/emulsion texture for spot treatment
- Oil-in-water lightweight sensation for comfortable day/night application without feeling greasy
- Moisturising actives to reduce possible irritation
- Botanical mixture with anti-oxidant effects to synergise with additives
- Stored at room temperature
- 2-3 years stability
- Powder form, water-soluble actives readily dissolved at room temperature for customisation process
- Good cosmetic acceptability
  - Non-allergenic fragrance (suitable for problem skin)

The common base is used for the leave-on masking treatment with the polysaccharide sheet material. The difference in formulation of the spot vs leave-on mask is

- Higher concentrations of actives used in spot treatment i.e. <5% leave on overnight formula vs 5-10% spot formula

Both are packaged in syringes which allow for

- Controlled extrusion of product (minimises wastage)
- Minimal air-gap, reduces oxidation
- Hygienic application

Application technique with the *POLYSACCHARIDE MEMBRANE SYSTEM:* the cream mask formulations are applied as follows:
- 5ml per application over entire face
- Hydrate reusable polysaccharide mask (100% plant derived, freeze-dried chemical-additive free membrane system)
- Apply over cream mask and leave on for minimum 15 mins
- Massage excess product onto neck/décolleté area

What is the *POLYSACCHARIDE MEMBRANE SYSTEM?*

This is our proprietary novel reusable mask system which utilises a patent pending hydrophilic mask that enhances transdermal absorption. The membrane creates mini-reservoirs that attract and keep moisture within the top most layers of skin, resulting in enhanced barrier function. One of the major causes of dull skin that can be addressed instantly with this system is this— efficient hydration of the skin barrier.

The process
- **STAGE 1 Leave on cream mask applied on damp skin**
  - Stratum corneum (top-most layer) begins process of absorption
- **STAGE 2 Polysaccharide membrane (rehydrated) instantly creates mini-reservoirs around skin pores i.e. *"second skin"* micro-climate**
  - **Creation of ideal skin micro-climate**
  - **Regulates cell functions**
    - Sebum production
    - Rebalancing moisture
    - Directly inhibits transepidermal water loss
    - Microbiome stabilising

The key difference between traditional sheet masks and the POLYSACCHARIDE MEMBRANE SYSTEM

Traditional sheet masks
- Standardised skin essence pre-infused into mask packets
- High volume of wastage due to large quantity of MOQ
- Environmental impact: non-biodegradable synthetic fabrics
- Additives and preservatives required
- May require refrigeration
- One time use—high costs
- Standard cosmetic shelf life 2-3 years

POLYSACCHARIDE MEMBRANE SYSTEM (Advantages for businesses)
- Highly adaptable to dermatology practices
- Customised skin essences based on in-house formulation system
- Especially suited for sensitive/reactive skin types that do not tolerate traditional sheet masks i.e. used for rosacea, eczema
- 100% additive free, biomimetic components engineered for medical biocompatibilty to simulate ideal skin environment for healthy functioning
- Freeze-dried formula in sterile packing with 5 year shelf life
- Reusable up to 7 applications, reduced costs and environmental impact
- Separation of mask and essence allows for tailored regimens, multiple SKUs with just 1 product

These are the actives used in our pharmacy—all are considered OTC without need for prescription. The raw materials are from our in-house EURO22716 accredited pharmaceutical division. Details of each ingredient included in dictionary section.

Acne
Berberine

Pigmentation/Skin Brightening
Sea kelp
Goji berry
Arbutin

Oily skin/oil-rebalancing
Organic green tea extract
Grape seed oil
Organic honey

2. Mask Peel (exfoliate and intensive treatment mask)
Acne/aging/scars
Spongila lacustris

Sensitive/dry/irritated skin
Lessonia nigrescens

Dull skin/uneven skin tone
Euglena Gracilis
Carrageenan polysaccharides

3. Rebalancing propolis-infused masks for glass skin
Glass skin is a term popularised by K-beauty which refers to a state of flawlessness—objectively defined as:
- Even skin tone
- Smooth without surface irregularities i.e. texture
- Absence of dark spots (other blemishes linked to dermatological conditions beyond scope of discussion)
- Glass-like translucency
    - Hydration factors
    - Skin cell renewal rates
    - No/minimal risk of skin irritation (vs retinoid/retinol "glow" which is not glass skin)

To achieve these effects with an over-the-counter skincare product, the formulation must contain actives that have cosmceutical (quasi-drug effects)

- Retinoid/retinol alternatives
    - Enhance skin cell renewal rates without damaging the skin barrier
- Multiple hydrating actives that act on various layers of skin
    - Moisture sandwiching effect
    - AKA skin flooding
    - Mix of humectants, occlusives, emollients and biomimetic natural moisturising factors
    - MUST-HAVES: polyglutamic acid, hyaluronic acid, botanical antioxidants, vitamin C
- Delivery method: the key is enhancing dermal absorption via
    - Sonic technology
    - Hydrodermabrasion
        - The K-beauty facial scene came into prominence with the *Aquapeel*, a medi-facial system designed with a handpiece that delivers gentle, vacuum pressure focused via a vortex design
        - Simultaneous infusion of antioxidants and gentle skin-resurfacing acids like lactic, salicylic acids
- Enhancing skin cell renewal with immediate effects
    - Microdermabrasion
        - Traditional microdermabrasion involved either crystal-based or crystal-free systems i.e. diamond microdermabrasion both of which did cause irritation to skin—albeit to a lesser extent than medium/deep chemical peels—and were performed in-clinic
        - Novel microcrystalline system for home use:

In 2019, our biomaterials arm created the copper oxide based microcrystalline handpiece as a home use device for microdermabrasion—the propolis infused mask was designed as the ideal gel mask base which forms a physical protective barrier between skin and the minimally abrasive handpiece.

DERM'S PRO TIP: GLASS SKIN VS RETINOID GLOW

Glass skin reflects a state of skin health. The retinoid glow is a sign of alteration of physiological pathways—not necessarily benefiting skin health.
The key is preservation of the skin barrier which is not the case with traditional cosmeceuticals like retinoid/retinol-based products.

The formulation of our propolis-infused mask base was designed to meet the following criteria:
- Ideal vehicle for botanical actives
- High dose of vitamin C (sodium ascorbyl phosphate) for instant skin brightening effects
- Solvent/carrier for freeze-dried extracts
- 2-3 years stability/shelf life for storage at room temperature
- Powder form, water-soluble actives readily dissolved at room temperature for customisation process
- Good cosmetic acceptability
  - Non-allergenic fragrance (suitable for problem skin)
- Cooling gel texture for anti-inflammatory effect

Cosmetic indications and actives used
The propolis-infused masks are marketed as an adjunct daily treatment model for long term maintenance, in addition to the intensive spot treatment/mask peel products. The key difference is in
- Mechanism of action

- intensive spot regimen designed for targeted treatment in a ultra-moisturising vehicle
- maintenance treatment focuses on overall regulation of the skin microclimate for medium to long term results
- Effects
  - intensive spot treatment for specific dermatological conditions i.e. rosacea, acne, sensitivity
  - maintenance focus on *"skin-clarifying"* results for improvement of general skin tone/irregularities associated with photoaging i.e. pigmentation spots, aging, dull skin, uneven skin tone which addresses pain points

These are the actives used in our pharmacy—all are considered OTC without need for prescription.

Skin tone/pigmentation
Carthamus Tinctorius, Poria Cocos, Atractyloides Macrocephala Bletilla Striata, Glycyrrhiza Uralensis, Phaseolus Radiatus, Panax Ginseng, Ampelopsis Japonica

Sebum control/inflammation/acne-prone
Salvia Miltiorrhiza, Sophora Flavescens, Ligusticum Chuanxiong, Panax Notoginseng, Phaseolus Radiatus, Scutellaria Baicalensis

4. Jelly peeling gels
These are the easiest to formulate on a small scale basis and also the most cost-effective.
At our pharmacy we compound these based on 100% chemical additive free based on the following raw materials:
- Cosmetic grade xanthan gum
- Sodium alginate powder

Both of which are natural sources of polysaccharides which are well suited as hydrogels in dermatologic therapeutics:

- Stored and sold as powder form

- o high stability without need for preservatives/additives
- o for all custom compounded recommend labelling at 6 months from time package is opened
- o note to formulators: refrigerate for extended shelf-life
- o rehydrate by adding water when needed
- Wet: Gel/jelly like texture
- Applied on skin and allowed to dry naturally
  - o Polysaccharides activated by sebum
  - o Bind to the superficial dead skin cells (corneocytes)
  - o Form a string-like polymer that is rubbed off skin
- Advantages
  - o Automatically adjusts to different skin types (dry, oily, combination)
  - o No risk of sensitisation (2-ingredient formula)
  - o Suitable for daily use
  - o 2-in-1 hydration and exfoliation effect
- Dr.TWL's Apothecary Secret:
  - o Another source of polysaccharide is a carrageenan extracted from red seaweed
  - o Xanthan gum also contains bacterial ferments that are beneficial for the microbiome and release additional micronutrients
  - o Sodium alginate derived from brown algae sources contain additional skin benefits such as
    - ▪ Sebum regulation
    - ▪ Antioxidant
    - ▪ Anti-inflammatory effects

    These properties make it ideal for problem skin types such as acne, rosacea, sensitive skin which usually do not take well to traditional exfoliation formulations.
  - 30 grams of powder make up about 100mls of product
    - o Advise to compound only 2-3 days worth of what is necessary, store in the refrigerator
  - INGREDIENT PAIRING: papain, bromelain enzymes (powder form)

- ○ Fruit enzymes at concentrations of 1-5% added to the powder formula
- ○ Hydrogel formulation enhances effectiveness of absorption via the skin barrier

CHAPTER TEN

Custom Skincare Business: Learn Pharmaceutical Compounding

☐ *A Professional Skincare System*
☐ *Dermatologist Designed*
☐ *Functional Dermatology*
☐ *For Real Results*

In this segment, I'm going to teach you how to set up a customised skincare service. As part of the Custom Medi-Essence service we offer at Dr.TWL Pharmacy, the very specifics of how to titrate cosmeceutical skincare actives using the system I developed. The notes are designed to accompany a video workshop included as part of your paperback and hardback purchases.

What you will learn:
- What are cosmeceuticals?
- Importance in dermatology and skincare
- Mechanisms of action: how cosmeceuticals work
- Why skincare products take time to work, how long and how to make your service stand out from other skin experts
- Skincare Plus Accelerate Program
  - Ways to enhance cosmeceutical absorption to accelerate results
  - 5 pillars of the instant glow
  - Inside-out, outside-in approach
  - Handheld microdermabrasion and hydrodermabrasion systems
- Dr.TWL Skin Physiotype:
  - A new, efficient way of skin subtyping for cosmeceutical use
  - Emphasis on skin concerns for higher client satisfaction rates

The science behind Dr.TWL's secret recipe:
- The *7 key cosmeceuticals that set you up for success*
- Setting up a customised skincare service

Learn how the *Dr.TWL Medi-Essence Formulation System* allows you to provide a complete personalised skincare service for your clients from the comfort of your own home.
- Custom Medi-Essence System
- Client consultation process
- Compounding at home without a facility
- Reference chart for customised compounding for skin concerns
- Raw materials/sourcing
- Additional downloadables:
  - Lecture notes with full color visuals
  - Client consultation templates
  - Client progress monitoring: skincare planner template

Skin typing is traditionally implemented by beauty brands and facialists as a quick guide to skincare routines. There are some clear disadvantages with such a system, i.e.

Disadvantages of traditional skin typing
- Oily/combination/dry skin model
- Does not fully address subjective skin concerns
- Based on out-dated skin models

Dr.TWL's Skin Physiotype Model
- Updated according to latest in skin micro-climate research
- Helpful guide for incorporation of cosmeceuticals

Cosmeceuticals are now the standard of skincare recommended by dermatologists—the term is well-defined within the realm of dermatology research; as per the original Kligman criteria largely based on retinoids, long considered the gold standard of cosmeceuticals.

- Identifiable molecular/physiological targets; established mechanism of action that alters skin function
- Evidence-based with clinical trials/peer-reviewed studies

- Able to penetrate the skin barrier (stratum corneum)

Modern perspectives on cosmeceuticals
- Cosmetic preparation with pharmaceutical benefits
- Pharmaceutical activity, usable on universal skin types
- Defined benefit for minor skin disorders i.e. cosmetic indications
- Quasi-drug effect with low/minimal risk profile

Problems with skin toxicity:
Not in cosmeceuticals *per se* but as stabilisers/preservatives/additives
- 1,4-dioxane (shampoos, endocrine disrupter)
- Formaldehyde (shampoos, carcinogen)
- Parabens (endocrine disruptor)

Now that you have a basic understanding of cosmeceuticals, we move on to the Skin Physiotype model.

Dr.TWL Skin Physiotype Model is designed with the 7 key cosmeceuticals, identified as ideal bioactives which are
- Present no/minimal risk of allergenicity/toxicity
- Well-defined mechanism of action
- Clear cosmetic indications for common skin concerns typically managed OTC:
  - Photoaging signs (pores, texture, radiance)
  - Mild/moderate acne (alone or adjunct to medical therapy)
  - Pigmentation

You may already be familiar with the skin typing convention of oily/combination/dry skin—but you may have already learnt from personal or professional experience that this is overly simplistic. For instance, many experience the oily-dehydrated skin phenomenon, especially those with acne-prone skin when they are prescribed astringent skincare.

Dry skin types can also develop acne—this category is particularly difficult to manage; for e.g. when we examine the underlying cause of acne, we realise quickly that it is what we determine as multi-factorial, rather than due to hyperseborrhea alone.

- Microbiome disruption is a form of dysbiosis—an imbalance in what constitutes healthy flora on skin.
- Underlying inflammation, driven by one's genetics as well
- Seborrhea

Skin typing however provides a practical, accessible method for
- laypersons to "self-diagnose"
- receive certain guidance on products to use
- empowers skincare providers
- offers a reliable template for non-medical consultations

The Skin Physiotype model builds on this. It is a dermatologist created tool for professional skin typing. More than that, it lays the foundation for recommendation of cosmeceuticals, backed by the latest in dermatology research. Unlike the traditional skin typing models, it takes into consideration factors such as the skin microclimate and microbiome.

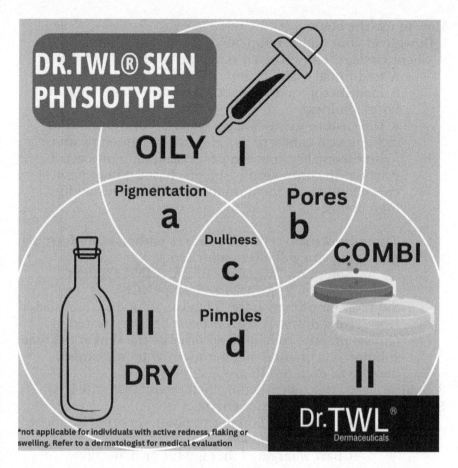

The 4 subcategories are added to this new skin typing model based on *top cosmetic skin concerns presenting at a dermatology practice—pigmentation, pores, pimples and dullness—which were addressed with a cosmeceutical skincare regimen. The Venn diagram approach rightly encapsulates the complex, overlapping nature of cosmetic skin concerns but also associates certain conditions such as enlarged pores with oily/combination skin types. It is created as a visual record for both skincare providers and clients, as a communication tool that represents the core values of the Dr.TWL ethos—cosmeceuticals created to address client/patient concerns, tailored to the individual, based on the latest research on the skin microenvironment.
*survey/audit tool

How to use the chart

1. Download your digital template
2. Client circles their perceived skin type based on
   A-traditional classification i.e. oily, combination, dry
   B-identify top# skin concern i.e. pigmentation, pimples.
   Pores, dullness
   # The custom medi-essence system is best tailored to
   tackling skin concerns in a step-wise manner, to advise
   focus on one key concern per consultation process. 3.
   Provider to compound based on chart 3. Subsequent
   consultations can focus on increasing dosages/adding
   ingredients.

   There are 2 main types of essences both in 80ml formula
   packaging you will offer your clients:
   o Solution 1 "MEDI-REBALANCING ESSENCE"
   o Solution 2 "MEDI-PEEL ESSENCE"
   Solution 1 is offered at the first visit, solution 2 is available
   from visit 2 onwards. This process has been tested in a
   clinical practice to help to acclimatise the skin to the base
   solution in a gradual manner in order to maximise
   benefits of each product.
3. Skincare provider matches the client record with the 2
   Dr.TWL Skin Expert reference charts
   o Chart 1: based on permutation reported by client
     for *base formulation*
   o Chart 2: targeted therapy for primary skin
     concern, for *titration of dose*
   o Chart 3: provider record up to 7 consultations for
     liquid additives (CICA, arnica, grape seed, green
     tea, yeast peptide)
     Compounding Rules:
     ESSENCE 1
     ▪ Visit 1 refer to standard base formulation
       chart 1 for identified 1 primary concern
     ▪ Visit 2 refer to chart 2 for titration of dose
       for 2 primary concerns (including concern
       identified at visit 1)
     ▪ Visit 3: repeat chart 2 for up to 3 concerns
     ▪ Visit 4 onwards: depending on concerns,
       double dose to 2 drops per visit for up to 2
       ingredients maximum 3 drops

ESSENCE 2 (separately compounded)
- From Visit 2 onwards add bakuchiol OR berberine OR papain powder to second 80 ml essence depending on concern:
  - Pimples/scars: berberine
  - Pores/Pigmentation: bakuchiol
  - Dullness: papain

EXERCISE
- We are going to take this case study as an example. Your client presents with multiple skin concerns such as pigmentation, enlarged pores and dullness. You are to zoom in on just 1 chief concern at the first visit. You can counsel the patient this way by telling them:

Script

"This dermatologist formulated system is designed to target the commonest skin concerns—the base vehicle contains hyaluronic, polyglutamic acids and 17 botanicals which are proven to help address these skin problems. As part of the protocol, we need to follow certain steps in order to help you achieve maximum results. The first visit we will compound a specialised formula that directly addresses all your concerns based on our reference chart. That means we need to focus on 1 main concern at the first visit and then gradually at the subsequent consultations we can up the dose and start targetting other problem areas."

This helps to build rapport, enhance client retention and also facilitates positioning as a trusted skin expert for your client's needs.

What you actually do

Visit 1 So for example your client zooms in a primary concern of pigmentation and oily skin, the base formulation guide in chart 1 teaches you to compound a base with 1 drop of yeast peptide and 2 drops of grape seed.

Visit 2 (1 month after first visit)
- Refill: Solution 1 Medi-Essence

Your client now prioritises enlarged pores on top of the primary concern of hyperpigmentation. That leads you to chart 2, which recommends grape seed oil for management of enlarged pores.

You fill in chart 3 with "1" indicating 1 drop of grape seed oil added to the formulation at this visit (1 month after initial, which is also time to replenish second bottle." Remember, this chart is also your record so in the event that the client feels that the formulation is already ideal and would like subsequent top-ups or refills, you can simply use this as a formulation record.

- Upsell: Solution 2 Medi-Peel

You are now ready to market ESSENCE 2, which is a product focussing on peeling and resurfacing to improve scars and overall skin texture. This is a separately compounded 80ml solution which utilises the same base vehicle as solution 1, N.B. you do not need to alter the formulation as per chart 1 base formulation for the medi-essence formula. For this, you directly add the powder extract in *tsp* measurement to the vehicle provided. I.e. you add bakuchiol OR berberine OR papain powder to second 80 ml essence depending on concern, recording down the concentration you dispensed on chart 3. One important point to remember is that if at any point of time, symptoms of sensitivity such as redness or flaking occurs, you should not dispense the peel essence and also refer to a dermatologist for management. This is usually a sign that the client has a underlying medical condition that needs to be treated with oral medications/prescription steroids although solution 1 can be continued as adjunct therapy.

- Pimples/scars: berberine
- Pores/Pigmentation: bakuchiol
- Dullness: papain

Visit 3 At visit 3, you are ready to address a third concern i.e. pimples or acne, which according to chart 2–the recommended extract is green tea.

The Science Behind the CUSTOM MEDI-ESSENCE SYSTEM

7 Key Cosmeceuticals
☐ Papain Enzyme [Exfoliation & anti-inflammatory]
☐ Berberine [Targets acne via multiple pathways]
☐ Centella Asiatica [Rich in amino acids and antioxidants]
☐ Grape Seed Oil/ Resveratrol [Stabilizes Oily Skin, Tighten Pores]
☐ Yeast Peptide [Anti-Ageing and Brightening]

☐ Green Tea [Treats acne and oily skin]
☐ Arnica Montana [Reduces redness and inflammation]

Traditionally, compounding of topicals in dermatology practices represents a significant part of patient therapeutics, it allows dermatologists to titrate doses, concentrations and mix prescription actives according to indications. Commonly titrated topicals are steroids and retinoids.

Cosmeceuticals represent a relatively uncharted territory within dermatology practices, given the conventional focus on prescription topicals. It however should not be ignored, as it is rapidly gaining ground in the beauty industry. The term "Prescription Emollient Device" coined by Eichenfield as the gold standard moisturiser for treatment of eczema is an example of a cosmeceutical directly relevant to dermatology practice i.e. an anti-inflammatory topical formulated with botanical actives (without steroids, traditional anti-inflammatory agents) and biomimetic molecules such as ceramides for barrier repair.

Dermatologists can take into consideration the current research on quasi-drugs as the basis for formulation of cosmeceutical skincare regimens.

There are some challenges which present in a dermatologist's office which I shall cover

Provider-related:
- Storage of raw material i.e. cosmeceutical additive (temperature, stability) at small scale
- Universal formulation vehicle i.e. bulk carrier must support overall cosmeceutical function, be biochemically compatible, readily soluble at room temperature and provide barrier repair/antioxidant/anti-inflammatory properties
- Access to hygienic packaging that does not require machine processing, readily put together by clinic assistants

Patient/consumer-related:
- Cosmetic acceptability

347

- Texture for universal skin types (water-based vs cream/ointment)

Traditional:

Conventional topical therapy is delivered via cream/ointment for enhanced absorption rates/permeability via these vehicles. However, such textures are suitable for spot therapy rather than whole-face delivery which is the recommended application method when it comes to cosmeceuticals. Cream/ointment formulas may feel uncomfortable on combination/oily skin and/or those living in humid climates and may affect compliance.

Cosmeceuticals:

Cosmeceuticals designed for universal skin types are ideally water-based i.e serum, mist or lotion/emulsion-based. Water-based is my preference due to ease of handling, packaging within small-scale dermatology practices, i.e. texture allows for easy decanting into containers, excellent solvent. A specifically formulated vehicle is used for the customising process which includes natural moisturising factors with high bioactivity i.e. polyglutamic acid and hyaluronic acid in combination with several plant-derived stabilisers/antioxidants that boost product shelf-life.

- Scent

Traditional prescription topicals are unscented and the experience may be slightly unpleasant for some users. Dermatologist prescribed cosmeceuticals must offer a pleasant user experience in-line to encourage compliance; in keeping with mass market standards of a sensorial skincare experience. Hypoallergenic or minimally allergenic fragrances can be used to enhance the skincare experience.

- Application method:

Compounded **creams** are typically dispensed in tubs. However this increases environmental exposure i.e. oxidation may occur leading to rapid degradation and loss of efficacy. The use of a water-based formulation allows for relatively low-cost bottle packaging (airless pumps-aerosol method) which also minimises user handling/contamination.

I present a small-scale titratable cosmeceutical system adapted for the physician's office with 7 key cosmeceutical actives for universal skin types. It includes a chart that allows physician assistants to record patient-reported concerns and a standardised titration method to facilitate compounding. The universal vehicle contains well-established cosmeceuticals that address the skin micro-climate such as polyglutamic acid and hyaluronic acid in water using ethoxydiglycol as a solubiliser and to enhance barrier penetration. Using such a system, a medicine bottle dropper method can be used to titrate additives in a standardised manner. The above chart references dilutions for pure concentrates in an 80ml vehicle. Where water-soluble powder additives are used, i.e. berberine, papain a *tsp* measurement is used.

The Medi-Essence System is a small-scale custom compounding protocol created with the following in mind:
- **Quality assurance: EUROISO22716 standard Polyglutamic acid/hyaluronic acid based vehicle**
- **Free of top 3 toxic chemicals in OTC cosmeceutical preparations**
- **Suitable for universal skin types**
- **Organic, USDA certified cosmeceutical additives**
- **Time-saving, 3-step process for efficiency**
- **Specially designed airless packaging to optimise provider/user experience**
-

Benefits
- **Leverage on well-established cosmeceutical skincare brand name**
- **Mentorship under an internationally renowned dermatologist**
- **30 min one-on-one online training included with specialist physician assistant**
- **Low MOQ for start-up with opportunity to scale up**
- **Flexible setup: home-based, salon or clinic**

DR.TWL® SKIN PHYSIOTYPE
Custom Cosmeceutical System
*Prefix 1 or 2 refers to number of drops using our dropper titration method

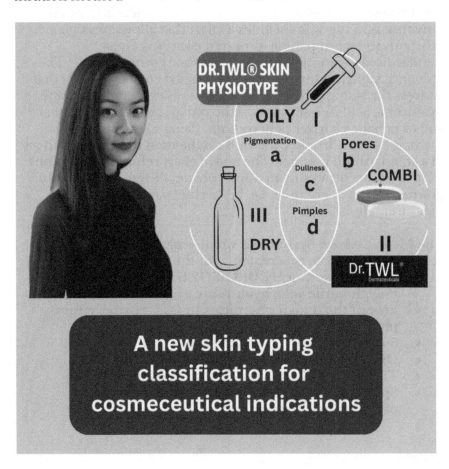

DR.TWL®
PRESCRIPTIVE APPROACH

SKIN PHYSIOTYPE

FUNCTIONAL ACTIVES

SKIN PHYSIOTYPE		FUNCTIONAL ACTIVES
I	a	Ia 1Yeast Peptide, 2Grape Seed
	b	Ib 1Papain Enzyme, 1Green Tea
	c	Ic 1Centella Asiatica, 1Yeast Peptide
	d	Id 2Papain Enzyme, 1Green Tea, 1Grape Seed, 1berberine
II	a	IIa 1Yeast Peptide, 1Grape Seed, 1Centella Asiatica
	b	IIb 1Papain Enzyme, 1Green Tea, 1Grape Seed
	c	IIc 1Centella Asiatica, 1Yeast Peptide, 1Arnica Montana
	d	IId 2Papain Enzyme, 1Green Tea, 2Grape Seed, 1berberine
III	a	IIIa 1Arnica Montana, 1Yeast Peptide, 1Grape Seed
	b	IIIb 1Papain Enzyme, 1Grape Seed, 1Arnica Montana
	c	IIIc 1Centella Asiatica, 1Yeast Peptide, 1Arnica Montana, 2Grape Seed
	d	IIId 1Papain Enzyme, 1Green Tea, 1Yeast Peptide, 1berberine, 1Arnica Montana

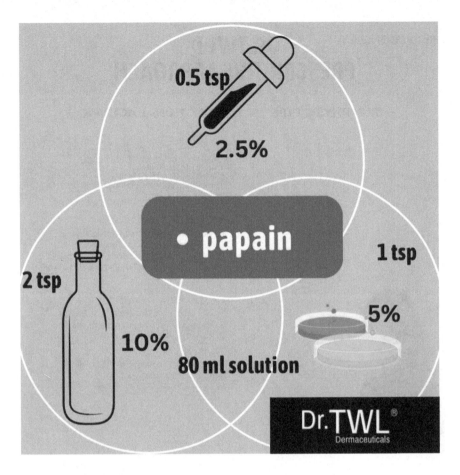

Protocol variations
Instructions for skin expert:

- Add additive depending on skin concern
  Amount/concentrations specified
  - Papain enzyme 2.5% EOD for combi/oily skin, 3X week for dry skin
- 2nd visit onwards:
  - Conduct review in 1 month
  - Increase papain frequency if no irritation: combi/oily skin *daily*; *EOD* for dry skin
  - Follow week 2 schedule frequency of use
- Conduct review in 1 month
  - Increase enzyme concentration if no irritation 5%
  - Check client progress/satisfaction
  - Replenish solutions +1 *additional active*

- ○ Start retinol alternative depending on concern:
Preventative anti-aging regimen (early to mid 20s)
  - ■ Sea buckthorn oil
    - Combi/oily skin 1 drop on fingers lightly tap over entire face EON
    - Dry skin 2 drops lightly tap over entire face nightly

Active anti-aging regimen (late twenties onwards)
  - ■ Sea buckthorn regimen
  - PLUS
  - ■ +Bakuchiol ⅛ Tsp
  - ■ ⅛ tsp only
    - Dry sensitive skin *EON*
    - Combi oily skin *nightly*

Advantages of system
- One-time purchase of copper peel set (2-year warranty) per client
- Customised facial system for long-term client retention
- Proprietary dermatologist-formulated 17-botanical face essence base

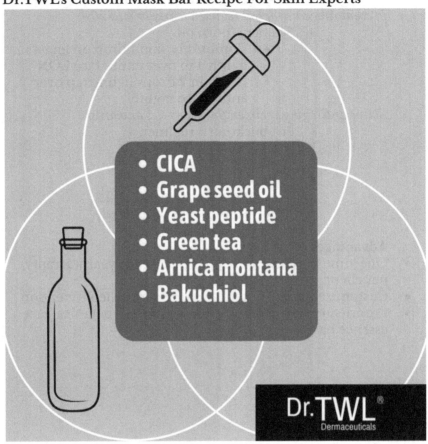

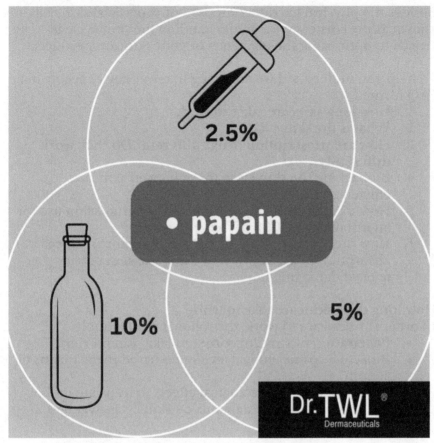

- Premixed solution base (storage at room temperature)
- Titrated dropper method for skin experts
- Additives provided
- Quick and efficient customisation process
- For more B2B support www.twlskin.com/dictionary/

Biohacking the skin cycle with the Skincare Plus Accelerate Program

The major limiting factor of skincare regimens is absorption—while you may have already heard of the skin barrier in the context of repair; it's also the physical barrier skincare has to cross in order to exert its effects on deeper layers of skin.

Besides the physical barrier composed of superficial skin cells known as the corneocytes, understanding the skin cycle is crucial to optimising the efficiency of your skincare products.

To help you understand we are going to cover key concepts in an FAQ format:
1. How long skincare takes to work
2. What is the skin cycle
3. **How are prescription drugs different? Do they work differently?**
4. Biohacking the skin cycle for enhanced skincare efficiency
5. How to adapt clinical procedures for home/salon use for an instant glow 100% of the time
6. How the Skincare Plus Accelerate Program enhances absorption of actives by breaching the skin barrier *without* damaging it

How long does skincare take to work?
In order for skincare to work, the following rules apply:
- Penetration of stratum corneum (aka skin barrier)
- Bioactive cosmeceutical (evidence-based mechanisms of action)
- Time taken for physiological effects to translate into visible skin changes: depends on skin cycle averages 27 days in adults.

The general consensus is that measurable skin outcomes for active cosmeceuticals such as retinol/retinoids take about 4-6 weeks.

Why skincare products take time to work

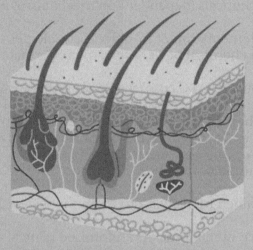

THE SKIN BARRIER

IS A PHYSICAL BARRIER THAT ACTIVES MUST CROSS

What is the skin cycle?

When skin cells grow, they do so from the inside. The top-most layer of cells known as the corneocytes begin life on average 27 days before they reach the surface—they migrate through layers of skin from the bottom most known as the stratum basale. By the time it reaches the skin surface, they are actually ready to be shed, which is what concludes the entire skin cycle. When we grow older, the skin cycle lengthens, which is the reason skin becomes dull. Our goal with a cosmeceutical regimen is to increase cell turnover so we can reveal new skin cells which makes skin appear more radiant—as it is with youthful skin.

How are prescription drugs different? Do they work differently?

This does **not** take into consideration prescription topicals which work immediately when absorbed by skin

- Topical steroids
- Tyrosinase inhibitors aka hydroquinone
- Cosmeceuticals (dependent on mechanism, molecular targets)

As well as implementation of in-office technologies such as skin resurfacing via chemical peels, lasers, microdermabrasion etc.

The beauty of using OTC cosmeceuticals is that we are able to incorporate benefits of prescription topicals into cosmetic formulations that are accessible without a physician's prescription. This brings us to the original Kligman criteria defining the properties a cosmeceutical possesses:

- Ability to penetrate the stratum corneum AKA the skin barrier
- Well defined molecular targets in the deeper layers of skin
- Evidence in the form of randomised clinical trials that back it up

So as you can see, the key lies in the selection of the cosmeceutical—not all actives qualify. For instance when we are discussing retinol alternatives such as peptides, bakuchiol and sea buckthorn, you will discover how and why these are well-positioned as cosmeceuticals compared to the gold standard retinol. The added benefit is that when these quasi-drugs are incorporated as a cosmetic and made available OTC, it usually means that the actives have also been assessed to be highly tolerable and have low irritation potential, compared to prescription topicals which have to be used under medical supervision.

Biohacking skincare

Beyond that, dermatologists are also interested in how we can enhance the absorption of actives—so that we can improve efficiency of the skincare.

The Dr.TWL Skincare Plus Accelerate Program is designed to overcome limitations in traditional cosmeceutical skincare routines by addressing skin permeability by enhancing transdermal delivery. This section is accompanied by a video workshop on custom skincare compounding available at https://www.twlskin.com/dictionary/.

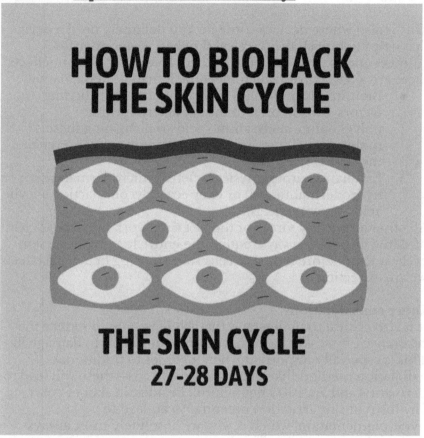

This brings us to:

The 5 pillars of the Skincare Plus Program
Dr.TWL Copper Peel Microdermabrasion

How to adapt clinical procedures for home/salon use for an instant glow 100% of the time

For skin experts and aestheticians, the key to success is really to deliver a product or a service that guarantees an instant glow-up. The question is, how do you achieve that? Well, it's not possible if you are relying on skincare products alone because even cosmeceuticals take time to work—they have to first penetrate the skin barrier and the bioactivity is something that is also dependent on the skin cycle. The latter, if you are in the 30 plus age group, by default will lengthen as compared to a younger person.

This is also where devices come in. You definitely need a device that helps to breach the physical skin barrier in order for cosmeceuticals to work fast. If you are looking at "instant effects" there are a few actives which meet the 2 main criteria, namely:

- Biomimetic molecules such as natural moisturising factors already present in skin i.e. hyaluronic, polyglutamic acids, amino acids replenishing these molecules will instantly plump up skin cells and repair the skin barrier
- Exfoliants: either physical (such as microdermabrasion or hydrodermabrasion) or chemical (glycolic, lactic, salicylic acids, enzyme peels)

All other actives, by virtue of the fact they work in deeper layers of skin will almost always require the entire length of one skin cycle at least before new skin cells start showing beneficial effects we are expecting.

Other considerations
It is also critical to understand that while we aim to reduce the resistance of the skin barrier, we also do not want to damage it. This is especially important when it comes to traditional exfoliation methods like using abrasive beads—these will lead to dermatitis and are 100% not helpful. Besides, in skin of color, any form of skin irritation potentially can lead to hyperpigmentation, which is why we absolutely must always respect the skin barrier. This brings us to the next segment, which is how the Skincare Plus Accelerate Program enhances absorption of actives and delivers instant results, based on the principles of medifacial protocols by breaching the skin barrier *without* damaging it.

Results in 1 Day—modelled after in-clinic facial protocols
Designed to be implemented for universal skin types including
sensitive skin for
- Inside-out approach: increased transdermal absorption
- Infusion: cosmeceuticals
- Outside-in: enhanced epidermal permeability

The key here is a single device that can achieve all of the above
PLUS the following
- Suited for universal skin types with adjustable modes for
  dry, combination and oily skin
- Portable, usb rechargeable

The result is a handheld facial device with duo modes modeled
after technologies that are proven to deliver instant results in a
clinical setting:
- Hydrodermabrasion with infusion of antioxidants
- Microdermabrasion with microcrystalline copper and a
  peptide gel

The protocol emphasises efficiency and is best thought of as a
way to shorten the number of steps in your skincare routine
rather than as an additional step.

This is how the 5 step skincare routine of
Cleanse, tone, 2-step serum (HA + Vita C), moisturise can be
compressed into just 2 steps with the copper peel device.

Hydrodermabrasion (cleanse, tone, infuse, moisturise)
- Method of cleansing with vacuum pressure
- Using water as a solvent (universal solvent) rather than a
  lathering agent
- Medi-facial essence composition:
  - Natural cleansers i.e. rice bran
  - Antioxidant botanicals
  - Barrier repair actives i.e. natural moisturising
    factors, amino acids, hyaluronic acid,
    polyglutamic acid

Step 1 Application of the water-based medifacial essence as a
spray on mist
Step 2 Glide hydrodermabrasion handpiece over skin surface

N.B. There is an removable filter sponge within the device which should be rinsed with gentle soap and water once a week for maintainence.

Duration 1-3 minutes
Recommended as *AM* skincare routine

3 Min Hydro Peel
THE SCIENCE
- Enhance epidermal permeability vacuum microdermabrasion cleansing
- Remove outer layer of corneocytes with enzyme peel
- Step-wise infusion of tailored cosmeceutical actives (functional dermatology)
  - Antioxidant
  - Anti-inflammatory
  - Antimicrobial/microbiome stabilising

Microdermabrasion (cleanse, exfoliate, mask)

For the evening routine, the copper microcrystalline head is used instead.
Step 1: Apply lifting peptide mask
Step 2: Glide microdermabrasion handpiece over skin surface

Duration 1-3 minutes
Recommended as *PM* skincare routine

3 Min Copper Peel
- Gel mask peel for targeted delivery
- Copper peel for collagen stimulation and peptide infusion

SKINCARE PLUS ✚ BY DR.TWL®

REVOLUTIONISING IN-CLINIC TECHNOLOGIES FOR HOME USE

STANDARD SKINCARE ROUTINE	SKINCARE PLUS
STANDALONE ACTIVES	SYNERGY
LIMITED BY SKIN BARRIER PERMEABILITY	ENHANCED DELIVERY
DOES NOT ADDRESS MICROBIOME	MICROBIOME FRIENDLY
MONOTHERAPEUTIC	ENCOURAGES CELL TALK
SLOW EFFECTS 2-6 WEEK SKIN CYCLE	INSTANT EPIDERMAL RESULTS

✚A PRESCRIPTIVE APPROACH

DR.TWL® SKINCARE PLUS
ACCELERATION PROGRAM

**Professional Skincare System
Dermatologist Designed
Based on Functional Dermatology
For Quick Results**

- *Personalised to skin concern*
- *Instant results *guaranteed*
- *Builds a long term client relationship*
- *Easy review + adjust titration system with skincare planner template*
- *Utilises latest technology in facial care systems*

Dr.TWL®
Dermaceuticals

What's in each kit:

✓ **2 X Customisable medifacial solutions**

✓ **1 X Customisable face peel mask**

✓ **3 X Reusable polysaccharide barrier repair face mask**

1 MONTH SUPPLY

✓ **Copper peel microcrystalline Microdermabrasion Device**

Dr.TWL®
Dermaceuticals

364

CONSULTATION STRATEGY TEMPLATE
QUASI-DRUG

PRESCRIPTION RETINOIDS HYDROQUINONE

- In-person
- Salon overheads
- Time/staffing inefficiencies
- No access to prescription creams
- Skin irritation side effects with peels

- Online
- Home-based
- Client concerns
- Targeted cosmeceutical actives identified
- Irritation-free

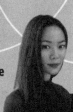

Dr.TWL®
Dermaceuticals

NEW ERA OF FUNCTIONAL DERMATOLOGY

BOTANICALS

QUASI-DRUG
RETINOID-LIKE

- CICA
- Grape seed oil
- Yeast peptide
- Green tea
- Arnica montana
- Bakuchiol

BARRIER FUNCTION

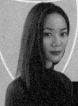

Dr.TWL®
Dermaceuticals

Review in 1 week

- Increase papain frequency if no irritation: combi/oily skin daily; EOD for dry skin
- Follow week 2 schedule frequency of use
- Conduct review in 1 month
- Increase enzyme concentration if no irritation 5%
- Check client progress/satisfaction
- Replenish solutions +1 additional active
- Start retinol alternative depending on concern:

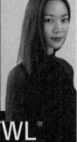

Dr.TWL®
Dermaceuticals

DERMATOLOGIST'S NOTES

Review in 1 month

- Increase enzyme concentration if no irritation 5%
- Check client progress/satisfaction
- Replenish solutions +1 additional active
- Start retinol alternative depending on concern

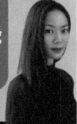

Dr.TWL®
Dermaceuticals

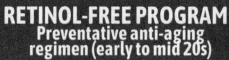

RETINOL-FREE PROGRAM
Preventative anti-aging regimen (early to mid 20s)

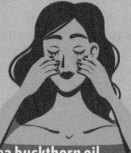

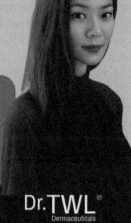

- Sea buckthorn oil
- Combi/oily skin 1 drop on fingers lightly tap over entire face EON
- Dry skin 2 drops lightly tap over entire face nightly

Dr.TWL®
Dermaceuticals

RETINOL-FREE PROGRAM
Active anti-aging regimen (late twenties onwards)

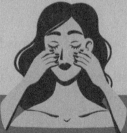

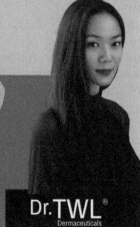

- Sea buckthorn regimen
- PLUS
- Bakuchiol
- Dry sensitive skin EON
- Combi oily skin nightly

Dr.TWL®
Dermaceuticals

Managing Client Expectations
Is there such a thing as an instant glow?
Yes. Though not from a a single skincare product alone especially after a single use. Usually this is associated with in-office procedures such as chemical peels, microdermabrasion and lasers. These technologies on its own or when paired with cosmeceuticals create a breach the skin barrier which changes the surface appearance of skin. This affects texture, pore size, skin tone which are all objectively measurable.

What can you do to accelerate the process?
Office-based procedures can be adapted in home use devices.

For skin tightening, lifting (linked to collagen production)
For instance, LED light can be harnessed as a portable treatment device without sacrificing energy delivery. Microcurrent on its own or combined with enzymatic peels can rapidly rejuvenate the skin surface by stimulating collagen production with low level electrical current. Radiofrequency is another clinic technology that is effectively harnessed in hand-held devices.

These technologies have been examined in scientific research that show measurable histological changes in skin after each treatment.

For instant glow
The key is to address these criteria which affect **transdermal delivery**
- Penetrate the skin barrier with microdermabrasion
- Select bioactive cosmeceuticals
- Moisture sandwich i.e. skincare layering creates an occlusive microclimate

*Access to actual formulations provided in **Skin Masters Advanced Partner Program,** available as opt-in at the sign-up link https://www.twlskin.com/dictionary/ (detailed percentages of actives, base used, optimal concentrations, raw ingredient supply sources), course fee fully redeemable for the first partner skincare set including supplies for starting your affiliate custom skincare business.

CHAPTER ELEVEN

Case Study of a Retinol-Free Anti-Aging Serum

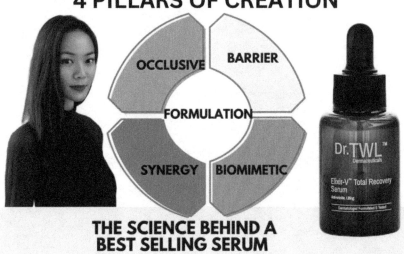

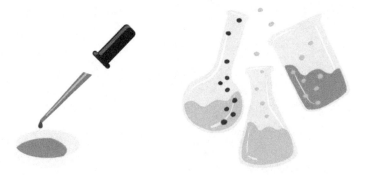

www.twlskin.com

In this tutorial, we go through the core ingredients and formulation of a gold standard antiaging serum for universal skin types.

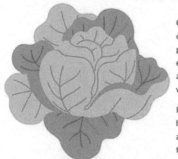

BEST FACE SERUM
PLANT-BASED SKINCARE

Contains Larecea™ our trademarked extract of Brassica oleracea (a botanical extract from cruciferous family plants) and a super-power Japanese Knotweed plant extract which is a source of trans-resveratrol, a potent anti-oxidant that enhances cellular regeneration at night, without the irritation effects of traditional retinoids.

Integrated humectant formula with polyglutamic acid & hyaluronic acid for intensive hydration and reducing appearance of pores. Polyglutamic acid is 5x more potent than hyaluronic acid in trapping moisture under the skin.

LARECEA + POLYGLUTAMIC ACID
Brassica oleracea

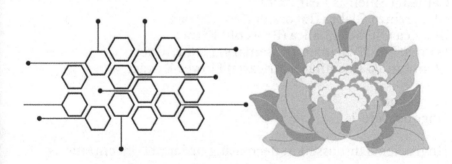

www.twlskin.com

Barrier repair actives and stabilising vehicle
- Glycerin
- Glyceryl Glucoside, Leaf Water
- Panthenol
- Betaine
- Sodium Hyaluronate

- Polyglutamic Acid
- Serine, Methionine, Histidine

The first category of actives we shall discuss are those that work on the superficial layers of skin. Humectants like hyaluronic acid, polyglutamic acid, amino acids and glycerin which trap moisture under the stratum corneum and prevent transepidermal water loss. Soothing actives like panthenol and amino acids also double up as building blocks for the skin's own reserve of natural moisturising factors.

Glycerin
Glyceryl Glucoside, Leaf Water
Panthenol
Betaine
Sodium Hyaluronate
Polyglutamic Acid
Serine, Methionine, Histidine

Centella Asiatica
Belamcanda Chinensis Root Extract
Scutellaria Baicalensis Root Extract
Polygonum Cuspidatum Root Extract

Camellia Sinensis Leaf Extract
Glycyrrhiza Glabra (Licorice) Root Extract
Brassica Oleracea Italica (Broccoli) Extract
Rosmarinus Officinalis (Rosemary) Leaf Extract
Chamomilla Recutita (Matricaria) Flower Extract

Beta-Glucan
Oligopeptide-1

*Ingredients discussed in decreasing order of concentrations.

BASE/VEHICLE: POLYGLUTAMIC ACID VS HYALURONIC ACID
The ideal serum vehicle is water-based which allows for a lightweight texture fit for the skincare layering technique. Polyglutamic acid is my choice for the combination serum base as it enhances the synergistic effects of the other additives. It holds 5X more water than hyaluronic acid but is significantly more expensive. Hence, it is best formulated with other actives

rather than as a pure serum for cost-efficiency. Higher concentrations of polyglutamic acid do not necessarily translate into increased efficacy and can increase the stickiness sensation of the product.

HUMECTANT/BARRIER REPAIR: AMINO ACIDS
The serum includes a mixture of amino acids (methionine, serine, histidine) both in synthetic and derivative form. For instance, whole plant extracts contain naturally occurring methionine, also known as Vitamin U, which is essential for wound healing and has additional UV-protective properties. Glycerin is a well-known traditional humectant and is part of ideal serum formulations to enhance effect of actives.

Humectants are not just barrier repair actives, glycerin for instance actually creates a micro-climate within the formulation itself that enhances the activity of other ingredients.

BOTANICAL ACTIVES/ADAPTOGENS
Adaptogens help skin to "adapt" to environmental stressors. When UV damage occurs, free radicals generated cause a form of physiological stress to the skin, known as oxidative stress. Plant actives are the most effective form of adaptogens as plants are innately selected to adapt to their environment. Different plant parts possess varying properties—the roots, stems, leaves and flowers contain varying actives that can be incorporated to strengthen skin. Skin resilience respects the entire skin eco-system, encouraging beneficial cell talk activity and improving skin immunity. A key function of adaptogens is to enhance skin resilience, which means it is able to repair DNA damage from daily stressors such as UV radiation, carcinogens and airborne pollution. In addition, adaptogens increase the skin's natural reserve of antioxidants that combat the effects of cell inflammaging, caused by biological aging processes.

The Science Behind the Ideal Face Serum

CASE STUDY: ELIXIR-V SERUM

This week's lecture goes into the formulation of our bestselling face serum, the Elixir-V. Learn all about what how gold standard practices in cosmeceutical formulation makes all the difference in the final product.

The end result? A serum that actually works.

RESVERATROL
LEARNING OBJECTIVES
- ☐ SOURCES (NATURAL VS SYNTHETIC)
- ☐ MECHANISM OF ACTION/HOW IT WORKS
- ☐ WHAT IS IT USED FOR
- ☐ DR.TWL FORMULATION SECRET: JAPANESE KNOTWEED

SOURCES (NATURAL VS SYNTHETIC)
Resveratrol was made prominent in 1992 as researchers unraveled the "French Paradox" which associated health benefits with moderate wine consumption. Turns out, grapes contain this key ingredient resveratrol which has potent physiological effects throughout the body.
- Polyphenols (stilbenoid group)
- Two forms (active *trans*-isomer, inactive *cis*-isomer)
- Natural sources (>70 plant sources)
- Dietary (grape seeds/skin, red wine, peanuts, soy)

MECHANISM OF ACTION/HOW IT WORKS
- **Antioxidant**

Protect cells against hydrogen peroxide-induced oxidative stress, UV-damage
- Direct: Free radical scavenger
- Indirect: Modulates cell antioxidant pathways

- **Anti-inflammatory**

Helps auto-immune and chronic inflammatory diseases
- NFKB, IL6, eicosanoids

- TLR2, TLR3, TLR4 signalling
- Reduces TLR7, TLR8, TLR9-mediated inflammation (psoriasis)

- **Anti-cancer effects**
- **Regulate metabolism (whole body fat and blood sugar levels)**
- **Specific skin targets:**
  - Wound healing
  - Scarring
  - Photoaging

WOUND HEALING

Wound healing involves a complex interplay of factors that requires sufficient blood vessel formation, antimicrobial activity that prevents skin infection and a balance of inflammatory responses that result in wound closure. Problems arise when the tissue is either too little or too much—leading to improper wound healing.

Resveratrol promotes wound healing by exerting the following effects:
The 4 'A's of Resveratrol
- Anti-inflammatory
- Anti-oxidative
- Angiogenesis (blood vessel formation)
- Anti-microbial (fights infections)

How it works
- Protects collagen-producing cells (fibroblasts)
- Stabilise skin structure
- Promote blood vessel formation (VEGF)
- Antibacterial effects (Staph aureus, Pseudomonas aeruginosa, Candida albicans, superior to commercial antimicrobial ointments)
- Special medical applications: treat non-healing wounds i.e. diabetic ulcers

Skincare benefits
- Anti-scarring
Prevents development of abnormal scars in laboratory studies
- Photoprotection

- Barrier function (moisture delivery)

Crucial to a solid grasp of this aspect of how reseveratrol works is the understanding of UV-related skin damage. You may have heard of oxidative stress, as well as the term antioxidant. These terms are meaningful only when you understand how UV-damage actually occurs. Here is a step-by-step explanation.

RESVERATROL SKIN BENEFITS

HOW FREE RADICAL DAMAGE OCCURS

1. UV rays reach skin
2. Free radicals are produced
3. These highly unstable molecules cause oxidative stress at the skin surface
4. Skin produces antioxidants to neutralize free radicals

www.twlskin.com

- UV rays reach skin

- Free radicals are produced
- These highly unstable molecules cause oxidative stress at the skin surface
- Skin produces antioxidants to neutralize free radicals

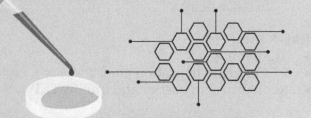

RESVERATROL SKIN BENEFITS

The balance of free radicals and antioxidants is what determines if cell damage occurs:

- Free radicals > antioxidant reserve →cell damage
- Free radicals < antioxidant reserve →cell protected

www.twlskin.com

The balance of free radicals and antioxidants is what determines if cell damage occurs:
- Free radicals > antioxidant reserve →cell damage

- Free radicals < antioxidant reserve →cell protected

How UV damages skin:
Chronic UV exposure results in activation of 3 major aging cascades known by the acronym MIA

- **Reactive oxygen species (ROS) production**
  - Metalloproteinases MMP-1 mediated
  - Inflammaging IL-6, 8 mediated
  - Apoptosis-induced via NFKB, caspase 3

How resveratrol works:
- Antiaging by targeting 3 main pathways of ROS-induced aging pathways

Clinical studies
- Beneficial effects on all signs of photoaging after minimum 30 days of application

Farris et al
  - Luminosity
  - Hydration
  - Elasticity

Igielska-Kalwat et al
- Tightening
- 20% increase hydration after 2 weeks
- Replenish skin barrier and inhibit TEWL

Dr.TWL's Formulation Secrets

Proanthocyanidins: Nature's Anti-aging Fingerprint

The best-selling Elixir-V Serum contains Japanese Knotweed, also known as polygonum cuspidatum. It is a source of trans-resveratrol which is an active form of the compound. It is lesser known in western pharmacology but is well established in ethnobotanical applications. Biochemical analysis has shown it to be a rich source of proanthocyanidins, a potent antioxidant, specifically found in the roots of the plant.

Native to East Asia, it is an invasive plant that also has medicinal properties.
Chromatographic studies have isolated the following

- Anthraquinones
- Flavanoids (rutin, apigenin, quercetin)
- Stilbenes (resveratrol)
- Catechin, epicatechin, epicatechin-gallate
- Procyanidin B12

By virtue of it being a whole plant extract rather than a chemically synthesised copy, there are additional benefits such as:

Holistic effects on skin physiology

- Antioxidant
- Antimicrobial (stilbenes, anthraquinones)
- Anti-inflammatory
- Inhibit pigment formation
- Anti-tumor
- Barrier repair

BEST FACE SERUM
INGREDIENT PAIRING

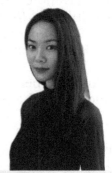

Centella Asiatica [Acne Scar Lightening]

Larecea™ [Regeneration]

Resveratrol [Anti-oxidant]

Potent Oligopeptides [Lifting] [Repair]

Polyglutamic Acid/Hyaluronic Acid [Humectant] [Pore Reduction]

INGREDIENT PAIRING
ANTIOXIDANT + PEPTIDE +HUMECTANT

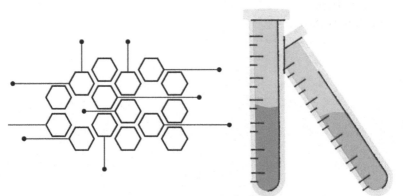

www.twlskin.com

The second core group of actives are a potent blend of our cosmeceutical actives—these are tested for tolerability on sensitive skin as well as efficacy. In a laboratory setting, these actives have been proven to penetrate the skin barrier and is absorbed into the deeper layers where it exerts its target cell effects.

- Centella Asiatica
- Belamcanda Chinensis Root Extract
- Scutellaria Baicalensis Root Extract

- Polygonum Cuspidatum Root Extract
- Camellia Sinensis Leaf Extract
- Glycyrrhiza Glabra (Licorice) Root Extract
- Brassica Oleracea Italica (Broccoli) Extract
- Rosmarinus Officinalis (Rosemary) Leaf Extract
- Chamomilla Recutita (Matricaria) Flower Extract

Elixir-V: the ideal face serum for oily skin that regulates sebum production from the inside out

These botanical actives also work on other aspects of skin physiology i.e. sebum regulation. Derived from traditional eastern medicine, the Elixir-V's key actives include Belamcanda Chinensis Root Extract, Scutellaria Baicalensis Root Extract and Polygonum Cuspidatum Root Extract. The trio regarded as the holy grail of ethnopharmacology.

BEST FACE SERUM
FORMULATION SECRETS

- BASE/VEHICLE
- HUMECTANT/BARRIER REPAIR
- AMINO ACIDS
- BOTANICAL ACTIVES/ADAPTOGENS

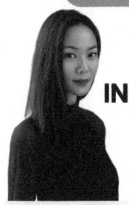

INGREDIENT PAIRING MASTERCLASS

By Dr.TWL®

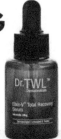

CASE STUDY: ELIXIR-V SERUM

www.drtwlderma.com

The best face serum is one that fulfils the following criteria:
- Highly tolerable even for sensitive skin types
- Non-sensitising i.e. no risk of skin irritation with long term use
- Synergistic blend of actives that boost efficacy
- Short term (immediate results) and longer term effects
- Evidence-based actives that qualify as cosmeceuticals

The Science of Skincare Layering: Face Serums First
The ideal face serum formulation can boost the results of your skincare routine. Dermatologists advocate skincare layering because it enhances absorption while maximising concentrations of skin actives. This is why an all-in-1 skincare product simply does not do as well as a more complex skincare layering regimen.

DR.TWL'S FACE SERUM FORMULATION SECRETS
The best face serum formulation includes ingredients from the following categories:
- Biomimetic actives that mimic natural skin molecules that work to repair damaged skin and protect from environmental damage
- Not just 1 or 2 actives, but a combination of actives in lower concentrations that synergise and boost antioxidant activity
- Emphasis on fundamentals of skincare —barrier repair
- Creating an occlusive microenvironment with humectants to enhance absorption and delivery of molecules

BEST FACE SERUM
4 PILLARS OF CREATION

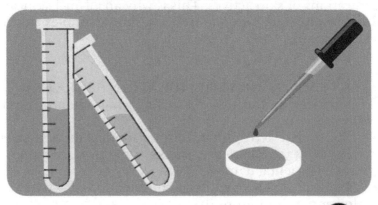

Glycerin
Glyceryl Glucoside, Leaf Water
Panthenol
Betaine
Sodium Hyaluronate
Polyglutamic Acid
Serine, Methionine, Histidine

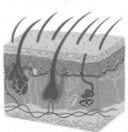

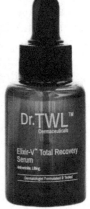

BARRIER REPAIR HYDRATION

www.drtwlderma.com

There are 3 important things to bear in mind when it comes to how effective an over-the-counter cosmeceutical skincare product is.

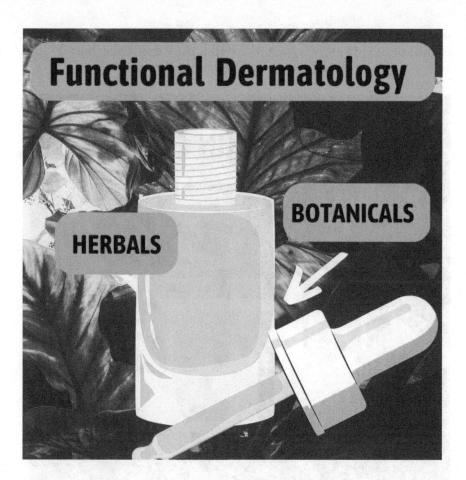

Functional Dermatology

HERBALS

BOTANICALS

1. Tolerability for universal skin types including sensitive skin
Firstly, whether it can be used long term, for all skin types. The main issue with traditional OTC cosmeceuticals like retinol is that many develop sensitivity after decades of use, or in the shorter term. While retinol does work, it does not appear to be as well tolerated by skin of color i.e. asian skin types compared to Caucasian skin—which was what most western brands were conducting product testing on. Add to that the fact that in certain climates such as Singapore's, there is high UV radiation year round which means there is a heightened risk of photosensitivity.

2. Bioactivity of ingredients
The definition of a cosmeceutical means that the ingredient must have pharmacologically active properties when tested on

skin cells. The Elixir-V serum was designed based on extensive ethnobotanical research to ensure that only evidence-based actives with synergistic properties were included in the formulation.

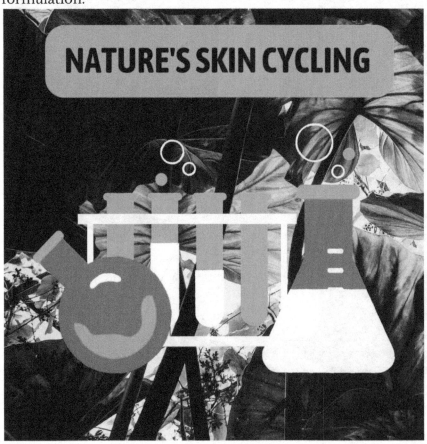

3. Ability to penetrate the skin barrier
The best face serum would be of no effect if it was not formulated to penetrate the skin barrier—the outermost layer of skin known as the stratum corneum. This is one of the original criteria set by the father of cosmeceuticals Albert Kligman. The Elixir-V serum is ideally formulated in a vehicle based on glycerin, polyglutamic acid and amino acids that increase absorption via an microocclusive effect. In dermatologist speak— we call this the vehicle. Essentially referring to the texture as well as the carrier of the active ingredients.

CASE STUDY: *Vitamin C face serums are the holy grail of any skincare routine.*

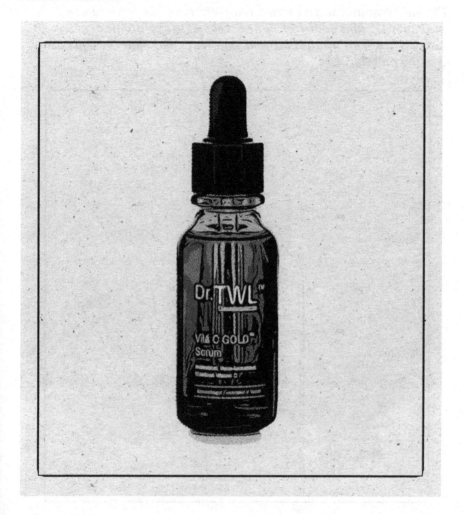

The creation of a gold standard formula involves the following criteria:

1. Suitability for sensitive skin and active skin conditions i.e. rosacea, acne, dermatitis
2. Ingredient pairing boost with Camellia Sinensis extract
3. Highly stable Sodium Ascorbyl Phosphate (SAP) formula to ensure optimal delivery and minimal environmental oxidation/degradation.

CASE STUDY: Hyaluronic acid serum

The ideal hyaluronic acid serum is a 100% pure HA formula at a minimum 1%, sans additives. When it comes to hyaluronic acid serums, purity is key. This means that your skin reaps maximum benefits while layering on skincare.

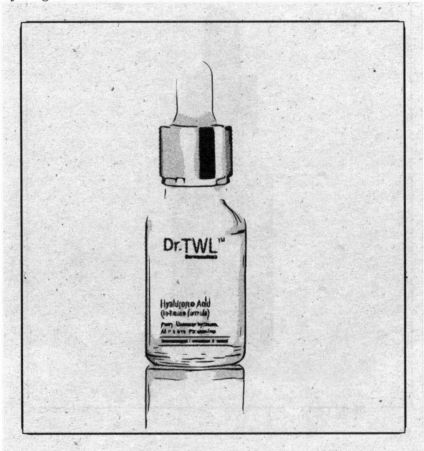

The in-house pharmacy formulation contains a unique blend of multi weighted molecular hyaluronic acid actives that ensure a well-rounded effect on skin physiology. First by functioning as a humectant at the superficial cell layers i.e. the corneocytes. Second, by penetrating deeper into the dermal layers to activate beneficial cell talk.

Dermatologist's Top Tips:
Why you should use always include a serum in your skincare regimen
The benefits of a serum are
- Delivers highest concentrations of actives
- Essential part of skincare layering technique
- Preserves maximum efficacy with minimal environmental loss/degradation

SECTION 4

Ingredient Mastery Learning Tools

download textbook resources and printables*

*https://www.twlskin.com/dictionary/ register account and receive download access in your welcome email

Ingredient Mastery
Learning Tools

<u>FLASH LEARNING METHOD SET A WITH MIND MAP</u>

We will now move on to the actual mastery of skincare actives which is the most daunting aspect of the course. I'll be coaching you in the exact methods I use to learn these myself, so you can easily develop your own system as you come across new ingredients.

I've selected here a list which we shall call SET A. The features of each ingredient has been summarised in just 2-3 sentences, from scientific papers which are quoted (most of the original papers are accessible behind a paywall but I have already extracted the essential details here for you.)

A. Learn 3-5 ingredients per day

Skincare Ingredient Mastery
How to use mind maps

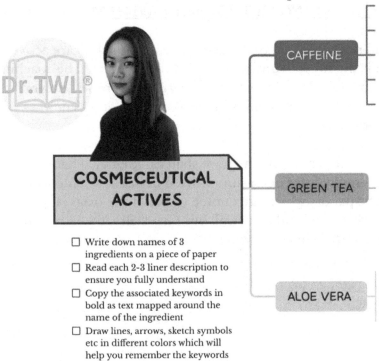

COSMECEUTICAL ACTIVES

CAFFEINE

GREEN TEA

ALOE VERA

- ☐ Write down names of 3 ingredients on a piece of paper
- ☐ Read each 2-3 liner description to ensure you fully understand
- ☐ Copy the associated keywords in bold as text mapped around the name of the ingredient
- ☐ Draw lines, arrows, sketch symbols etc in different colors which will help you remember the keywords

Skincare Ingredient Mastery
How to use mind maps

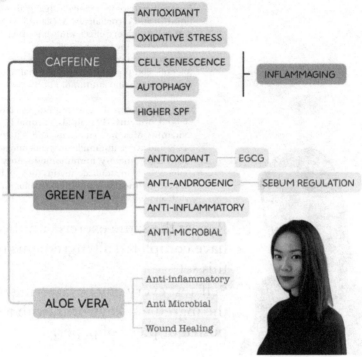

- **CAFFEINE**
  - ANTIOXIDANT
  - OXIDATIVE STRESS
  - CELL SENESCENCE — INFLAMMAGING
  - AUTOPHAGY
  - HIGHER SPF

- **GREEN TEA**
  - ANTIOXIDANT — EGCG
  - ANTI-ANDROGENIC — SEBUM REGULATION
  - ANTI-INFLAMMATORY
  - ANTI-MICROBIAL

- **ALOE VERA**
  - Anti-inflammatory
  - Anti Microbial
  - Wound Healing

C. Revise and self-test everyday

Skincare Ingredient Mastery
How to use mind maps

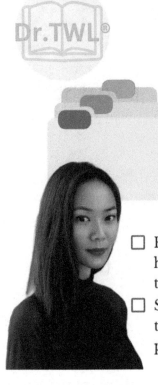

Licorice :
Contains active compounds such as **glabridin, liquirtin and Licochalcone A**. Glabridin has an **anti-inflammatory** effect, while liquirtin has been used for the treatment of **hyperpigmentation**. Licochalcone A is a phenolic compound with **antibacterial**, anti inflammatory, and **antitumor** effects.

Colloidal Oatmeal : Contains **polysaccharides** (~60%), **proteins** (~12%), **lipids, flavonoids, vitamins**. Most well known includes Vitamin A, B, E, and avenanthramides, potent antioxidants. **Anti-inflammatory, immunomodulatory** effects. Used in atopic dermatitis for **skin barrier repair**. **Oatmeal saponins** help to solubilize oil, dirt, and sebaceous secretions.

☐ Repeat the same exercise until you have completed all ingredients in this set

☐ Self-test every day by covering up the ingredient keywords (with a post-it or piece of paper)

D. Use post-its

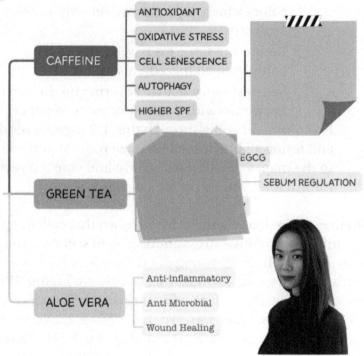

Skincare Ingredient Mastery
Self Testing

The key here is to

- [ ] Break down complex information into bite-sized, digestible format in just 2-3 sentences for the first few, before we introduce longer formats in 2-3 paragraphs of text
- [ ] Keyword method of learning (keywords have been bolded)
- [ ] Make your own 1-page mind map for set A ingredients with just 3 steps
  For each session
  - [ ] Write down names of 3 ingredients on a piece of paper

- ☐ Read each 2-3 liner description to ensure you fully understand
- ☐ Copy the associated keywords in bold as text mapped around the name of the ingredient
- ☐ Draw lines, arrows, sketch symbols etc in different colors which will help you remember the keywords
- ☐ Repeat the same exercise until you have completed all ingredients in this set
- ☐ Self-test every day by covering up the ingredient keywords (with a post-it or piece of paper)

I recommend going through this, 1-3 ingredients daily and fitting all into a single A4 size page. When you add on to the map, you will instinctively find yourself reviewing information you learnt the day before.

Caffeine: Antioxidant: studies have shown that caffeine protects the skin from **oxidative stress**-induced **senescence** through activating **autophagy** (cleaning out damaged cells).
Effective in sunscreen formulations to achieve **higher SPF** values. Active against **hair loss** i.e. androgenetic alopecia.

- Li, Y. F., Ouyang, S. H., Tu, L. F., Wang, X., Yuan, W. L., Wang, G. E., Wu, Y. P., Duan, W. J., Yu, H. M., Fang, Z. Z., Kurihara, H., Zhang, Y., & He, R. R. (2018). Caffeine Protects Skin from Oxidative Stress-Induced Senescence through the Activation of Autophagy. *Theranostics, 8*(20), 5713–5730.
- Rosado, C., Tokunaga, V. K., Sauce, R., de Oliveira, C. A., Sarruf, F. D., Parise-Filho, R., Maurício, E., de Almeida, T. S., Velasco, M., & Baby, A. R. (2019). Another Reason for Using Caffeine in Dermocosmetics: Sunscreen Adjuvant. *Frontiers in physiology, 10*, 519.
- Völker, J. M., Koch, N., Becker, M., & Klenk, A. (2020). Caffeine and Its Pharmacological Benefits in the Management of Androgenetic Alopecia: A Review. *Skin pharmacology and physiology, 33*(3), 93–109.

Green tea: Catechins: **antioxidant, anti-inflammatory**, and **antibiotic** properties. **EGCG**, a catechin found in high amounts in green tea has been shown to be a potent **photoprotectant** and **antioxidant**. Research has also found that ECGC lowers lipid levels, and is **anti-androgenic**, making it effective at **regulating sebum** (oil) production in the skin. One study showed **decreased total lesion count** in **acne** patients treated with green tea as compared to treatment with a placebo.

- Fowler, J. F., Jr, Woolery-Lloyd, H., Waldorf, H., & Saini, R. (2010). Innovations in natural ingredients and their use in skin care. *Journal of drugs in dermatology : JDD*, *9*(6 Suppl), S72–s83.

Tea Tree Oil : Contains **antiseptic** and **anti-inflammatory** effects for treating acne. In one study of 60 patients with mild to moderate acne, 30 patients were treated with tea tree oil, and the other 30 were treated with a placebo. Tea tree oil gel was found to be **3.55x more effective than placebo** for total acne lesion count, and 5.75x more effective than placebo in the acne severity index.

- Fowler, J. F., Jr, Woolery-Lloyd, H., Waldorf, H., & Saini, R. (2010). Innovations in natural ingredients and their use in skin care. *Journal of drugs in dermatology : JDD*, *9*(6 Suppl), S72–s83.

Colloidal Oatmeal : Contains **polysaccharides** (~60%), **proteins** (~12%), **lipids, flavonoids, vitamins**. Most well known includes Vitamin A, B, E, and avenanthramides, potent antioxidants. **Anti-inflammatory, immunomodulatory** effects. Used in atopic dermatitis for **skin barrier repair. Oatmeal saponins** help to solubilize oil, dirt, and sebaceous secretions.

- Fowler, J. F., Jr, Woolery-Lloyd, H., Waldorf, H., & Saini, R. (2010). Innovations in natural ingredients and their use in skin care. *Journal of drugs in dermatology : JDD*, *9*(6 Suppl), S72–s83.

Aloe vera: Exhibits potent **anti-inflammatory effects**, used to accelerate **skin healing** and as a **bactericidal** agent. In a study of 30 patients, 83.3% demonstrated significant improvements in **psoriasis** area and severity index score after treatment with aloe vera as compared to a placebo. Used to treat psoriasis.

- Fowler, J. F., Jr, Woolery-Lloyd, H., Waldorf, H., & Saini, R. (2010). Innovations in natural ingredients and their use in skin care. *Journal of drugs in dermatology : JDD*, 9(6 Suppl), S72–s83.

Indigo Naturalis: Used to treat **psoriasis.** In a study, 42 patients underwent treatment of indigo naturalis to one lesion compared to a control lesion for 12 weeks. The lesion treated showed reduced scaling, redness and thickening of the skin. Overall, there was a 74% clearance rate of lesions treated with indigo naturalis.

- Fowler, J. F., Jr, Woolery-Lloyd, H., Waldorf, H., & Saini, R. (2010). Innovations in natural ingredients and their use in skin care. *Journal of drugs in dermatology : JDD*, 9(6 Suppl), S72–s83.

Coffee berry: Polyphenols that prevent damage from **free radical** exposure and **oxidative stress.** Also protect against **UVA and UVB.**

- Fowler, J. F., Jr, Woolery-Lloyd, H., Waldorf, H., & Saini, R. (2010). Innovations in natural ingredients and their use in skin care. *Journal of drugs in dermatology : JDD*, 9(6 Suppl), S72–s83.

Treating Hyperpigmentation
Soy: Lipids, lecithins, and phytosterols** enhance the normal skin barrier. **Isoflavones** have an antioxidant effect. Study of hairless mice showed that after treatment of soy isaflavone extract, after exposure to UVB radiation, treated mice showed **decrease in skin redness,** and UVB-induced keratinocyte death. Also displayed **less transepidermal water loss** and **less wrinkles.**

The **fatty acid** component, which is about **15 percent**, provides some **anti- inflammatory** properties, while the phytosterols and vitamin E provide moisture and barrier protection, as well as antioxidative benefit.

Small soy proteins such as **soybean trypsin inhibitor (STI)** and Bowman-Birk inhibitor (BBI), function to **inhibit pigmentation** in the skin. In a 12-week randomized, double-blind, vehicle controlled study comparing moisturizer with soy and vehicle in Fitzpatrick skin types I–III ages 31–60 years old with mottled hyperpigmentation, lentigines, blotchiness, tactile roughness and dullness, there was significant improvement in pigmentation, blotchiness, dullness, fine lines, overall texture, skin tone and appearance

- Fowler, J. F., Jr, Woolery-Lloyd, H., Waldorf, H., & Saini, R. (2010). Innovations in natural ingredients and their use in skin care. *Journal of drugs in dermatology : JDD*, *9*(6 Suppl), S72–s83.

Licorice: Contains active compounds such as **glabridin, liquirtin and Licochalcone A**. Glabridin has an **anti-inflammatory** effect, while liquirtin has been used for the treatment of **hyperpigmentation**. Licochalcone A is a phenolic compound with **antibacterial**, anti inflammatory, and **antitumor** effects.

In a study, 12 subjects were treated with **0.05% Licochalcone A** extract after being exposed to UV light. Results showed a significant decrease of redness, compared to the control group. Finding support anti-inflammatory and photoprotective effect of licorice. Liquirtin was compared to vehicle in a blinded controlled split-face study of 20 women aged 18–40 years with melasma in which they received treatment twice daily for four weeks. 70% of patients reported an "excellent' response (75-100%) in pigmentation, and 60% experience a reduction in lesion size.

Well documented to **inhibit melanogenesis,** has **anti-inflammatory effects**. In a study with 62 subjects with mild to moderate redness, there was a significant improvement in redness after 4-8 weeks. Showed that licorice improved the appearance of **persistent facial redness**. Effective in treatment of **rosacea**.

- Fowler, J. F., Jr, Woolery-Lloyd, H., Waldorf, H., & Saini, R. (2010). Innovations in natural ingredients and their use in skin care. *Journal of drugs in dermatology : JDD, 9*(6 Suppl), S72–s83.

Niacinamide: Niacinamide is a form of **vitamin B3**, an essential nutrient. Although it is derived from **niacin**, it does not cause the same side effects such as flushing and low cholesterol. It has **anti-inflammatory** properties, helps to **regulate oil**, and protects against **oxidative stress,** all of which are beneficial in the treatment of **acne**.

It can help to **minimize redness** and **treat inflammatory acne** such as pustules and papules. Niacinamide also helps to build and strengthen the **skin barrier**, which can help to retain moisture. This is beneficial for all skin types as it helps to regulate the amount of oil produced by sebaceous glands, and helps to boost moisture if you have eczema or mature skin.

Additionally, it is a potent **antioxidant**, protects from environmental aggressors such as sunlight and pollution. In a trial of 76 patients, treatment of **4% niacinamide gel** showed reduction in acne lesions and acne severity in 82% of participants. .Inhibits transfer of melanosomes to keratinocytes. In a clinical study, **3.5% niacinamide/retinylpalmitate** demonstrated significantly decreased **hyperpigmentation** and increased skin lightness compared with vehicle alone after four weeks of use in Asian women.

- Fowler, J. F., Jr, Woolery-Lloyd, H., Waldorf, H., & Saini, R. (2010). Innovations in natural ingredients and their use in skin care. *Journal of drugs in dermatology : JDD*, 9(6 Suppl), S72–s83.

Mushrooms: Contains **antioxidants**, including phenolic acids, flavonoids, tocopherols, ascorbic acid, carotenoids.
E.g *Codyceps taii* and *Sparassis crispa* show promise for treatment in photoaging. ***Codyceps*** most commonly utilized in Chinese medicine. Exhibit antioxidant properties, reduced oxidative stress in mice and enhance natural antioxidant production. **Polysaccharides** in *C. taii* also promoted our body's natural antioxidant activity, scavenging free radicals and **inhibiting lipid peroxidation** (cell damage to the lipids in our skin).
E.g **Veratric acid**, a phenolic acid found in *Sparassis Crispa*. After exposure to UVB, some cells were treated with veratric acid, while others received no post-UV treatment. Veratric acid treated cells showed **reduced DNA damage**, and overall photoprotective effects.

- Fowler, J. F., Jr, Woolery-Lloyd, H., Waldorf, H., & Saini, R. (2010). Innovations in natural ingredients and their use in skin care. *Journal of drugs in dermatology : JDD*, 9(6 Suppl), S72–s83.

Feverfew: Asteraceae family, includes daisies and chrysanthemums. Originally used as a fever reducer, has anti-inflammatory, anti-irritant, and antioxidant properties. Contains a compound called **parthenolide**, which induces allergic response. Parthenolide-depleted feverfew extracts have been developed, shown to enhance **DNA repair** activity, increase production of **antioxidants**, and significantly reduce both UVA and UVB induced **DNA damage** of human keratinocytes (skin cells) after UV exposure, thus reducing oxidative damage.

- Fowler, J. F., Jr, Woolery-Lloyd, H., Waldorf, H., & Saini, R. (2010). Innovations in natural ingredients and their use in skin care. *Journal of drugs in dermatology : JDD*, 9(6 Suppl), S72–s83.

Olive Oil: Considered one of the healthiest forms of dietary fat, has anti-inflammatory effects. One study showed that mice treated with olive oil after UVB radiation exposure had delayed onset of and **reduced** the incidence of **skin cancer** development.

Also believed to protect against **oxidative stress** via upregulation of **antioxidants**. Human skin keratinocytes and fibroblasts treated with olive oil displayed increase production of enzymes that monitor and repair damage caused by oxidative stress.

- Fowler, J. F., Jr, Woolery-Lloyd, H., Waldorf, H., & Saini, R. (2010). Innovations in natural ingredients and their use in skin care. *Journal of drugs in dermatology : JDD, 9*(6 Suppl), S72–s83.

Alpha mangostin: Alpha mangostin is a **xanthathoid** extracted from the certain parts of the mangosteen tree. Alpha mangostin has shown to have **anti-inflammatory, antioxidant, antibacterial** properties that can be effective in the treatment of acne. It has shown to tamp down inflammation through inhibition of the TAK1–NF-κB inflammatory pathway. Additionally, studies have shown that it exhibits antioxidant activity through upregulating the body's natural antioxidants such as **superoxide dismutase** (SOD). Film-forming solutions comprising alpha mangostin rich extract has also shown to **inhibit *P. acnes*** growth.

- Soleymani, S., Farzaei, M. H., Zargaran, A., Niknam, S., & Rahimi, R. (2020). Promising plant-derived secondary metabolites for treatment of acne vulgaris: a mechanistic review. *Archives of dermatological research, 312*(1), 5–23.

Ampelopsin: Ampelopsin is a type of flavonoid that has **neuroprotective**, and hepatoprotective activities, regulating plasma lipids and blood glucose. It decreased inflammation by suppressing inflammatory pathways activated by oxidative stress. It also helped to **protect against oxidative stress** by inhibiting ROS production.

- Soleymani, S., Farzaei, M. H., Zargaran, A., Niknam, S., & Rahimi, R. (2020). Promising plant-derived secondary metabolites for treatment of acne vulgaris: a mechanistic review. *Archives of dermatological research, 312*(1), 5–23. https://doi.org/10.1007/s00403-019-01968-z

Apple polyphenols: Apple polyphenols are purified and extracted from **unripe apples**, and are composed of **catechins, phenol carboxylic acids, and procyanidins**. It is a potent **antioxidant**, exhibiting better free radical scavenging activities than vitamin E and C.

- Soleymani, S., Farzaei, M. H., Zargaran, A., Niknam, S., & Rahimi, R. (2020). Promising plant-derived secondary metabolites for treatment of acne vulgaris: a mechanistic review. *Archives of dermatological research, 312*(1), 5–23. https://doi.org/10.1007/s00403-019-01968-z

Berberine: A traditional eastern herb medicine, berberine is an **isoquinone alkaloid** extracted from various plants. Berberine has **bactericidal, anti-inflammatory, antioxidant** effects, and can also **reduce androgen/sebum** production that has been shown effective in the treatment of acne. Berberine enhances bacterial killing in macrophages, through inflammasome activation. It has also demonstrated anti-inflammatory activities by inhibiting important proinflammatory proteins such as IL-6 and TNF-α proteins, and modulating inflammatory pathways. Additionally, it also prevents additional oxidative damage by decreasing mitochondrial ROS (free radical molecules), decreasing the effects of oxidative stress, and increasing the production of natural antioxidants in the body. Lastly, it has shown that it can prevent androgen synthesis (hormones that lead to increased sebum production in the body), decreasing sebum production by suppressing lipogenesis of sebaceous glands.

- Soleymani, S., Farzaei, M. H., Zargaran, A., Niknam, S., & Rahimi, R. (2020). Promising plant-derived secondary metabolites for treatment of acne vulgaris: a mechanistic

review. *Archives of dermatological research*, *312*(1), 5–23.
https://doi.org/10.1007/s00403-019-01968-z

Curcumin : Is a **polyphenol** extracted from *Curcuma Longa* L and has a wide range of pharmacological benefits. One study found that Curcumin loaded vehicles could accumulate significantly in the skin, prohibiting the growth of *P acnes*. Furthermore, it has shown potent **antioxidant** and **anti-inflammatory** effect through regulation of inflammatory pathways in the body.

- Soleymani, S., Farzaei, M. H., Zargaran, A., Niknam, S., & Rahimi, R. (2020). Promising plant-derived secondary metabolites for treatment of acne vulgaris: a mechanistic review. *Archives of dermatological research*, *312*(1), 5–23. https://doi.org/10.1007/s00403-019-01968-z

Ellagic Acid : Abenzopyran derivative **polyphenol** present in various medicinal plants like *Punica granatum*, and *Rubus spp*. One study showed that a combination of **ellagic acid and tetracycline** made *P. acnes* more susceptible to antibiotics and the human immune system's natural defenses. It has also demonstrated **anti-inflammatory** activity, decreasing the expression of various proinflammatory proteins. It is also a potent antioxidant that exhibits suppression of **oxidative stress** through free radical scavenging activity, and decreasing of ROS production.

- Soleymani, S., Farzaei, M. H., Zargaran, A., Niknam, S., & Rahimi, R. (2020). Promising plant-derived secondary metabolites for treatment of acne vulgaris: a mechanistic review. *Archives of dermatological research*, *312*(1), 5–23. https://doi.org/10.1007/s00403-019-01968-z

Epigallocatechin-3-gallate (EGCG) is the main **flavonoid** found in **green tea**, of ***Camellia Sinensis***. It has **anti-sebum** and oil control effects, and has shown to decrease sebum by modulating sebum-producing pathways in the sebocyte cell line. EGCG has also demonstrated inhibiting the testosterone-induced sebum synthesis in sebocytes and suppressed androgen-related pathogenesis of **acne**. It also has **anti-inflammatory** and **antioxidant** effects.

- Soleymani, S., Farzaei, M. H., Zargaran, A., Niknam, S., & Rahimi, R. (2020). Promising plant-derived secondary metabolites for treatment of acne vulgaris: a mechanistic review. *Archives of dermatological research, 312*(1), 5–23. https://doi.org/10.1007/s00403-019-01968-z

Arbutin: A naturally occuring **b-glucopyranoside, hydroquinone derivative,** found in bearberry and other trees. It is a botanical **bleaching** agent that works via reversible **tyrosinase inhibition** (enzyme that catalyzes production of melanin). In an open label study, a gel formulation containing arbutin was given to 10 subjects with **melasma**, in which all 10 subjects showed a significant improvement compared to the control.

- Ertam I, Mutlu B, Unal I et al. Efficiency of ellagic acid and arbutin in melasma: a randomized, prospective, open-label study. J Dermatol 2008; 35: 570–574

Kojic acid: A popular botanical ingredient found in cosmetics to block the formation of pigment by melanocytes. Kojic acid's **anti-melanogenic** effect is mainly through the inhibition of NF-κB activity in human keratinocytes. It also **inhibits tyrosinase** by capturing the **copper ion** that is crucial in tyrosinase activation.

- Saeedi, M., Eslamifar, M., & Khezri, K. (2019). Kojic acid applications in cosmetic and pharmaceutical preparations. *Biomedicine & pharmacotherapy = Biomedecine & pharmacotherapie, 110*, 582–593. https://doi.org/10.1016/j.biopha.2018.12.006

Goji berry: Goji berry root extract can result in **depigmentation** via suppression of **oxidative stress**, and MAPK and PKA signalling pathways, which are key pathways linked to the inhibition of melanin synthesis.

- Huang, H. C., Huang, W. Y., Tsai, T. C., Hsieh, W. Y., Ko, W. P., Chang, K. J., & Chang, T. M. (2014). Supercritical fluid extract of Lycium chinense Miller root inhibition of melanin production and its potential mechanisms of action. *BMC complementary and alternative medicine, 14,* 208. https://doi.org/10.1186/1472-6882-14-208

Ganoderma lucidum polysaccharides: Reduce melanogenesis by inhibiting cAMP/PKA signalling pathways, and inhibiting paracrine effects. Paracrine regulates melanogenesis as it secretes hormones that induce melanin synthesis.
- Hu, S., Huang, J., Pei, S., Ouyang, Y., Ding, Y., Jiang, L., Lu, J., Kang, L., Huang, L., Xiang, H., Xiao, R., Zeng, Q., & Chen, J. (2019). Ganoderma lucidum polysaccharide inhibits UVB-induced melanogenesis by antagonizing cAMP/PKA and ROS/MAPK signaling pathways. *Journal of cellular physiology, 234*(5), 7330–7340. https://doi.org/10.1002/jcp.27492
- Jiang, L., Huang, J., Lu, J., Hu, S., Pei, S., Ouyang, Y., Ding, Y., Hu, Y., Kang, L., Huang, L., Xiang, H., Zeng, Q., Liu, L., Chen, J., & Zeng, Q. (2019). Ganoderma lucidum polysaccharide reduces melanogenesis by inhibiting the paracrine effects of keratinocytes and fibroblasts via IL-6/STAT3/FGF2 pathway. *Journal of cellular physiology, 234*(12), 22799–22808. https://doi.org/10.1002/jcp.28844

C. songaricum extract : C. songaricum enhanced cognitive behaviour, increased resistance to stress and extended female mean lifespan of flies, indicating that *C. songaricum* **flavonoids** acted as **free radical scavengers** (Yu *et al*. 2010; Liu *et al*. 2012)

Echinacoside: Derived from *Cistanche tubulosa*, it is a potent **antioxidant** that shows anti-aging effects. In a study involving D-galactose aged mice, it has been shown to repair cell damage and **delay cell senescence**. This is done via enhancing the activities of GSH-Px and SOD (both natural antioxidants in the body), reducing the content of MDA (marker of oxidative stress, causes damage to the body).

Ginseng: is one of the most popular eastern herbs known for its medicinal benefits. In a study done on mice, the results showed that dietary supply containing red ginseng extract significantly inhibited **wrinkle** formation caused by chronic UVB irradiation. Its leaves have been found to be effective in **moisturizing**, anti-aging, **depigmenting**, evening out **skin tone**.

Additionally, red ginseng byproduct **polysaccharides** (RGBP) when combined with an enzyme linked to a high pressure process, inhibits solar ultraviolet MMPs (enzymes that break down collagen). Hence, indicating that enzyme modified Panax ginseng inhibits UVB-induced skin aging through the regulation of **procollagen**-I, and MMP-1 expression.

- Kang, T. H., Park, H. M., Kim, Y. B., Kim, H., Kim, N., Do, J. H., Kang, C., Cho, Y., & Kim, S. Y. (2009). Effects of red ginseng extract on UVB irradiation-induced skin aging in hairless mice. *Journal of ethnopharmacology, 123*(3), 446–451. https://doi.org/10.1016/j.jep.2009.03.022
- Jiménez-Pérez, Z. E., Singh, P., Kim, Y. J., Mathiyalagan, R., Kim, D. H., Lee, M. H., & Yang, D. C. (2018). Applications of *Panax ginseng* leaves-mediated gold nanoparticles in cosmetics relation to antioxidant, moisture retention, and whitening effect on B16BL6 cells. *Journal of ginseng research, 42*(3), 327–333. https://doi.org/10.1016/j.jgr.2017.04.003
- Hwang, E., Lee, T. H., Park, S. Y., Yi, T. H., & Kim, S. Y. (2014). Enzyme-modified Panax ginseng inhibits UVB-induced skin aging through the regulation of procollagen type I and MMP-1 expression. *Food & function, 5*(2), 265–274. https://doi.org/10.1039/c3fo60418g

Althaea rosea flower extract Antimicrobial, anti-inflammatory, antioxidant properties. Contains plant compounds **quercetin, anthocyanin, kaempferol, linoleic** etc.

- Fahamiya, N., Shiffa, M., & Aslam, M. (2016). A Comprehensive Review on Althaea rosea Linn. *Journal of Pharmaceutical Research*, 6(11).
- Al-Snafi, A. E. (2013). The pharmaceutical importance of Althaea officinalis and Althaea rosea: A review. *Int J Pharm Tech Res*, 5(3), 1387-1385.

Plankton: While there is no research specifically on plankton extract, it is a type of **marine algae**. Marine algae has **moisture** binding properties, are potent **antioxidants**, and has skin **anti-aging** properties. It is also **anti-melanogenic** to combat pigmentation.

- Kim, J. H., Lee, J. E., Kim, K. H., & Kang, N. J. (2018). Beneficial Effects of Marine Algae-Derived Carbohydrates for Skin Health. *Marine drugs, 16*(11), 459. https://doi.org/10.3390/md16110459

Nymphea alba flower (Lotus): **antioxidant**, contains **tannins, alkaloids, flavonoids, polysaccharides** which have **moisturizing** effects

- Cudalbeanu, M., Ghinea, I. O., Furdui, B., Dah-Nouvlessounon, D., Raclea, R., Costache, T., Cucolea, I. E., Urlan, F., & Dinica, R. M. (2018). Exploring New Antioxidant and Mineral Compounds from *Nymphaea alba* Wild-Grown in Danube Delta Biosphere. *Molecules (Basel, Switzerland), 23*(6), 1247. https://doi.org/10.3390/molecules23061247

Caprylic triglyceride: derived from **coconut oil** and **glycerin**. Works as an **antioxidant, emollient,** dispersing agent. Mix of fatty acids that skin can use to prevent **transepidermal water loss.**

- K.A Traul, A Driedger, D.L Ingle, D Nakhasi.Review of the toxicologic properties of medium-chain triglycerides, Food and Chemical Toxicology, Volume 38, Issue 1,
- 2000, Pages 79-98, ISSN 0278-6915, https://doi.org/10.1016/S0278-6915(99)00106-4.

Macademia seed oil: high in **monounsaturated fatty acids**, and contains **vitamin E** (tocotrienol and tocopherol) which are natural antioxidants. These antioxidants can reduce **inflammation** and **oxidative stress** of the skin. This vegetable oil can penetrate the skin because the components in it are very similar to the skin's natural oils, and serve to maintain moisture and nourish the skin.

- Hanum, T. I., Laila, L., Sumaiyah, S., & Syahrina, E. (2019). Macadamia Nuts Oil in Nanocream and Conventional Cream as Skin Anti-Aging: A Comparative Study. *Open access Macedonian journal of medical sciences, 7*(22), 3917–3920. https://doi.org/10.3889/oamjms.2019.533

Sunflower seed oil: The components of sunflower oil mainly consist of **oleic** and **linoleic acids**. Linoleic acid serves as an agonist at peroxisome proliferator-activated receptor-alpha (PPAR-α), which enhances keratinocyte proliferation and lipid synthesis. This in turn enhances **skin barrier repair**. This property makes sunflower oil a suitable ingredient in skin products due to the positive benefits of linoleic acid

- Lin, T. K., Zhong, L., & Santiago, J. L. (2017). Anti-Inflammatory and Skin Barrier Repair Effects of Topical Application of Some Plant Oils. *International journal of molecular sciences, 19*(1), 70. https://doi.org/10.3390/ijms19010070

Sunflower seed oil preserves stratum corneum integrity, did not cause erythema, and improved hydration in the same volunteers.

- Danby, S. G., AlEnezi, T., Sultan, A., Lavender, T., Chittock, J., Brown, K., & Cork, M. J. (2013). Effect of olive and sunflower seed oil on the adult skin barrier: implications for neonatal skin care. *Pediatric dermatology, 30*(1), 42–50. https://doi.org/10.1111/j.1525-1470.2012.01865.x

Shea butter: Shea butter is composed of **triglycerides** with **oleic, stearic, linoleic, and palmitic fatty acids**, as well as unsaponifiable compounds. Shea butter is frequently used in the cosmetic industry due to its high percentage of the unsaponifiable fraction (e.g., **triterpenes, tocopherol, phenols, and sterols**), which possesses potent **anti-inflammatory** and **antioxidant** properties. In the study of lipopolysaccharide-activated macrophage cells, shea butter exhibited anti-inflammatory effects through inhibition of iNOS, COX-2, and cytokines via the NF-κB pathway. Additional research on AD has shown that the cream containing shea butter extract had the same efficacy as ceramide-precursor product.

- Danby, S. G., AlEnezi, T., Sultan, A., Lavender, T., Chittock, J., Brown, K., & Cork, M. J. (2013). Effect of olive and sunflower seed oil on the adult skin barrier: implications for neonatal skin care. *Pediatric dermatology*, *30*(1), 42–50. https://doi.org/10.1111/j.1525-1470.2012.01865.x

The cream containing shea butter extract did not differ in acceptability or efficacy from a ceramide-precursor product.

- Hon, K. L., Tsang, Y. C., Pong, N. H., Lee, V. W., Luk, N. M., Chow, C. M., & Leung, T. F. (2015). Patient acceptability, efficacy, and skin biophysiology of a cream and cleanser containing lipid complex with shea butter extract versus a ceramide product for eczema. *Hong Kong medical journal = Xianggang yi xue za zhi, 21*(5), 417–425. https://doi.org/10.12809/hkmj144472

Beeswax: Beeswax is mainly used as an emulsifying agent. In cosmetics, beeswax is used as a stiffener, a substance providing elasticity, plasticity and increasing skin adhesiveness. Beeswax is the base for lipsticks, sticks and creams. Beeswax has lubricating, softening activities and **reduces transepidermal water loss** from skin. **Sterols**, which are also components of intercellular space, provide these characteristics of beeswax. **Squalene,**

10-hydroxy-*trans*-2-decenoic acid and **flavonoids** (chrysin) provide **antiseptic** properties to this product, and protect the skin against pathogenic microorganisms. Beeswax constitutes a protective barrier against many external factors by forming a film on the skin surface. **β-carotene** present in beeswax is a valuable source of **vitamin A**, into which it is converted. Vitamin A delays **collagen** degradation, stimulates mitotic division in the epidermis, thus leads to sooner regeneration of the skin after damage

- Kurek-Górecka, A., Górecki, M., Rzepecka-Stojko, A., Balwierz, R., & Stojko, J. (2020). Bee Products in Dermatology and Skin Care. *Molecules (Basel, Switzerland)*, *25*(3), 556. https://doi.org/10.3390/molecules25030556

Corylus avellana(hazelnut): anti-inflammatory activity, skin conditioning ingredient, emollient.

- Final Report on the Safety Assessment of Corylus Avellana (Hazel) Seed Oil, Corylus Americana (Hazel) Seed Oil, Corylus Avellana (Hazel) Seed Extract, Corylus Americana (Hazel) Seed Extract, Corylus Rostrata (Hazel) Seed Extract, Corylus Avellana (Hazel) Leaf Extract, Corylus Americana (Hazel) Leaf Extract, and Corylus Rostrata (Hazel) Leaf Extract. (2001). International Journal of Toxicology, 20(1_suppl), 15–20. https://doi.org/10.1080/109158101750300928

Simmondsia Chinensis (jojoba): The review of literatures suggest that jojoba has **anti-inflammatory** effect and it can be used on a variety of skin conditions including skin infections, skin aging, as well as wound healing. Moreover, jojoba has been shown to play a role in cosmetics formulas such as sunscreens and moisturizers and also enhances the absorption of topical drugs.

- Pazyar, N., Yaghoobi, R., Ghassemi, M. R., Kazerouni, A., Rafeie, E., & Jamshydian, N. (2013). Jojoba in dermatology: a succinct review. *Giornale italiano di dermatologia e venereologia : organo ufficiale, Societa italiana di dermatologia e sifilografia, 148*(6), 687–691.

Snail Secretion Filtrate: Daily application of topical products containing SCA proved effective and well tolerated for improvement in coarse **eye wrinkles** (rhytides) and fine facial rhytides.Important biological effects on cell proliferation and migration.

- Fabi, S. G., Cohen, J. L., Peterson, J. D., Kiripolsky, M. G., & Goldman, M. P. (2013). The Effects of Filtrate of the Secretion of the Cryptomphalus Aspersa on Photoaged Skin. *Journal of drugs in dermatology : JDD, 12*(4), 453–457.
- Trapella, C., Rizzo, R., Gallo, S., Alogna, A., Bortolotti, D., Casciano, F., Zauli, G., Secchiero, P., & Voltan, R. (2018). HelixComplex snail mucus exhibits pro-survival, proliferative and pro-migration effects on mammalian fibroblasts. *Scientific reports, 8*(1), 17665. https://doi.org/10.1038/s41598-018-35816-3

Bambusa Vulgaris: extract from the bamboo plant, **antioxidant** accelerates **wound healing, anti-inflammatory**

- Lodhi, S., Jain, A. P., Rai, G., & Yadav, A. K. (2016). Preliminary investigation for wound healing and anti-inflammatory effects of Bambusa vulgaris leaves in rats. *Journal of Ayurveda and integrative medicine, 7*(1), 14–22. https://doi.org/10.1016/j.jaim.2015.07.001
- Panee J. (2015). Potential Medicinal Application and Toxicity Evaluation of Extracts from Bamboo Plants. *Journal of medicinal plant research, 9*(23), 681–692. https://doi.org/10.5897/jmpr2014.5657

Inulin : **prebiotics** for skin, reduces the growth of **bacteria**, maintains skin **microbiome**, naturally occurring fructose **polysaccharide** found in **chicory root**

- https://www.news-medical.net/whitepaper/20200923/Is-There-Evidence-for-Topical-Prebiotics-for-a-Balanced-Skin-Microbiome.aspx

Rosa Damascena Flower Oil: Often used as a **fragrance** in cosmetics, it is **antibacterial**, **antiseptic**, and an **antioxidant**.

- Boskabady, Mohammad Hossein et al. "Pharmacological effects of rosa damascena." *Iranian journal of basic medical sciences* vol. 14,4 (2011): 295-307.

Boswellia Carterii Resin Extract (Frankincense): Contains Boswellic acid (BA), which are pentacyclic **triterpenes** with strong **anti-inflammatory** activity. We registered a significant improvement of **roughness** and **fine lines** in the half side of the face treated with BAs; noninvasive instrumental diagnostic investigations showed an improvement of elasticity, a decrease of sebum excretion, and a change of echographic parameters suggesting a reshaping of dermal tissue

- Pedretti, A., Capezzera, R., Zane, C., Facchinetti, E., & Calzavara-Pinton, P. (2010). Effects of topical boswellic acid on photo and age-damaged skin: clinical, biophysical, and echographic evaluations in a double-blind, randomized, split-face study. *Planta medica*, 76(6), 555–560. https://doi.org/10.1055/s-0029-1240581

Betula Alba Juice (Birch): Results show that **flavonoid** and phenolic acid rich CRB possesses **antioxidant** activity and stimulates dermal fibroblast proliferation at low concentration.

- Boroduškis, M., Kaktiņa, E., Blāķe, I., Nakurte, I., Dzabijeva, D., Kusiņa, I., ... & Ramata-Stunda, A. Chemical characterization and in vitro evaluation of birch sap and a complex of plant extracts for potential use in cosmetic anti-ageing products.

Vanilla planifolia fruit extract: antioxidant, source of **catechins**. Consists mostly of **vanillin** (80%)

- https://www.cir-safety.org/sites/default/files/vanill042018 slr.pdf

Honey: Contains several unique **antibacterial** components. These components are believed to act on diverse bacterial targets, are broad spectrum, operate synergistically, and decrease production of virulence factors. Moreover, honey has the ability to block bacterial communication, and therefore, it is unlikely that bacteria will develop resistance against honey, unlike conventional antibiotics.

Honey only targets pathogenic bacteria without disturbing the growth of a normal gut microbiome when taken orally. It also contains **prebiotics**, **probiotics**, and **zinc** and enhances the growth of beneficial gut flora.
- Hussain M. B. (2018). Role of Honey in Topical and Systemic Bacterial Infections. *Journal of alternative and complementary medicine (New York, N.Y.)*, *24*(1), 15–24. https://doi.org/10.1089/acm.2017.0017

Lactic acid bacteria: Topical application of lactic acid is effective for **depigmentation** and improving the surface roughness and mild wrinkling of the skin caused by environmental photo-damage. The oral administration of Lactobacillus delbrueckii and other lactic acid bacteria has been reported to inhibit the development of atopic diseases.
Mechanism: Previous studies have reported the beneficial effects of lactic acid bacteria, their extracts or ferments on skin health, including improvements in skin conditions and the prevention of skin diseases. Lipoteichoic acid isolated from Lactobacillus plantarum was reported to **inhibit melanogenesis** in B16F10 melanoma cells. In particular, lipoteichoic acid also exerted **anti-photoaging** effects on human skin cells by regulating the expression of matrix metalloproteinase- 1.
- Huang, H. C., Lee, I. J., Huang, C., & Chang, T. M. (2020). Lactic Acid Bacteria and Lactic Acid for Skin Health and Melanogenesis Inhibition. Current pharmaceutical biotechnology, 21(7), 566–577. https://doi.org/10.2174/1389201021666200109104701

Bifidobacterium longum lysate: Using a probiotic lysate, Bifidobacterium longum sp. extract (BL), applied to the skin was able to *improve **sensitive** skin.*

Significant decrease in skin dryness after 29 days for volunteers treated with the cream containing the 10% bacterial extract.

- Guéniche, A., Bastien, P., Ovigne, J. M., Kermici, M., Courchay, G., Chevalier, V., Breton, L., & Castiel-Higounenc, I. (2010). Bifidobacterium longum lysate, a new ingredient for reactive skin. *Experimental dermatology*, *19*(8), e1–e8. https://doi.org/10.1111/j.1600-0625.2009.00932.x

Paeonia lactiflora root extract (peony): the **depigmenting** potential of **paeoniflorin** in cosmetic applications for treating hyperpigmentation.

Resveratroloside (trans-resveratrol-4'-O-beta-d-glucopyranoside) was found to be the main metabolite of P. officinalis subsp. officinalis seeds and its tyrosinase inhibiting activity was confirmed via an enzymatic assay.

- Qiu, J., Chen, M., Liu, J., Huang, X., Chen, J., Zhou, L., Ma, J., Sextius, P., Pena, A. M., Cai, Z., & Jeulin, S. (2016). The skin-depigmenting potential of Paeonia lactiflora root extract and paeoniflorin: in vitro evaluation using reconstructed pigmented human epidermis. *International journal of cosmetic science*, *38*(5), 444–451. https://doi.org/10.1111/ics.12309
- Rainer, B., Revoltella, S., Mayr, F., Moesslacher, J., Scalfari, V., Kohl, R., Waltenberger, B., Pagitz, K., Siewert, B., Schwaiger, S., & Stuppner, H. (2019). From bench to counter: Discovery and validation of a peony extract as tyrosinase inhibiting cosmeceutical. *European journal of medicinal chemistry*, *184*, 111738. https://doi.org/10.1016/j.ejmech.2019.111738

Sea Buckthorn extract: anti-inflammatory and **anti-psoriatic** efficacies of a neutraceutical sea buckthorn oil (SBKT) derived from the fruit pulp of *Hippophae rhamnoides*. Chemical analysis of the SBKT showed the presence of 16 major saturated, mono-, and polyunsaturated fatty acids components, imparting significant nutritional values.

- Balkrishna, A., Sakat, S. S., Joshi, K., Joshi, K., Sharma, V., Ranjan, R., Bhattacharya, K., & Varshney, A. (2019). Cytokines Driven Anti-Inflammatory and Anti-Psoriasis Like Efficacies of Nutraceutical Sea Buckthorn (*Hippophae rhamnoides*) Oil. *Frontiers in pharmacology, 10*, 1186. https://doi.org/10.3389/fphar.2019.01186

A balanced composition of fatty acids give the number of vitamins or their range in this oil and explains its frequent use in cosmetic products for the care of dry, flaky or rapidly aging skin. Moreover, its unique unsaturated fatty acids, such as palmitooleic acid (**omega-7**) and gamma-linolenic acid (**omega-6**), give sea-buckthorn oil its **skin regeneration** and cell repair properties.

Sea-buckthorn oil also improves blood circulation, facilitates oxygenation of the skin, removes excess toxins from the body and easily penetrates through the epidermis. Because inside the skin the gamma-linolenic acid is converted to **prostaglandins**, sea-buckthorn oil protects against **infections**, prevents allergies, eliminates inflammation and inhibits the aging process.

- Zielińska, A., & Nowak, I. (2017). Abundance of active ingredients in sea-buckthorn oil. *Lipids in health and disease, 16*(1), 95. https://doi.org/10.1186/s12944-017-0469-7

Safflower Seed (*Charthamus tinctorius* L., SSO): Anti-wrinkle, protect against skin photoaging. Contains significantly high levels of **unsaturated fatty acids** and phytochemicals. SSO has been traditionally used in China, Japan, and Korea to improve skin and hair. Taken together, these results indicate that SSO and its active compound **acacetin** can prevent UVB-induced MMP-1 expression, which leads to skin **photoaging**, and may therefore have therapeutic potential as an **anti-wrinkle** agent to improve skin health.

Antioxidant, antibacterial, antifungal
A notable antioxidant capacity was demonstrated for the tested oil that exhibited high antibacterial effects by both bacteriostatic and bactericidal pathways including lysozyme activity.

- Khémiri, I., Essghaier, B., Sadfi-Zouaoui, N., & Bitri, L. (2020). Antioxidant and Antimicrobial Potentials of Seed Oil from *Carthamus tinctorius L.* in the Management of Skin Injuries. *Oxidative medicine and cellular longevity*, *2020*, 4103418. https://doi.org/10.1155/2020/4103418

Almond: antibacterial, antiviral
Here, we tested the antibacterial and antiviral effect of a mix of **polyphenols** present in natural almond skin. Amongst the isolated compounds, the **aglycones, epicatechin** and **catechin** showed the greatest activity against *S. a*ureus but were not active against all the other strains.

- Musarra-Pizzo, M., Ginestra, G., Smeriglio, A., Pennisi, R., Sciortino, M. T., & Mandalari, G. (2019). The Antimicrobial and Antiviral Activity of Polyphenols from Almond (*Prunus dulcis* L.) Skin. *Nutrients*, *11*(10), 2355. https://doi.org/10.3390/nu11102355

Anti-inflammatory, promotes lipolysis aka breakdown of fat cells.

- Huang, W. C., Chen, C. Y., & Wu, S. J. (2017). Almond Skin Polyphenol Extract Inhibits Inflammation and Promotes Lipolysis in Differentiated 3T3-L1 Adipocytes. *Journal of medicinal food*, *20*(2), 103–109. https://doi.org/10.1089/jmf.2016.3806

Flaxseed Oil: FFSO can alleviate symptoms of **eczema** such as epithelial damage, redness, swelling, and pruritus.

- Yang, J., Min, S., & Hong, S. (2017). Therapeutic Effects of Fermented Flax Seed Oil on NC/Nga Mice with Atopic Dermatitis-Like Skin Lesions. *Evidence-based complementary and alternative medicine : eCAM, 2017,* 5469125. https://doi.org/10.1155/2017/5469125

Panax ginseng: prevent skin wrinkles through **polysaccharide** content - **antioxidant, anti-aging** effects
- **Ginsenosides** have been proposed to account for most of the biological activities of ginseng. Sabouri-Rad, S., Sabouri-Rad, S., Sahebkar, A., & Tayarani-Najaran, Z. (2017). Ginseng in Dermatology: A Review. *Current pharmaceutical design, 23*(11), 1649–1666. https://doi.org/10.2174/1381612822666161021152322

Hair growth - a wide variety of structurally diverse classes of phytochemicals, including those present in ginseng, have demonstrated hair growth-promoting effects in a large number of preclinical studies.
- Choi B. Y. (2018). Hair-Growth Potential of Ginseng and Its Major Metabolites: A Review on Its Molecular Mechanisms. *International journal of molecular sciences, 19*(9), 2703. https://doi.org/10.3390/ijms19092703

Also has **antimelanogenesis** properties and skin-protective properties through regulation of activator protein 1 and cyclic adenosine monophosphate response element-binding protein signaling. Used as a skin-improving agent, with **moisture** retention and **whitening** effects.
- Lee, J. O., Kim, E., Kim, J. H., Hong, Y. H., Kim, H. G., Jeong, D., Kim, J., Kim, S. H., Park, C., Seo, D. B., Son, Y. J., Han, S. Y., & Cho, J. Y. (2018). Antimelanogenesis and skin-protective activities of *Panax ginseng* calyx ethanol extract. *Journal of ginseng research, 42*(3), 389–399. https://doi.org/10.1016/j.jgr.2018.02.007
- Kim, J. E., Jang, S. G., Lee, C. H., Lee, J. Y., Park, H., Kim, J. H., Lee, S., Kim, S. H., Park, E. Y., Lee, K. W., & Shin, H. S. (2019). Beneficial effects on skin health using polysaccharides from red ginseng by-product. *Journal of*

food biochemistry, *43*(8), e12961.
https://doi.org/10.1111/jfbc.12961

Dianella Ensifolia: Effective for **hyperpigmentation**, reduction of **discoloration**, and inhibition of free radicals and lipid oxidation. Produced an increase in the rate of depigmentation compared to two pharmaceutical treatments containing hydroquinone.

- Mammone, T., Muizzuddin, N., Declercq, L., Clio, D., Corstjens, H., Sente, I., Van Rillaer, K., Matsui, M., Niki, Y., Ichihashi, M., Giacomoni, P. U., & Yarosh, D. (2010). Modification of skin discoloration by a topical treatment containing an extract of Dianella ensifolia: a potent antioxidant. *Journal of cosmetic dermatology*, *9*(2), 89–95. https://doi.org/10.1111/j.1473-2165.2010.00491.x

St. John's wort (Hypericum perforatum): **antioxidant, anti-inflammatory,** anticancer, and **antimicrobial** activities.

- Wölfle U, Seelinger G, Schempp CM. Topical application of St. John's wort (Hypericum perforatum). Planta Med. 2014 Feb;80(2-3):109-20. doi: 10.1055/s-0033-1351019. Epub 2013 Nov 8. PMID: 24214835.

Black elder (Sambucus nigra L): antiviral and **antimicrobial** properties have been demonstrated in these extracts, against **photoaging** and **inflammation**
Potential to ameliorate UVB-induced skin **photoaging** and **inflammation.** Mechanism: EB notably decreased UVB-induced **matrix metalloproteinase-1** (MMP-1) expression and inflammatory cytokine secretion through the inhibition of mitogen-activated protein kinases/activator protein 1 (MAPK/AP-1) and nuclear factor-κB (NF-κB) signaling pathways, blocking extracellular matrix (ECM) degradation and inflammation in UVB-irradiated HaCaTs.

- Lin P, Hwang E, Ngo HTT, Seo SA, Yi TH. Sambucus nigra L. ameliorates UVB-induced photoaging and inflammatory response in human skin keratinocytes.

Cytotechnology. 2019 Oct;71(5):1003-1017. doi: 10.1007/s10616-019-00342-1. Epub 2019 Sep 11. PMID: 31512082; PMCID: PMC6787119.

Artocarpus lakoocha: high nutritional and antioxidant values, reduction of **melanin** in combination with **licorice**, skin **whitening**. In combination with Licorice, *Artocarpus lakoocha* (Al) and *Glycyrrhiza glabra* (Gg) extracts have been reported to show **tyrosinase** inhibitory activity and melanin pigment reduction.

- Panichakul T, Rodboon T, Suwannalert P, Tripetch C, Rungruang R, Boohuad N, Youdee P. Additive Effect of a Combination of *Artocarpus lakoocha* and *Glycyrrhiza glabra* Extracts on Tyrosinase Inhibition in Melanoma B16 Cells. Pharmaceuticals (Basel). 2020 Oct 14;13(10):310. doi: 10.3390/ph13100310. PMID: 33066628; PMCID: PMC7602378.

The A. lakoocha extract was the most effective agent, giving the shortest onset of significant whitening effect after only 4 weeks of application

- Tengamnuay P, Pengrungruangwong K, Pheansri I, Likhitwitayawuid K. Artocarpus lakoocha heartwood extract as a novel cosmetic ingredient: evaluation of the in vitro anti-tyrosinase and in vivo skin whitening activities. *Int J Cosmet Sci.* 2006;28(4):269-276. doi:10.1111/j.1467-2494.2006.00339.x

Artocarpus altilis (Moreceae): photoprotection i.e. suppresses structural alterations in skin damaged by ultraviolet radiation B irradiation. Mediated by decrease in MMP-1 production in fibroblasts and TNF-α and IL-6 productions in keratinocytes.

- Tiraravesit N, Yakaew S, Rukchay R, Luangbudnark W, Viennet C, Humbert P, Viyoch J. Artocarpus altilis heartwood extract protects skin against UVB in vitro and in vivo. J Ethnopharmacol. 2015 Dec 4;175:153-62. doi: 10.1016/j.jep.2015.09.023. Epub 2015 Sep 18. PMID: 26387741.

Turmeric (Curcuma longa): anti inflammatory, antimicrobial, antioxidant, and anti-neoplastic properties, mainly due to **Curcumin.**
Ten studies noted statistically significant improvement in skin disease severity in the turmeric/curcumin treatment groups compared with control groups.

- Vaughn, A. R., Branum, A., & Sivamani, R. K. (2016). Effects of Turmeric (Curcuma longa) on Skin Health: A Systematic Review of the Clinical Evidence. *Phytotherapy research : PTR, 30*(8), 1243–1264. https://doi.org/10.1002/ptr.5640

Lithospermum erythrorhizon: anti-inflammation, antioxidant, **antiaging,** moisturizing properties. By inhibiting glycation, modulating oxidative stress, suppressing inflammation and UV-absorptive properties

- Glynn, K. M., Anderson, P., Fast, D. J., Koedam, J., Rebhun, J. F., & Velliquette, R. A. (2018). Gromwell (Lithospermum erythrorhizon) root extract protects against glycation and related inflammatory and oxidative stress while offering UV absorption capability. *Experimental dermatology, 27*(9), 1043–1047. https://doi.org/10.1111/exd.13706

These results suggest that LE-derived extracts may protect oxidative-stress-induced skin aging by inhibiting degradation of skin collagen, and that this protection may derive at least in part from the antioxidant phenolics present in these extracts.

- Yoo, H. G., Lee, B. H., Kim, W., Lee, J. S., Kim, G. H., Chun, O. K., Koo, S. I., & Kim, D. O. (2014). Lithospermum erythrorhizon extract protects keratinocytes and fibroblasts against oxidative stress. *Journal of medicinal food, 17*(11), 1189–1196. https://doi.org/10.1089/jmf.2013.3088

Taken together, our data demonstrate that LES is more effective in increasing skin humidity and decreasing the TEWL values,

- Chang, M. J., Huang, H. C., Chang, H. C., & Chang, T. M. (2008). Cosmetic formulations containing Lithospermum erythrorhizon root extract show moisturizing effects on human skin. *Archives of dermatological research*, *300*(6), 317–323. https://doi.org/10.1007/s00403-008-0867-9

Squalane (olive): is commonly harvested from plant sources like olives, wheat germ oil, and rice bran. Used as an **emollient** and **antioxidant**, good for skin hydration as reduces water loss. An added advantage of squalane is that even though it is technically an oil, it does not have a greasy feel, is odorless, **non comedogenic**, **antibacterial**, and is safe for sensitive skin.

- Sethi, A., Kaur, T., Malhotra, S. K., & Gambhir, M. L. (2016). Moisturizers: The Slippery Road. Indian journal of dermatology, 61(3), 279–287. https://doi.org/10.4103/0019-5154.182427

Bakuchiol: Bakuchiol is derived from the seeds and leaves of the plant **psoralea corylifolia**. It is claimed that it is a "**functional analogue of retinol**" based on its effects on gene expression profiles of skin cells in vitro. Studies have shown functional similarities to retinoids without the limiting side effects, such as erythema, burning, and stinging. Not enough evidence to show superiority to retinol.
- Wang, J. V., Schoenberg, E., & Saedi, N. (2019). Bakuchiol as a Trendy Ingredient in Skincare: Recent Evidence. *Skinmed*, *17*(3), 188–189.
- Spierings NMK. Cosmetic commentary: Is bakuchiol the new "skincare hero"? Journal of Cosmetic Dermatology. 2020 Dec;19(12):3208-3209. DOI: 10.1111/jocd.13708.

Citrus Aurantium Dulcis (orange) Peel Oil: Often used as fragrance, contains antioxidants but high methanol content may cause **irritation**.

Lactobacillus Ferment Lysate: Production of cytokines such as

IL-10, IL-12, IFN-γ, and TNF-α was significantly increased. These have **anti-inflammatory** effects on the skin.

Bisabolol: It is also referred to as alpha-bisabolol, is a monocyclic **sesquiterpene** alcohol or a natural component of **essential oils. Anti-inflammatory** as it inhibits proinflammatory cytokines. Also possesses **bactericidal** and **fungicidal** properties against certain strains of fungus and bacteria. **Antioxidant** properties.

Camellia Oleifera (Tsubaki) Seed oil: oleic acid rich, **inhibits melanogenesis** via inhibition of **tyrosinase, antioxidant** activity.
- Chaikul P, Sripisut T, Chanpirom S, Sathirachawan K, Ditthawuthikul N. Melanogenesis Inhibitory and Antioxidant Effects of Camellia oleifera Seed Oil. Adv Pharm Bull. 2017;7(3):473-477. doi:10.15171/apb.2017.057

Opuntia Ficus-indica (Prickly Pear) Seed Oil: Contains high content of **linoleic acid**, helps to keep skin hydrated. Effective carrier oil, helps to deliver other ingredients (e.g Vit A) into skin, **antioxidant and antibacterial** effects
- AlZahabi S, Sakr OS, Ramadan AA. Nanostructured lipid carriers incorporating prickly pear seed oil for the encapsulation of vitamin A. Journal of Cosmetic Dermatology. 2019 Dec;18(6):1875-1884. DOI: 10.1111/jocd.12891.

Vitis Vinifera (grapeseed) Seed oil: Grape seed extract has the ability to release **endothelial growth factor** and its topical application results in contraction and closure of the skin wound. Furthermore, it possesses **antioxidant** and **antibacterial** properties.
- Hemmati, A. A., Foroozan, M., Houshmand, G., Moosavi, Z. B., Bahadoram, M., & Maram, N. S. (2014). The topical effect of grape seed extract 2% cream on surgery wound healing. *Global journal of health science*, 7(3), 52–58. https://doi.org/10.5539/gjhs.v7n3p52

Camelina Sativa Seed oil: rich in **omega 3 fatty acids - alpha linoleic acid,** high content of **vitamin E, alpha tocopherol,** rich in **antioxidants**

- Budin JT, Breene WM, Putman D. Some compositional properties of camelina (camelina sativa L. Crantz) seeds and oils. *Journal of the American Oil Chemists' Society.* 1995;72(3):309-315. doi:10.1007/BF02541088

Aesculus Hippocastanum (Horse chestnut) extract: contains **saponins** known as **aescin,** are potent **anti-inflammatory** compounds. Said to have more powerful antioxidant capabilities than vitamin E. Aescin also reduces capillary fragility, and therefore helps to prevent leakage of fluids into surrounding tissues, which can cause swelling. Can help to reduce swelling and puffiness.

- Wilkinson JA, Brown AM. Horse Chestnut - Aesculus Hippocastanum: Potential Applications in Cosmetic Skin-care Products. Int J Cosmet Sci. 1999 Dec;21(6):437-47. doi: 10.1046/j.1467-2494.1999.234192.x. PMID: 18503457.

***Alteromonas* ferment extract:** It is an **exopolysaccharide** produced by an extremophile that lives in deep-sea hydrothermal vents. In in vitro keratinocyte models they showed that it protected against UV-induced lipid peroxidation. In vitro it was shown to strongly chelate cadmium and lead. In vivo they showed that it created a protective film on the skin that limited fine particle adhesion and improved **barrier** function.

- Garre, A., Martinez-Masana, G., Piquero-Casals, J., & Granger, C. (2017). Redefining face contour with a novel anti-aging cosmetic product: an open-label, prospective clinical study. *Clinical, cosmetic and investigational dermatology, 10,* 473–482. https://doi.org/10.2147/CCID.S148597

Lavandula Angustifolia (lavender): Promotes healing of skin tissue, can also be an allergen as it contains **geranoil, linalool,** and **linalyl acetate** which are known contact allergens.

- Mori, H. M., Kawanami, H., Kawahata, H., & Aoki, M. (2016). Wound healing potential of lavender oil by acceleration of granulation and wound contraction through induction of TGF-β in a rat model. *BMC complementary and alternative medicine, 16,* 144. https://doi.org/10.1186/s12906-016-1128-7

Madecassoside: component of **Centella Asiatica,** used as **wound healing** agent, **non-sensitizing,** high antioxidant content.

- Bylka, W., Znajdek-Awiżeń, P., Studzińska-Sroka, E., & Brzezińska, M. (2013). Centella asiatica in cosmetology. *Postepy dermatologii i alergologii, 30*(1), 46–49. https://doi.org/10.5114/pdia.2013.33378

Helianthus annuus (sunflower) seed oil: primary function is an **emollient.** Contains fatty acids that help to restore skin's natural barrier function. A 2013 study examined the effects of sunflower seed oil on the adult **skin barrier** and found that the oil preserved stratum corneum integrity, did not cause erythema, and improved hydration in the volunteers.

- Danby SG, AlEnezi T, Sultan A, Lavender T, Chittock J, Brown K, Cork MJ. Effect of olive and sunflower seed oil on the adult skin barrier: implications for neonatal skin care. Pediatr Dermatol. 2013 Jan-Feb;30(1):42-50. doi: 10.1111/j.1525-1470.2012.01865.x. Epub 2012 Sep 20. PMID: 22995032.

Arnica Montana Flower Extract: topical treatment with *Arnica montana* reduced the UVB-induced **inflammatory** response, alleviates **oxidative damage** induced by UVB exposure. Mechanism of action is through inhibition of myeloperoxidase activation, decrease of nuclear factor kappa B levels and reduction of proinflammatory cytokines levels.

- da Silva Prade J, Bálsamo EC, Machado FR, Poetini MR,

Bortolotto VC, Araújo SM, Londero L, Boeira SP, Sehn CP, de Gomes MG, Prigol M, Cattelan Souza L. Anti-inflammatory effect of Arnica montana in a UVB radiation-induced skin-burn model in mice. Cutan Ocul Toxicol. 2020 Jun;39(2):126-133. doi: 10.1080/15569527.2020.1743998. Epub 2020 Mar 30. PMID: 32183539.

Gentiana Lutea Root Extract: Anti-inflammatory agent, with mechanisms related to regulation of pro-inflammatory cytokines such as TNF-α and IFN-γ.
In animal studies, topical application alleviated skin lesions such as surface roughness, excoriations and scabs on the skin of contact dermatitis.

- Yang B, Kim S, Kim JH, Lim C, Kim H, Cho S. Gentiana scabra Bunge roots alleviates skin lesions of contact dermatitis in mice. J Ethnopharmacol. 2019 Apr 6;233:141-147. doi: 10.1016/j.jep.2018.12.046. Epub 2019 Jan 7. PMID: 30630090.

SECTION 5

Course Workbook 1

download textbook resources and printables*

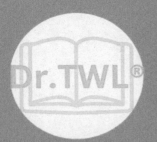

ACNE WORKBOOK

DERM'S ACNE CHEATSHEET
A Practical Guide

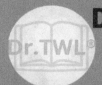

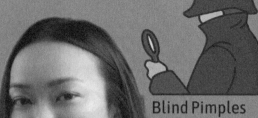

Blind Pimples

5 PILLARS

Acne Types
Comedones
Papules
Cysts

PRACTICAL TIPS

Pus?
Pain?
Conceal?
Rapid healing?
Injection?

ACNE TREATMENT

Whiteheads
Blackheads
Pustules

Skincare Routine Must-Haves

- Antibacterial skin cleanser
- I use a honey-based formula instead of chemical alternatives like triclosan or chlorhexidine (bad for the microbiome).
- Spot Treatment
- Berberine, chlorella vulgaris (an algae-extract) and botanical actives are my top choice
- Vitamin C serum
- Antioxidants improve acne–Oxidative stress worsens inflammation—this drives comedone formation. Vitamin C works by making the skin microenvironment inhospitable for germs like P.acnes (also known as cutibacterium acnes). If you have sensitive skin, avoid L-ascorbic acid formulations, use Sodium Ascorbyl Phosphate or Magnesium Ascorbyl Phosphate which are neutral salts instead.

CLEANSER

SERUM

SPOT CREAM

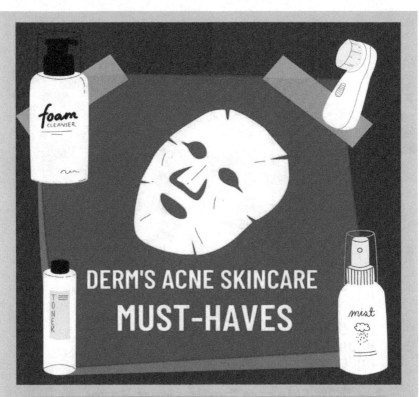

Skin Goals:

Skin Health Profile:

Skincare Recommendations:

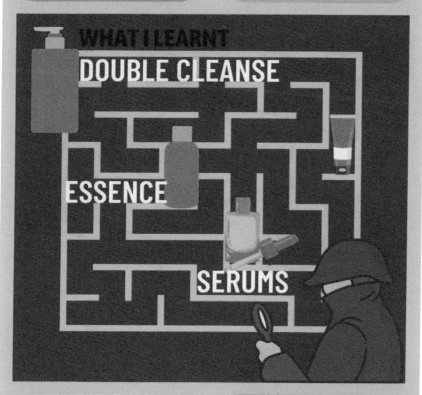

SERUMS

SPOT TREATMENT

CLEANSING NOTES

FACIAL ESSENCE

WHAT I WILL IMPLEMENT /CHANGE

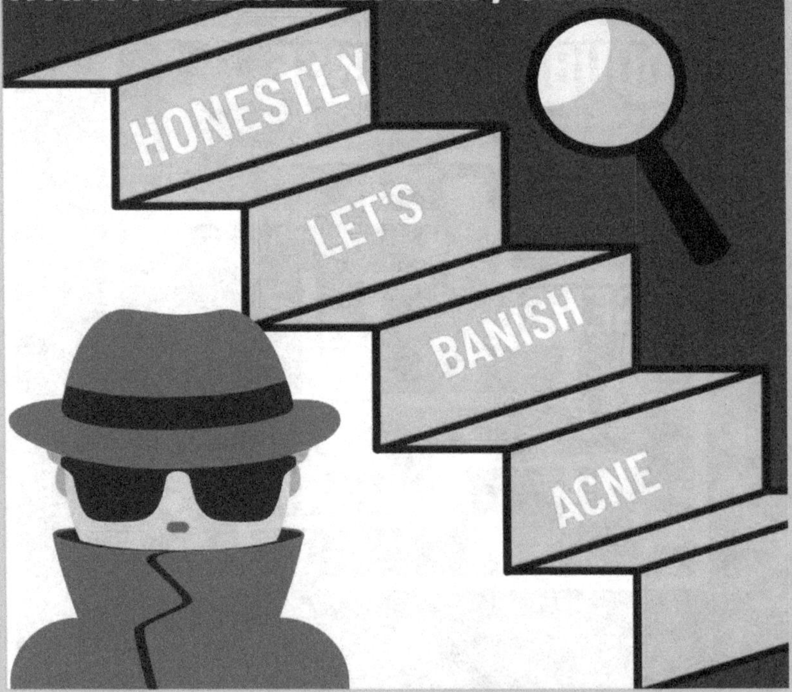

HONESTLY LET'S BANISH ACNE

SERUMS

SPOT TREATMENT

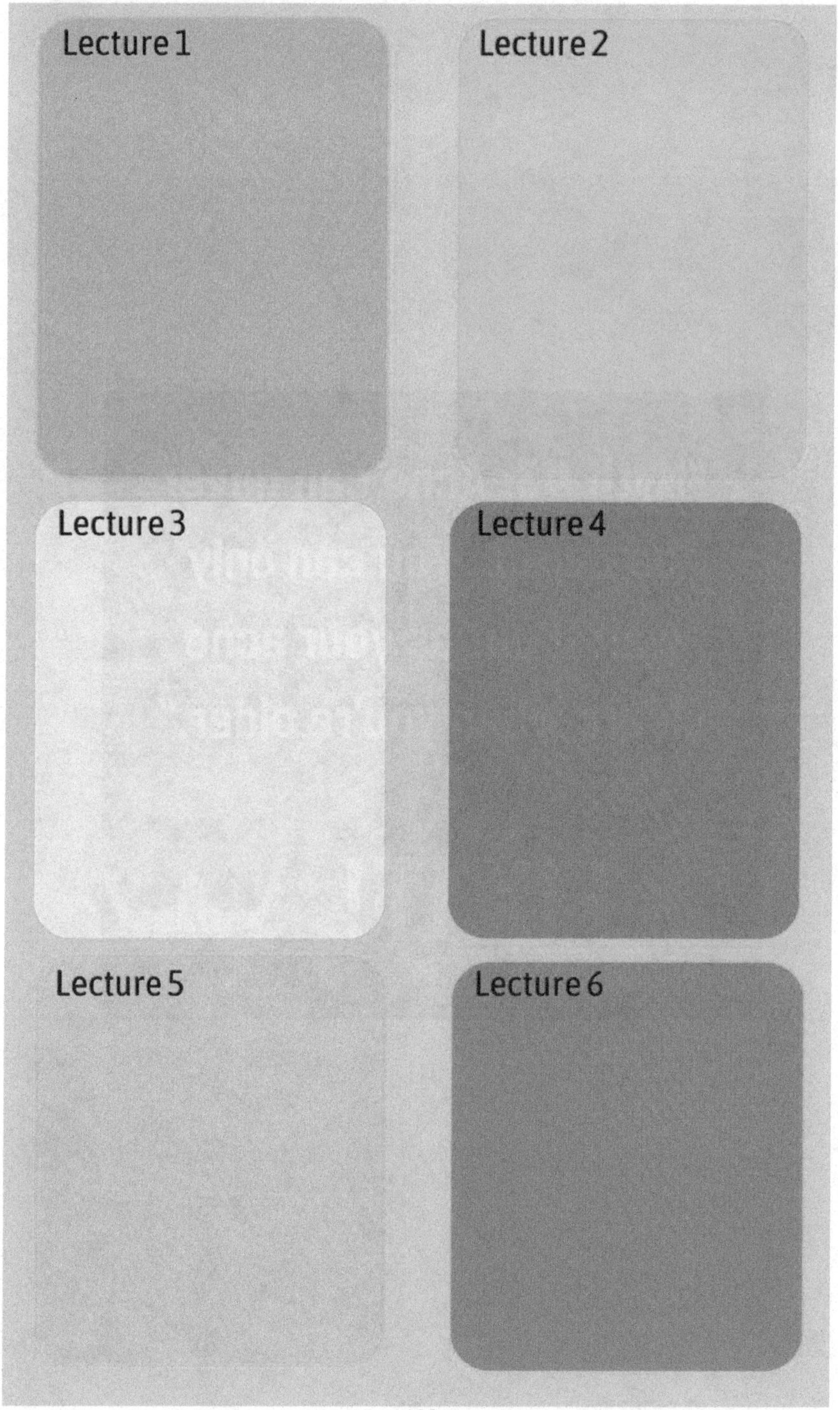

Lecture 1

Lecture 2

Lecture 3

Lecture 4

Lecture 5

Lecture 6

"Myth #3: Acne can never be cured. You can only wait it out as your acne clears when you're older."

FIX IT!

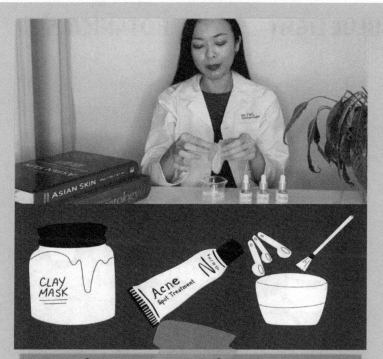

Ingredients For My Skin Type

BLUE LIGHT

BOTANICALS

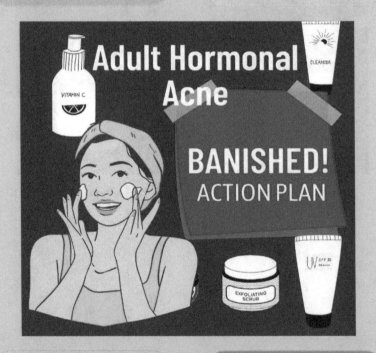

STOP PICKING

DIET

BREAKFAST

LUNCH

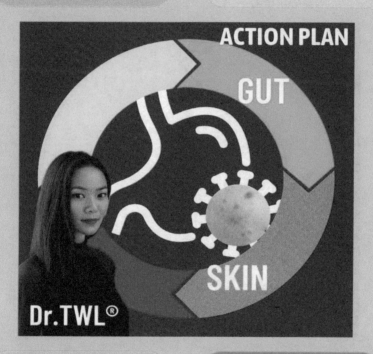

ACTION PLAN

GUT

SKIN

Dr.TWL®

TEA/SNACK

DINNER

JOURNALING

COLORING

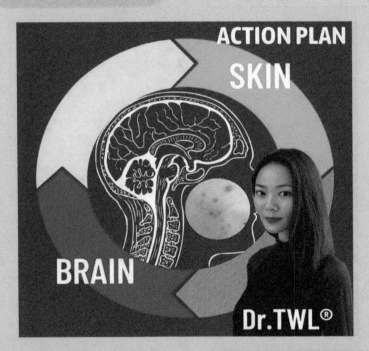

HOBBIES

FAV BOOKS

EMOTIONS

HAIR CHANGES

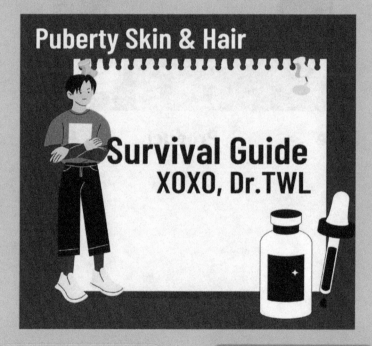

Puberty Skin & Hair

Survival Guide
XOXO, Dr.TWL

SKIN CHANGES

BODY CHANGES

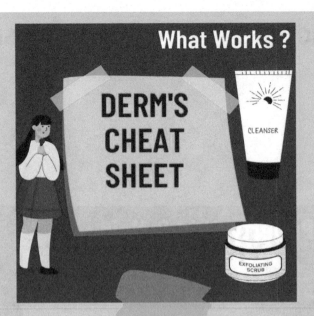

Date   **Product**   **Result**

DERM'S ACNE CHEATSHEET
A Practical Guide
Skincare Routine Must-Haves

- Sebum Regulation
- It's less about removing oil, but more how to regulate oil gland production.
- Cyst, Pustule Management
- A pustule is when you see pus at the tip of an acne bump—you may gently cleanse and extrude the pus with a warm compress. After a shower, when skin is slightly damp, it may be easier to express the fluid. The pus actually contains bacteria and dirt that the body is trying to express—but definitely don't squeeze. If the material doesn't drain readily, stop immediately and apply a hydrocolloid patch which can help the pus rise to the surface. Use patches without any active ingredients infused—especially drying ingredients like tea tree oil etc, by the time a pustule is formed this is not necessary and can in fact cause worsened inflammation. Definitely don't pick acne, this is when a pimple patch may be helpful—it forms a protective barrier between your pimple and pesky fingers!

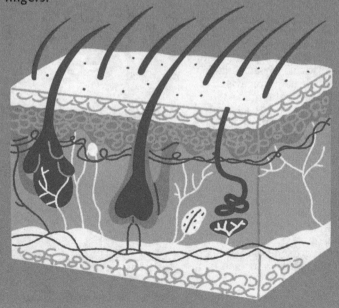

DERM'S ACNE CHEATSHEET
A Practical Guide
Skincare Routine Must-Haves

3 Things You Must Know About Acne

1. Genes and Acne
It's true—Acne is mainly genetic. This is why you find some people never get acne, or *gasp have perfect skin without a skincare routine. The gene PPPARy is a receptor that determines how your skin reacts to the increase in circulating testosterone levels when you hit puberty. Men and women alike. Increased testosterone causes an increase in sebum production and triggers inflammation. That's when mini whiteheads and blackheads begin to form under the skin.

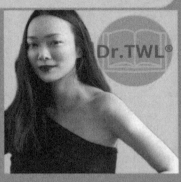

2. Gut-Skin Axis
Diet can most certainly worsen your skin overall, and acne too. While studies appear to pinpoint the role dairy plays in the inflammatory cascade of acne, the fact is that diet affects whole body processes. Saturated fat, highly processed (additive-laden) food isn't good at all for your health, and that makes it your skin health too.

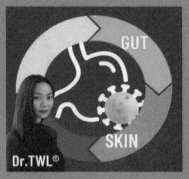

3. Brain-Skin Axis
Stress can cause acne-flare-ups in those who are prone. The brain-skin-axis highlights the role neuroendocrine systems play in modulating skin health. Acne, eczema, rosacea and perioral dermatitis are some dermatological conditions that are worsened by stress.

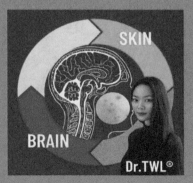

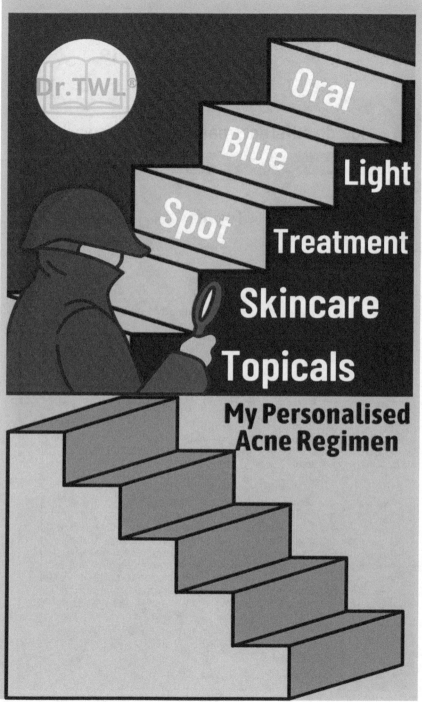

443

DERM'S ACNE CHEATSHEET
A Practical Guide
Acne Treatments

How do different treatment options work

Oral

Topical

Physical Therapy

Traditional prescription medications for moderate-severe acne, cystic acne
Oral antibiotic options include doxycycline, erythromycin, minocycline (less commonly used due to risk of blue-black pigmentation developing and also lung hypersensitivity/allergy issues). Persistent acne or cystic acne may require treatment with oral isotretinoin which is a vitamin A derivative that stops oil production completely—this is why it remains a highly effective "cure" for acne. It however can cause side effects of skin dryness, which means it is not recommended for those with eczema or other dry skin conditions. It can also affect cholesterol levels and liver enzymes, so you should consult with your dermatologist before deciding if it is the best for you. Oral contraceptive pills are also effective for treatment of hormonal acne—those who have PCOS will also find their symptoms improving with hormonal therapy.

Traditional acne creams
Benzoyl peroxide in high concentrations up to 60% are available over the counter—but I don't recommend it anymore because of the risk of irritant contact dermatitis. Most people who use it finds that it stops working after a while—or works only for those with mild acne who require spot treatment. Salicylic acid/sulfur based pimple creams are outdated and do not target the root cause of acne which is inflammation. Retinoids can be of use in those with predominantly comedonal acne, tretinoin tends to be less drying than adapalene, which is considered a newer generation retinoid. My preference is for tretinoin. Retinols in general are not as effective for acne and can instead cause irritant contact dermatitis with prolonged use. Always apply retinoid with moisturiser and under the supervision of a dermatologist.

DERM'S ACNE CHEATSHEET
A Practical Guide
Acne Treatments

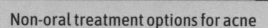

Non-oral treatment options for acne

Peels

Blue Light

Botanicals

Blue Light
This is my top recommendation for those who prefer not to be on oral medications. Blue light works by killing the acne bacteria Cutibacterium acnes. However hand-held devices do not deliver sufficient energies for a therapeutic outcome. In-clinic machines are used with goggles for eye-protection for effective treatment. My team and I last year created a home-based LED light delivery system that can work also for bacne with a strap included in the kit—based on our clinic LED light therapy model. Note of caution about face mask type LED light therapy —those without in-built eye protection are particularly concerning— there was a recall associated with the original neutrogena protoype because of the risk of retinal damage.

Chemical Peels for All Skin Types Including Skin of Color
AHAs like glycolic acid are effective for microscopic exfoliation. It targets superficial skin cells and helps in skin cell renewal. In acne, there is increased retention of dead skin cells around the follicules, which together with production of sebum at the start of puberty leads to follicular plugging— this is what is known as pore clogging. However, higher concentrations of AHAs must be applied under medical supervision as they require neutralisation and can cause side effects of irritant contact dermatitis which is a form of chemical burn. Salicylic acid is far gentler and works by regulating oil production— I recommend using glycolic acid, lactic acid and salicylic acid in rotation for optimal effects on skin.

Enzyme Peels are my top choice now because these are far gentler on skin and have additional anti-inflammatory effects beneficial for acne. Papain enzyme from papaya extract and bromelain from pineapples are available as home peels in my practice for instance, it is gentle enough to be used daily and does not have any risks of post-inflammatory hyperpigmentation.

Microdermabrasion
For acne skin types, I recommend hydrodermabrasion which utilises vacuum technology to gently exfoliate the skin and infuse antioxidants which improve acne by stabilising the microbiome. Handheld systems which are really pore vacuums can actually be used at home for a DIY Hydrodermabrasion experience but the key is using the ideal facial solution which makes all the difference to the effects of the facial experience.

In clinic, diamond microdermabrasion is used to exfoliate and resurface the skin for acne scarring—note of caution, not to be performed on areas of active acne.

Botanical creams
This is my top choice for treatment of active acne currently—I recommend berberine which is actually well known in eastern ethnobotany, dermatology research has also demonstrated its effects on acne. It is anti-inflammatory, regulates oil production, reduces post inflammatory hyperpigmentation and scarring. Algae extracts like chlorella are also helpful.

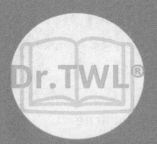

COSMECEUTICALS

DERM'S CHEATSHEET
A Practical Guide

Enhance absorption

Transdermal delivery

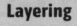
Layering

COSMECEUTICAL
SKINCARE GUIDE

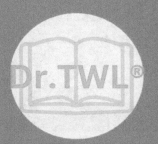

INSTANT GLOW

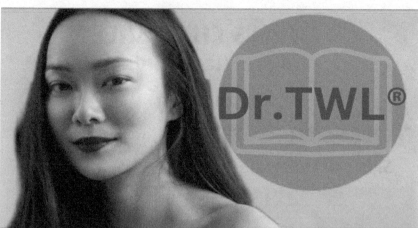

HERE ARE MY TOP FIVE TIPS

CLEANSE & PEEL IN 1 STEP

USE A VITAMIN C SERUM AFTER

USE A MOISTURISER THAT CONTAINS PEPTIDES, BOTANICALS AND NIACINAMIDE.

SPRITZ ON A FACIAL MIST THAT CONTAINS POLYGLUTAMIC ACID

USE A BB OR CC CREAM

WHAT MAKES SKIN GLOW?

DERM'S CHEATSHEET
A Practical Guide
Exfoliation

FACTORS AFFECTING SKIN RADIANCE

Skin cell renewal   **Inflammation**

Moisture levels

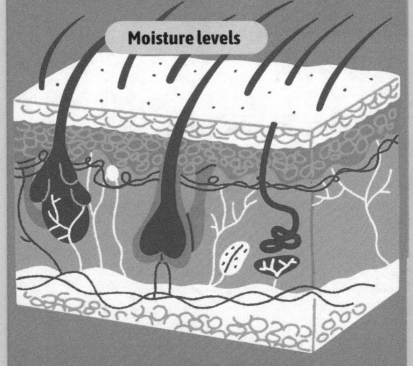

- Skin cell renewal rate (also associated with age)
- Moisture levels
- Existing dermatological conditions

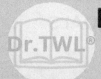

DERM'S 2-STEP HACKS
A Practical Guide
Glowing Skin

DRY

COMBI

OILY

Use a milk cleanser to cleanse and hydrate in 1 step
It's more an emulsion (oil in water) rather than a milk per se. But these cleansers look milky and are preferred over micellar formulations.

Moisturise immediately without drying your skin
Applying moisturiser to damp, wet skin enhances absorption a la the wet pajamas therapy described above. Use a palm-sized amount of moisturiser if you have dry skin—rather than the smaller amounts you are used to. If you are heading out, wait for it to absorb over half an hour or so and massage the excess onto your hands and rest of your body like your neck area.

Use a milk cleanser to cleanse and hydrate in 1 step

If you have combination skin,
Double cleanse if you wear makeup
The first step should be an emulsion-based moisturiser, the second a hydrating foaming cleanser. Choose honey or soy as natural emulsifiers.
Apply moisturiser on wet skin and leave on a larger amount over dry areas like the cheeks.

For oily skin types
Double cleanse with a hydrodermabrasion or microdermabrasion tool
Moisturise with hydrating face mists and a sleeping mask at night
Creams aren't comfortable on oily skin especially in summer or tropical weather like where I practice in Singapore. So if you have super greasy skin I won't blame you for disliking cream moisturisers. Instead, I advise my patients to use a facial mist that contains polyglutamic acid, hyaluronic acid and glycerin.

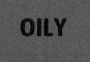

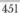

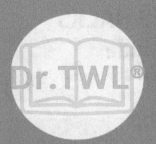

EXFOLIATION GUIDE

DERM'S CHEATSHEET
A Practical Guide
Exfoliation

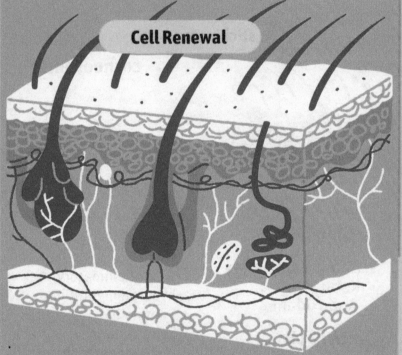

Target Comedones

Surface Irregularities

Cell Renewal

- Glycolic acid peels have antiinflammatory, keratolytic, and antioxidant effects.
- targets the corneosome by enhancing breakdown and decreasing cohesiveness, causing desquamation.

DERM'S CHEATSHEET
A Practical Guide
Chemical Exfoliation

Glycolic Acid

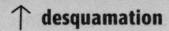

↑ **desquamation**   ↑**breakdown**

↓ **stickiness**

corneosome

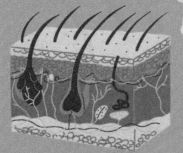

Skin Effects

- Anti-inflammatory
- Keratolytic
- Antioxidant

Quick Facts

- Sugarcane derived
- GA has the smallest molecular weight
- Penetrates skin easily
- very superficial (30%–50% GA, applied for 1–2 minutes); superficial (50%–70% GA, applied for 2–5 minutes); and medium depth (70% GA, applied for 3–15 minutes).

Benefits
- Acne
- Acne scars
- Melasma
- Postinflammatory hyperpigmentation
- Photoaging
- Seborrhea are indications for chemical peeling

DERM'S CHEATSHEET
A Practical Guide

Chemical Peels for Acne

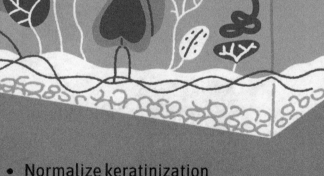

- retention hyperkeratosis
- sebum
- follicular plugging
- P.acnes

- Normalize keratinization
- Increase epidermal and dermal hyaluronic acid
- Increase collagen gene expression.

DERM'S ACNE CHEATSHEET
A Practical Guide
Skincare Routine Must-Haves

- Another method is to use a dermabrasion tool, or one of the pore vacuums to gently encourage the pus to drain—this is only recommended if the pus is already at the tip of the bump, not when it is "hidden".
- For acne cysts, you may need to visit a dermatologist if it does not drain on its own after 1-2 weeks, an injection with steroid may be necessary. If you get more than 3-5 cysts per month, you may need oral medication treatment to prevent it from becoming severe cystic acne—that can quickly progress and lead to scarring.

Skincare Hacks For Pores
Backed By Science!

Hydroderm abrasion

Dry Masking

Microderm abrasion

Pore Vacuums

Rose Extract Toner

Skin Icing

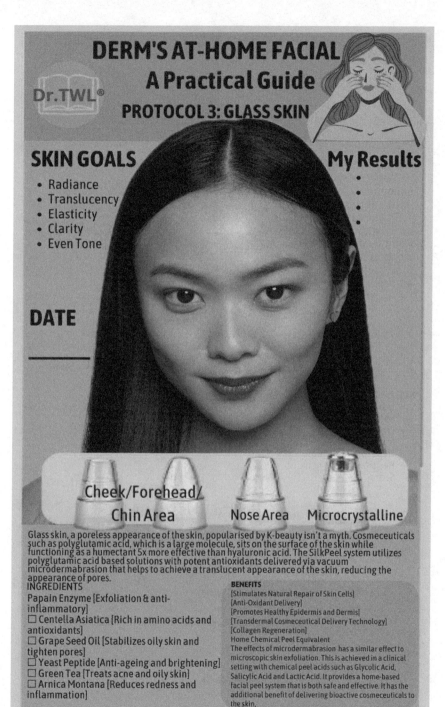

DERM'S AT-HOME FACIAL
A Practical Guide
PROTOCOL 3: GLASS SKIN

Dr.TWL®

SKIN GOALS

- Radiance
- Translucency
- Elasticity
- Clarity
- Even Tone

DATE

_____

My Results

-
-
-
-

Cheek/Forehead/Chin Area **Nose Area** **Microcrystalline**

Glass skin, a poreless appearance of the skin, popularised by K-beauty isn't a myth. Cosmeceuticals such as polyglutamic acid, which is a large molecule, sits on the surface of the skin while functioning as a humectant 5x more effective than hyaluronic acid. The SilkPeel system utilizes polyglutamic acid based solutions with potent antioxidants delivered via vacuum microdermabrasion that helps to achieve a translucent appearance of the skin, reducing the appearance of pores.

INGREDIENTS

Papain Enzyme [Exfoliation & anti-inflammatory]
☐ Centella Asiatica [Rich in amino acids and antioxidants]
☐ Grape Seed Oil [Stabilizes oily skin and tighten pores]
☐ Yeast Peptide [Anti-ageing and brightening]
☐ Green Tea [Treats acne and oily skin]
☐ Arnica Montana [Reduces redness and inflammation]

BENEFITS

[Stimulates Natural Repair of Skin Cells]
[Anti-Oxidant Delivery]
[Promotes Healthy Epidermis and Dermis]
[Transdermal Cosmeceutical Delivery Technology]
[Collagen Regeneration]
Home Chemical Peel Equivalent
The effects of microdermabrasion has a similar effect to microscopic skin exfoliation. This is achieved in a clinical setting with chemical peel acids such as Glycolic Acid, Salicylic Acid and Lactic Acid. It provides a home-based facial peel system that is both safe and effective. It has the additional benefit of delivering bioactive cosmeceuticals to the skin.

DERM'S ACNE FACIAL KIT
Dr.TWL® A Practical Guide

**PROTOCOL 2: ACNE, (ADULT HORMONAL, TEENAGER) ACNE SCARS
DULL SKIN, AGING SKIN, HYPERPIGMENTATION**

MICRODERMABRASION

HOW: Microcrystalline copper nanoparticles exfoliate the skin surface while stimulating collagen, combining effects with Hydrodermabrasion in your facial mist/essence works as solvent, vacuum pressure increases dermal absorption of active ingredients

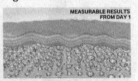
MEASURABLE RESULTS FROM DAY 1

RESULTS
- Instantly Brighter Skin
- Softer, Smoother
- Lighten Post-Inflammation Hyperpigmentation
- Resurface Deep Acne Scars

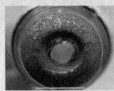
PATENTED COPPER OXIDE MICRODERMABRASION TIP

STEPS
Apply gel mask as barrier between skin and copper nanoparticle tip
Glide hand piece over T-zone first, then moving to the forehead, cheeks and chin

Gel Mask Ingredients for Glow
Vitamin C
Oligopeptides
Botanicals
Propolis

How to choose your kit
- Optimal pressure for sensitive skin <=60 kPa
- Choose device with at least 3 settings for dry, combination and oily skin
- Redness is normal, lasts < 5 seconds
- BONUS TIP: MICRODERMABRASION head with microcrystalline copper exfoliates skin effectively

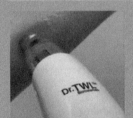

Frequency, Duration
- Dry, Sensitive—once a week
- Combination—twice a week
- Oily—thrice a week, step up to daily

Skin Health/Profile	Results	Skin Goals

Notes & Remarks

DERM'S ACNE FACIAL KIT
A Practical Guide

PROTOCOL 1: ACNE, (ADULT HORMONAL, TEENAGER) ACNE SCARS

TOOLS/EQUIPMENT

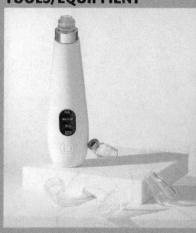

- **PORE VACUUM KIT**
- **DIFFERENT HANDPIECE SHAPES FIT FACIAL CONTOUR**
- **FACIAL ESSENCE/MIST ACTIVE INGREDIENTS:**
  - Glycerin
  - Sodium Hyaluronate
  - Vitamin C (L-ascorbic, Magnesium Ascorbyl Phosphate, Sodium Ascorbyl Phosphate)
  - Antioxidant plant extracts
  - Anti-inflammatory botanicals

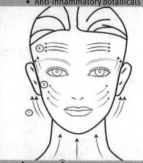

HYDRODERMABRASION
HOW: Water in your facial mist/essence works as solvent, vacuum pressure increases dermal absorption of active ingredients

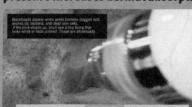

STEPS
1. Double cleanse face
2. Spray facial mist or pat on essence
3. Apply vacuum pore device over the entire face in the directions shown

CAUTION
1. Do not use over areas of inflamed painful acne bumps
2. Not for use on eczema skin, areas of broken skin
3. Wash hand pieces thoroughly with soap and water and let dry after each use

EFFECTS ON SKIN
1. LIFTING, TIGHTENING Increase collagen production
2. RADIANCE, GLOW UP Remove dead skin cells
3. REDUCE COMEDONES Reduce micro comedones formation
4. BUILD RESILIENCE Infuse antioxidants into skin
5. BARRIER REPAIR Deliver humectants, prevent water loss

Monthly Treatment Challenge

Date:

Result:

Visibly improved Keep Using

DERM'S AT-HOME FACIAL
A Practical Guide

Dr.TWL® Favorite Facial Tools

Favorite Mist

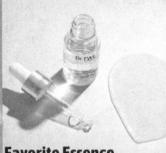

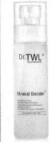

Favorite Essence

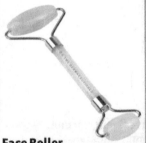

Face Roller

Start with the bottom of the face—specifically the center of the chin—and work your way up, rolling outward across the jaw and up toward the ear. Using light pressure, perform similar outward and upward strokes from the centre of the face and forehead towards the sides and work upwards from the décolleté.

For acne scars and pigmentation, use the small roller head to roll over the affected area for 30 seconds before application of serum.

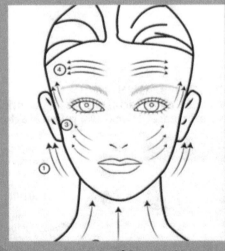

My Skincare Notes

DERM'S AT-HOME FACIAL
A Practical Guide

Dr.TWL®

PROTOCOL 4: ENLARGED PORES, REDNESS, SENSITIVITY, INFLAMED ACNE

CRYOTHERAPY, SKIN ICING

Reduces skin redness, inflammation and sensitivity. With regular use, it reduces skin reactivity and excess oil production. Use with your favorite serums to enhance absorption

TYPES
ICE-based
Metal alloy-based: Zinc has sebum regulating benefits

RESULTS
- Tighten Pores
- Reduce Swelling
- Reduce Redness
- Improve Sebum Regulation
- Anti-inflammation

DRY MASKING
- Improve Moisture
- Reduce Wrinkles
- Skin Texture
- Skin Environment

HOW TO

Freeze for 30 mins & Remove

Test on skin to ensure comfort

Lift, Massage
Use before applying skincare

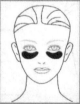 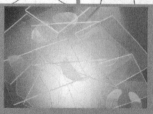

How It Works   **RESULTS**
- Hydrocolloid
- Silicone
- Biofunctional Textiles

DATE
_____

AM/PM
_____

Skin Health/Profile	Results	Skin Goals

461

DERM'S ACNE CHEATSHEET
Understand Your
Acne Type and Severity

CYST **OPEN COMEDONE (BLACKHEAD)** **CLOSED COMEDONE (WHITEHEAD)** **PAPULE**

Quantity/Severity

Mild: 3-5 pimples a month, mostly comedones and papules
Try plant-based OTC creams first—I stopped recommending benzoyl peroxide, salicylic acid and retinol-based acne creams 8 years ago. Plant-based alternatives like berberine work well. Switch to a skincare regimen targeting acne.

PUSTULE

Moderate: 5-20 pimples a month, comedones, papules and few cysts
LED light therapy and quasi-drug herbal formulations (refer chapter on quasi-drugs

Severe: More than 20 pimples a month, more than 5 cysts
Prescription medications like isotretinoin likely required for cystic acne conditions. Add on LED light therapy and cosmeceuticals/quasi drugs can reduce duration of treatment, improve flare-free periods.

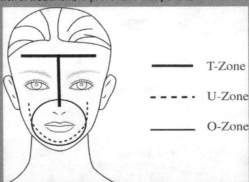

——— T-Zone
- - - - U-Zone
——— O-Zone

Facial pattern/distribution: O-zone, T-zone, U-zone
T-zone: The nose, forehead and chin most commonly affected for physiologic acne.
Remedy: Prescription retinoids like tretinoin and adapalene. Skincare regimen that includes anti-bacterial cleanser, spot treatment and use of antioxidant serums.
U-Zone: Oral medications and or blue light therapy is recommended, also visit a gynaecologist to rule out Polycystic Ovarian Disease if you also suffer from irregular periods and or experience increased facial hair growth, a condition known as hirsutism.
O-zone: O for maskne but also Overlap with other conditions like rosacea, eczema, perioral dermatitis
Remedy: The most cOmplex! See a dermatologist if your condition is persistent, it may not be acne. Most of these cases will require treatment with prescription oral medications and creams.

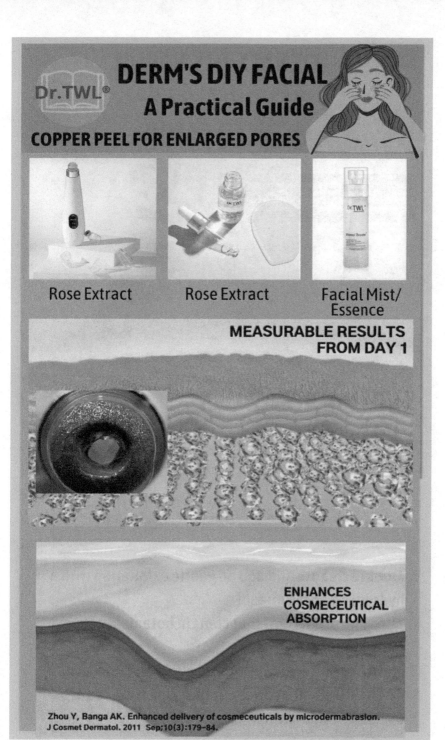

DERM'S DIY FACIAL
A Practical Guide

COPPER PEEL FOR ENLARGED PORES

Rose Extract   Rose Extract   Facial Mist/Essence

MEASURABLE RESULTS FROM DAY 1

ENHANCES COSMECEUTICAL ABSORPTION

Zhou Y, Banga AK. Enhanced delivery of cosmeceuticals by microdermabrasion. J Cosmet Dermatol. 2011 Sep;10(3):179–84.

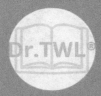

DERM'S DIY FACIAL
A Practical Guide

HOW TO GLOW

Blackheads appear when pores become clogged with excess oil, bacteria, and dead skin cells.
If the pore closes up, you'll see a tiny bump that looks white or flesh colored. These are whiteheads.

SKIN RADIANCE

1. **Double cleanse** and add on gentle exfoliation with a **hydrodermabrasion** tool
2. Use **skincare serums** that contain botanical actives and ubiquinone
3. **Moisturise** after cleansing and avoid air conditioning when I sleep—that dries out the skin barrier due to transepidermal water loss.

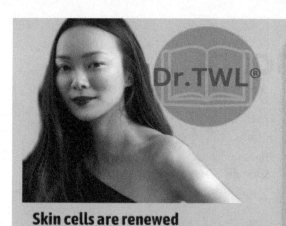

Skin cells are renewed

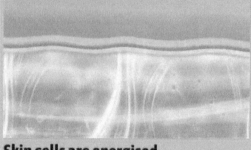

Skin cells are energised

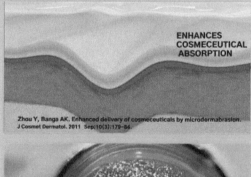

ENHANCES
COSMECEUTICAL
ABSORPTION

Zhou Y, Banga AK. Enhanced delivery of cosmeceuticals by microdermabrasion. J Cosmet Dermatol. 2011 Sep;10(3):179–84.

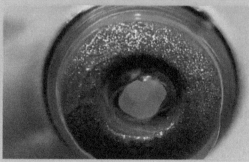

Skincare *Planner*

Skin Problems:

Date:

Skin Type:

Skin Goals:

Morning Routine

Step	Product	Schedule	Mon	Tue	Wed	Thu	Fri	Sat	Sun

Night Routine

Step	Product	Schedule	Mon	Tue	Wed	Thu	Fri	Sat	Sun

Notes

Dr.TWL®

download more sample templates www.twlskin.com

SECTION 5

Course Workbook 2

download textbook resources and printables*

*https://www.twlskin.com/dictionary/ register account and receive download access in your welcome email

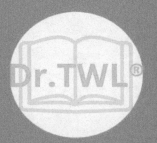

BARRIER REPAIR

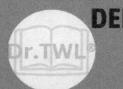

DERM'S SKIN BARRIER CHEATSHEET
A Practical Guide

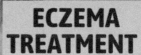

5 PILLARS

Redness
Flaking
Swelling
Oily-Dry
Bumps
Itch

ECZEMA TREATMENT

PRACTICAL TIPS

Applying concealer
Choose makeup
Sunscreen stinging
Sensitivity to
EVERYTHING!

Does layering
work?
Wet wraps
SENSITIVE OR
          REACTIVE SKIN?

Skin Decoder

Skin Barrier Repair
Red, dry and tight face? It could be eczema, rosacea or BOTH.
- Redness
Could be due to
Eczema (skin barrier damage) or Rosacea (hyperactive blood vessels)
- Thank Flaking
Eczema/Dermatitis NOT because you have too much dead skin!
DO NOT SCRUB!
STOP: all astringent acne products (alcohol-based, salicylic acid, AHA/BHA, tea tree oil, sulfur, benzoyl peroxide, retinols, retinoids)
- Swelling
Inflammation
Can occur in eczema, rosacea

GENTLE CLEANSER	SERUM	MOISTURISER
	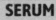	

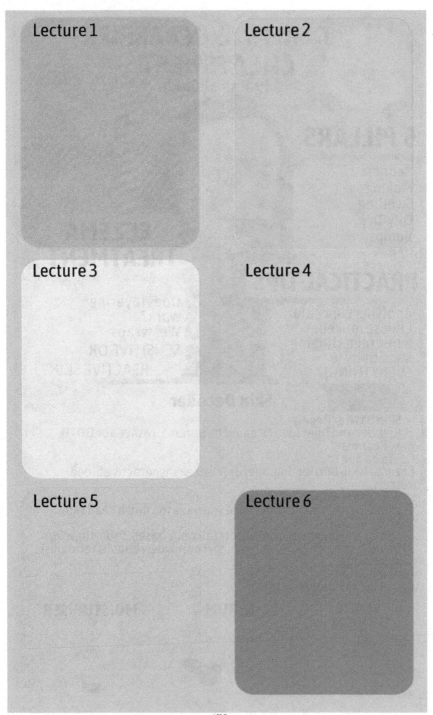

Lecture 1

Lecture 2

Lecture 3

Lecture 4

Lecture 5

Lecture 6

470

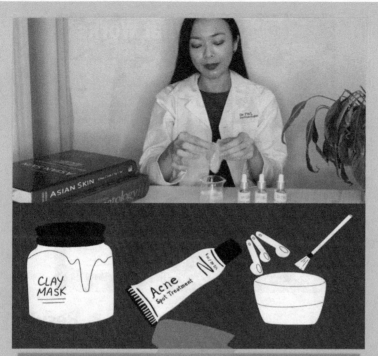

Ingredients For Barrier Repair

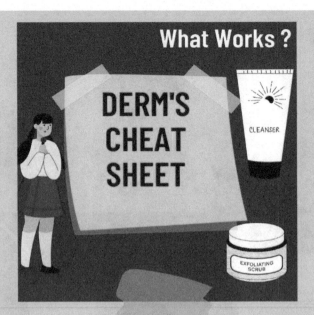

Date	Product	Result

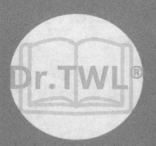

SKIN RESILIENCE

DERM'S SKIN RESILIENCE CHEATSHEET
A Practical Guide

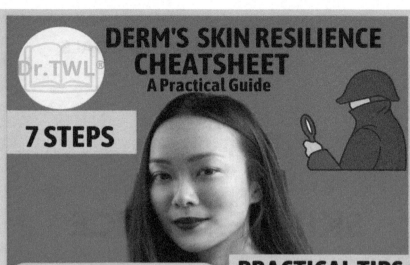

7 STEPS

PRACTICAL TIPS

Mind-Skin Connection
- The skin is the first to suffer the ill-effects of stress. Even with the perfect skincare regimen, your immune system has the final say. Mindfulness practice, meditation, reflective journaling, art therapy are practical activities that help you de-stress—make that part of your daily routine. Get a good night's rest with sleep hygiene and follow the circadian rhythm

Gut-Skin Axis
- Dairy and saturated fats acnegenic foods
- Gut microbiome affects immune system functioning
- Eat a plant-based diet which increases microbiome diversity.

Cut out retinoids
- retinoids disrupt the skin barrier

Use botanicals
- Purslane
- brassica
- multi-functional botanical actives
- anti-oxidant
- anti-inflammatory
- UV-protective
- aging skin exposome concept
- environmental damage affects biological aging

Layer skincare
- Serum
- Essence
- Emulsion
- Mist

Hydrodermabrasion
- vacuum technology
- sensitive skin
- korean glass skin appearance
- pair with the correct facial solutions.

LED Light Therapy
- Green, red and purple light
- enhancing cell mitochrondria activity
- cell repair

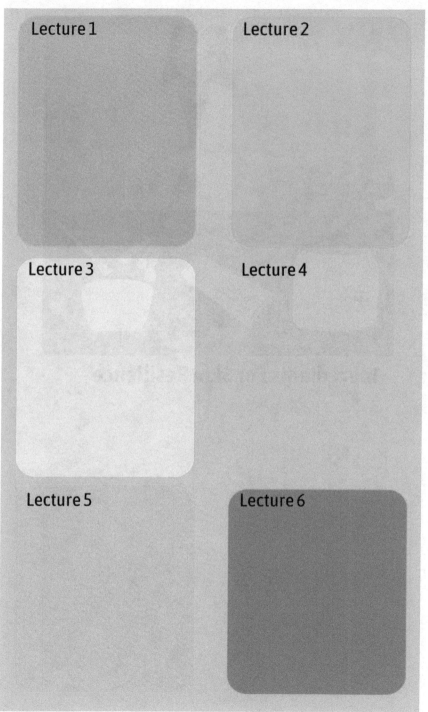

Lecture 1

Lecture 2

Lecture 3

Lecture 4

Lecture 5

Lecture 6

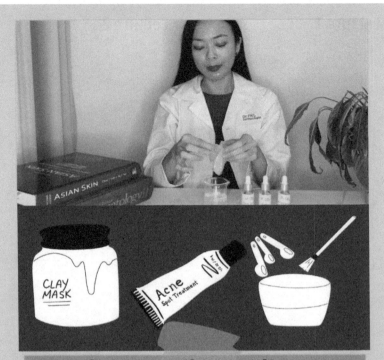

Ingredients For Skin Resilience

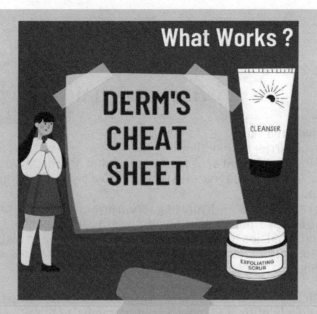

Date	Product	Result

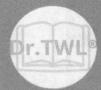

DERM'S CHEATSHEET
A Practical Guide
Barrier Repair

Oily-Dehydrated Skin
- Sign of barrier dysfunction
- STOP: all astringent acne products (alcohol-based, salicylic acid, AHA/BHA, tea tree oil, sulfur, benzoyl peroxide, retinols, retinoids)
- DO: Layer skincare—hydrating serum (hyaluronic acid), facial mist/essence (polyglutamic acid, glycerin, amino acids), lotion/emulsion (peptides, anti-inflammatory botanicals), cream (ceramides—plant-phytoceramides +synthetic vs bovine)

Bumps/Itch
- Acne/Folliculitis vs Eczema (Papular eczema, perioral dermatitis, allergic/irritant)
- PRO TIP: If itchy, more like eczema BUT both eczema + acne can co-exist
- DO: Use a botanical pimple cream, apply hyaluronic acid serum, ceramide-based moisturiser, if not better after 1 week, visit a dermatologist
- STOP: All facial treatments/shaving/waxing/threading

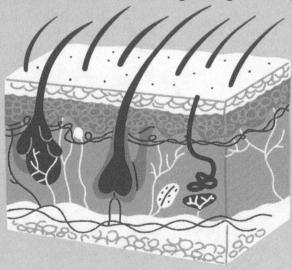

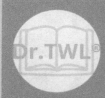

DERM'S CHEATSHEET
A Practical Guide
Barrier Repair

Applying makeup/concealer
Can be tricky over red flaky skin
PRO TIP:
For redness Use green color correctors (check ingredient base of corrector).
For flaky skin
1. Apply thin layer of moisturising lotion/cream, allow to fully absorb
2. After 5-10 mins, wipe off excess with a soft reusable microfibre cloth (dead skin flakes will come off too, don't rub too hard)
3. Spritz on hydrating facial mist (water based), allow to dry for 5 mins
4. For concealer: start with small amount (pea sized) to build thin layer on flaky area. Build on gradually for coverage.
5. Finish with facial mist, let it settle.

How to choose makeup for sensitive skin
Pure mineral makeup (without fillers, BMO Bismuth Oxychloride which gives the cut glass feeling—an experience you may have had with certain mineral makeup!)
For foundation, choose a BB or CC cream with hydrating, antioxidant and anti-inflammatory ingredients
In general: avoid mascara, eyeliner, dark pigments (hard to cleanse without friction to skin, bad for skin barrier)

Sunscreen stinging
• Due to chemical sunscreen component (avobenzones), choose pure physical blockers (zinc oxide, titanium dioxide)
• Damaged skin barrier (everything will sting, switch to physical blockers, apply copious moisturiser before sunscreen)
• Eczema (sweat allergy, acts as an irritant)

Sensitivity to everything—including water?
You may have cosmetic intolerance syndrome, visit a dermatologist

DERM'S CHEATSHEET
A Practical Guide
Barrier Repair

Enhance absorption

Transdermal delivery

Layering

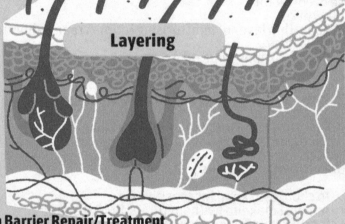

Skin Barrier Repair/Treatment
Layering ingredients

1. Layering skincare serum-lotion-emulsion-cream works because of higher concentrations of active ingredients in each product, vs an all-in-one formula
2. Wet masking increases dermal absorption which is the skin's ability to absorb actives
3. Transdermal Delivery* smaller molecules, multi-weighted hyaluronic acid etc.

Serum: Hyaluronic acid
Face Essence/Mist: Polyglutamic acid, Glycerin, Rice bran, Amino Acids
Emulsion/Creams: All of above plus ceramides, shea (phytoceramides)
Sheet Mask:
GOLD STANDARD: Polysaccharides are plant vegetal material with ultra-moisturising properties, form a reservoir that holds all the ingredients against your skin for optimal absorption
BUDGET HACK: You can apply a wet, ultra-soft microfibre towel over all the layered skincare)

Wet wrap hack
- Apply right after shower (damp skin, don't dry yourself)
- Slather on copious amounts (2 palm-sized amounts per limb)
- Wear comfortable cotton PJs that cover your limbs (thinner material so it does not absorb the creams which you want to be on your skin)

DERM'S CHEATSHEET

Skin Flooding
The Truth About Barrier Repair

sleeping mask	Switch off the A/C	face mist or essence

- Use your favorite moisturiser as a sleeping mask
- If you don't have patience for serums, just use a face mist or essence
- Forget slugging, choose ceramides
- Sheet masks? Use a moist microfibre towel instead
- Switch off the A/C

choose ceramides

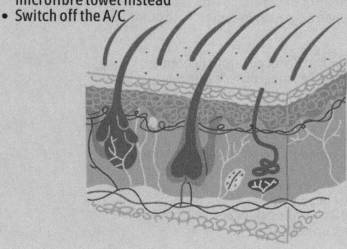

DERM'S ACNE CHEATSHEET
A Practical Guide
Barrier Repair

The Barrier Repair Sandwich by Dr.TWL

Perioral dermatitis

Rosacea

Eczema

Acne + eczema

Sensitive or Reactive Skin?
No clear medical definitions, but used in beauty lingo
Basically skin that gets red, stings, flakes, swells whenever there is a change in routine/environment/products used/psychological state

Can be eczema, rosacea, perioral dermatitis, severe acne with secondary eczema caused by inappropriate product use

Sensitive: History of atopy (eczema, rhinitis/sensitive nose/hay fever, asthma), long history of intolerance to harsh cleansing products

Reactive: May be episodic to environmental changes—spicy food, hot soup, hot summer weather, cold winters, well in-between
Most important to:
Use a hydrating skincare routine and layer on skincare

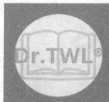

DERM'S CHEATSHEET
A Practical Guide

The Barrier Repair Sandwich ™ Dr.TWL

Transdermal absorption

Topical

Occlusion

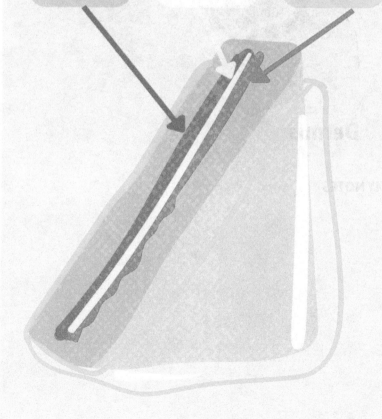

EPIDERMIS TALKS
A Practical Guide

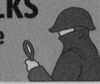

Epidermis

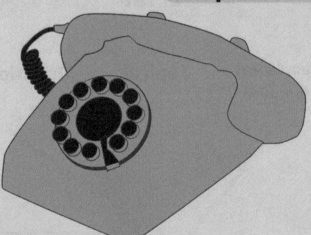

Dermis

MY NOTES

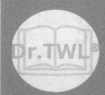

SKIN DETECTIVE
A Practical Guide

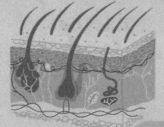

Epidermis

SKIN

CROSS-TALK

FLOODING

Dermis

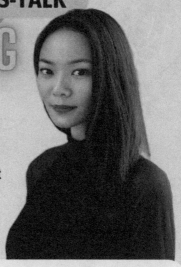

**Skin Barrier Repair/Treatment
Layering ingredients**

MY NOTES

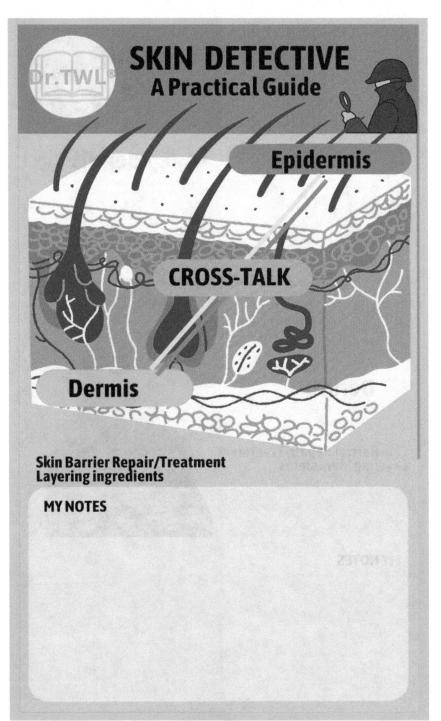

SKIN DETECTIVE
A Practical Guide

Epidermis

CROSS-TALK

Dermis

Skin Barrier Repair/Treatment
Layering ingredients

MY NOTES

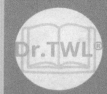

7 Steps to Resilience

Treating the Skin Ecosystem

1. **Mind-Skin Connection**
2. **Gut-Skin Axis**
3. **Cut out retinoids**
4. **Use botanicals**
5. **Layer skincare**
6. **Hydrodermabrasion**
7. **LED Light Therapy**

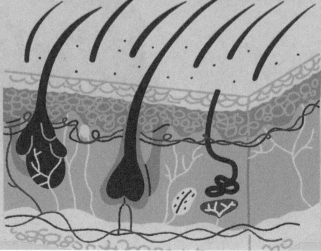

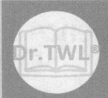

SKIN DETECTIVE
A Practical Guide

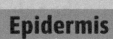

Epidermis

CROSS-TALK

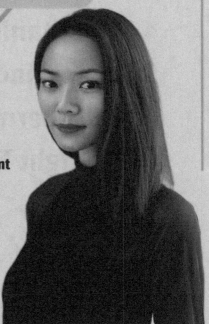

Dermis

Skin Barrier Repair/Treatment
Layering ingredients

SECTION 6

Skin Expert Mastery: Ingredient Dictionary

download textbook resources and printables*

*https://www.twlskin.com/dictionary/ register account and
receive download access in your welcome email

Ingredient Dictionary

The following actives are not exhaustive but represent a selection of must-know and good-to-know cosmeceuticals identified from an analysis of over 300 skincare brands.

This segment is created to facilitate comprehensive mastery of skincare actives that qualify as cosmeceuticals and have been found as common ingredients used based on our analysis of over 300 popular skincare brands. A different approach is taken with this set as the actives are now classified based on plant parts, their origin i.e. from microorganisms—it has been specially created in such a way that you will encounter actives you have already learnt about in the earlier chapters, as a way to help you revise and to consolidate what you have learnt. These actives are written about in a slightly different way while still presenting the key points and features—this process helps to facilitate true mastery in the learning process, as you learn how to convey knowledge you have acquired in your own words and in the context of a framework that makes sense to you.

Use these notes as a guide to create your own ingredient dictionary using the techniques you have learnt in the earlier sections. Create learning aides in the form of concept maps and flashcards.

Leaves

Aloe Barbadensis Leaf

Bladderwrack (Seaweed)

Brassica Oleracea Italica (Broccoli) Extract

Camellia Sinensis (Tea) Leaf Extract

Caffeine

Centella Asiatica (Cica)

Glycyrrhiza Glabra (Licorice) Leaf Extract

Salvia Officinalis (Sage) Leaf Extract

Spinacia Oleracea (Spinach) Leaf Extract

Artemisia vulgaris (Mugwort) Extract

Seeds

Cannabis Sativa (Hemp)

Oryza Sativa (Rice) Bran Extract

Zea Mays (Corn) Kernel Extract

Lens Esculenta (Lentil) Seed Extract

Avena Sativa (Oat) Kernel Extract

Psoralea corylifolia seed (Bakuchiol)

Vitis Vinifera (Grape) Seed Oil

Flowers

Arnica Montana Extract

Chamomilla Recutita (Matricaria) Flower Extract

Hamamelis virginiana (Witch Hazel) Flower Extract

Rosmarinus Officinalis (Rosemary) Flower Extract

Rosa Damascus (Rose) Flower Extract

Root

Daucus Carota Sativa (Carrot) Root Extract

Scutellaria Baicalensis Root Extract

Polygonum Cuspidatum Root Extract (Knotweed)

Salvia Miltiorrhiza (Red Sage) Root Extract

Derived from Microorganisms

Astaxanthin

Corthellus Shiitake (Mushroom) Extract

Spirulina

Glycine Max (Soybean) Seedcoat Extract

Others

Betaine

Salmon Roe

Olea Europea (Olive Oil)

Myrrh Oil

Sea Buckthorn Oil

Melaleuca alternifolia (Tea Tree Oil)

Cucumis Sativus (Cucumber) Fruit Extract

Plant Stem Cells

A section on other relevant skincare actives

Hyaluronic acid and its molecular weights

Natural Moisturizing Factors

- Methionine
- Polyglutamic Acid
- Serine

CHAPTER TWELVE

Leaves

Aloe Barbadensis Leaf (Aloe vera)
- high water content 99–99.5%
- 0.5–1.0% solid over 75 different potentially active compounds i.e. water- and fat-soluble vitamins, minerals, enzymes

- anti-inflammatory
- skin protection
- anti-bacterial
- anti-viral
- antiseptic
- wound healing

Skin barrier
- retain skin moisture
- structural integrity

UV protective effect
- radiation damage

Wound healing
- improve the wound healing process
- reduce inflammation.
- inhibit thromboxane (an inhibitor of wound healing)

Regenerative properties
- glucomannan
- polysaccharide rich i.e. mannose
- affects fibroblast growth factor receptors
- stimulates activity and proliferation

Effects on collagen
- increases collagen production
- change collagen composition
- increase collagen cross-linking —>promote wound

healing
- stimulates fibroblast, produces collagen + elastin fibers

Effects on skin appearance
- increases elasticity
- reduces wrinkles
- cohesive effects on superficial flaking epidermal cells
- skin softening: amino acids
- zinc: astringent, tighten pores

Cosmeceutical applications
- gel masks, moisturisers
- aloe vera gel gloves
- anti-acne treatment

Side effects
- generally well tolerated
- redness, burning, stinging sensation
- rarely: generalized dermatitis in sensitised individuals
  - anthraquinones (aloin, barbaloin—found in the outer rind of the plant)

Bladderwrack (Fucus Vesiculosus)
- brown seaweed
- bladder-like air pockets along leaves
- nutrient-dense
- free radical scavenger i.e. **neutralise free radicals**

SKINCARE EXPERT LINGO
Antioxidants neutralise free radicals, reducing oxidative stress on skin

Antioxidants
- phlorotannins
- fucoxanthin
- fucoidan
- vitamins A and C

Collagen production
- fucoidan stimulates collagen synthesis,
- 228% increase in collagen production

- reduced epidermal hyperkeratosis while improving elasticity
- mucopolysaccharides inhibit skin enzymes that break down collagen and elastin

SKINCARE EXPERT LINGO
Collagen is your skin's secret for staying firm and youthful. It's the protein that makes up 75-80% of your skin, and plays a big part in the way your skin looks and ages. As collagen diminishes with age, our skin loses its firmness and begins to sag, exposing wrinkles and fine lines.

Cosmeceutical applications
- shower soaps, bath salts and facial scrubs

What are free radicals?
Harmful compounds that can cause oxidative stress to skin
Oxidative stress:
- free radicals combine with oxygen
- free radicals greater than the body's ability to neutralise
- secrete enzymes that break down collagen and elastic fibres

Effects on skin appearance
- reduces inflammation
- prevents wrinkles and fine lines

Brassica Oleracea Italica (Broccoli) Extract
Brassica oleracea italica
- broccoli, kale and cabbage
- vitamins B1, B2, B3, B6, iron, magnesium, potassium, zinc, sulforaphane
- broccoli sprout extract (sulforaphane)
- omega 3 fatty acids (ALA) for the skin barrier
- natural source of vitamin A, C prevents premature aging
- arachidonic acid: anti-inflammatory effect

Targets key signs of photo-aging
- inhibits chemically-induced skin tumors
- reduce ultraviolet damage

- fight oxidative stress
- maintain collagen levels

Vitamin A (Retinol) in broccoli
- skin cell regeneration
- even skin tone
- no known toxicity
- non-irritating, suitable for sensitive skin

Sulforaphane
- sulfur-rich compound
- anti-carcinogenic (cancer fighting) effects
- UV protective

SKINCARE EXPERT LINGO
*UV radiation causes **oxidative stress** to our skin, **damaging** the elastic fibres that keep our skin firm. This makes wrinkles and fine-lines more prominent and cause hyperpigmentation.*

Sulforaphane
- protective enzymes repair damaged skin cells
- applied on the skin daily 3 days before UV exposure, cell damage declined by 37%
- potent antioxidant

Our bodies have natural antioxidant defense mechanisms against free radicals. However, these mechanisms decline with age.

BIMODAL ANTIOXIDANT ACTION
- stimulates body's natural antioxidant defense mechanisms
- directly neutralises free radicals

ANTI-ACNE
- natural retinol source
- anti-bacterial (AMP)
- anti-inflammatory

Study: 20 subjects for 4 weeks effective for mild-to-moderate acne without irritation.

Antimicrobial peptides (AMP) are part of your body's natural immune response to microorganisms. Studies have shown that brassica extracts helps to stimulate and strengthen the body's AMP response.

ANTI-AGING
- stimulates collagen production

Study: Effective in accelerating the wound closure process by stimulating production of collagen.

SKINCARE EXPERT LINGO
Collagen is the protein in your body that gives your skin structure. Loss of collagen is related to reduced production and increased breakdown due to aging and UV exposure. Choosing active ingredients that stimulate collagen production gives skin a firm, plumped appearance.

Camellia Sinensis Leaf Extract (Green Tea Plant)
When we talk about green tea as a skincare ingredient, we are typically referring to an extract from green tea leaves vs green tea oil which is derived from the seeds.

Epigallocatechin gallate (EGCG) is the most widely studied catechin in Camellia Sinensis.
- polyphenols
- catechins
- antioxidant
- anti-inflammatory
- anti-androgenic
- controls sebum production
- boosts collagen production

WHY EGCG IS AN ANTIOXIDANT SUPERPOWER
- protect the body's natural antioxidant reserve vitamin C, E
- neutralises free radicals
- UV protective
- inhibit collagenases (responsible for collagen breakdown)

To combat the effects of increased sun exposure, try looking for sunscreen products that contain green tea extract. Recent findings show that green tea extract should combine with zinc oxide and titanium dioxide in sunscreen preparations. This combination protects the skin against damage caused by both UVA and UVB rays. Clinical studies also showed that topical treatment with green tea extract reduced UVB-induced inflammatory response and oxidative stress, helping our skin look healthier, even after sun exposure.

Anti-ageing
Another benefit of green tea for skin is that it can improve the skin's texture, increase moisture, and decrease oiliness. Research has proved that green tea extract can improve microcirculation. This is the circulation of blood in the smallest blood vessels. It also improves the condition of blood vessels, resulting in better skin nutrition and oxygenation. A clinical study showed that 6% Camellia extract applied to forearm skin revealed significant increase in moisture and improved skin texture Furthermore, clinical trials also showed significant anti-sebum activity of green tea extract

Caffeine
Antioxidants are the number one way to combat oxidative stress by scavenging free radicals that directly causes photoaging due to UV damage. Caffeine is a rich source of antioxidants in skincare.

SKINCARE EXPERT LINGO
What is photoaging?
UV rays accelerate skin aging—dermatologists describe that as extrinsic aging which is caused by external factors. Another term for this is photoaging, which is skin aging caused by sun damage. Specifically, sun-exposed areas such as the face, the "V" area of the chest.

How does photoaging occur?
- UV-exposure stimulates skin inflammation
- cells secrete enzymes that break down collagen and elastic fibers

498

- increases production of free radicals leading to cell damage

Cosmeceutical applications
- eye creams
- cellulite creams

What causes puffy eyes and dark circles?
The skin under your eyes is one of the thinnest in the body. Hence, it is easy for blood vessels to show through the skin. This results in a swollen and dark appearance under the eyes. Skin of color may also be prone to developing hyperpigmentation under the eyes. If you suffer from eczema or dry skin, post-inflammatory hyperpigmentation can also occur.

How do caffeinated eye creams work?
- temporary effect:
  - vasoconstrictive
  - decrease redness, puffiness
  - reduce eye bags
- longer term benefits:
  - anti-inflammatory
  - improves microcirculation
  - decrease discoloration

DERM'S PRO TIP
☐ Refrigerate your eye creams
Lower temperatures have an anti-inflammatory effect and boosts the efficacy of caffeine by enhancing vasoconstriction i.e. blood vessel narrowing.

☐ Emphasise 4-6 weeks of use before results are seen
The active ingredients in eye creams require daily use for 4-6 weeks before visible results are seen.

What is cellulite?

Cellulite commonly affects the thighs, buttocks and hip area resulting in a dimpled, lumpy appearance of skin. This abnormal appearance is linked to structural changes in the fatty tissue under the skin. Specifically the fibrous bands linking skin to the underlying muscles tighten, resulting in fat being pushed to the surface of skin. It has also been linked to hormonal factors such as pregnancy, genetics as well as weight gain.

Role of caffeine

- prevents fat cell accumulation
- stimulates fat degradation
- slimming cream (3.5% caffeine) significant short term improvements in the thigh and upper-arm area

DERM'S PRO TIP

Typical 3% caffeine concentration for skincare. However, caffeine toxicity from cellulite cream can become a problem when high concentrations of caffeine are applied on larger areas of skin.

Centella Asiatica Extract

CICA is the colloquial term for the herb Centella asiatica, a popular ingredient in skincare. It is a species belonging to the flowering plant family *Apiaceae*. Cica is also known as gotu kola, Indian Pennywort and tiger grass. It was used as a culinary vegetable and medicinal herb for hundreds of years to treat small wounds, scratches, burns, scars and eczema. On top of that, C. asiatica provides a rich source of natural bioactive substances that can be used in cosmetics.

KEY BIOACTIVES

- triterpene compounds
  - asiaticoside
  - madecassoside
  - asiatic acid
- antioxidant

- anti-inflammatory
- anti-aging
- targets cellulite
- anti-acne

Anti-inflammatory
The anti-inflammatory properties of Centella asiatica extract are related to its saponins, i.e. asiaticoside. Research has shown that asiaticoside inhibits proinflammatory cytokines, reducing inflammation in the skin.

Centelloids/saponins for eczema/sensitivity
- calming effect
- reduces sensitivity to irritants
- reduced skin redness
- improves skin barrier function
  - decreased TEWL/ pH

Madecassoside for acne
Study
- madecassoside to human skin cells stimulated with P.acnes
- reduction in inflammation

Anti-aging: undereye wrinkles
One study published in the International Journal of Cosmetic Science detailed 27 women applying asiaticoside cream to one eye, and a control cream to the other eye twice a day for 12 weeks.
- significant improvement in wrinkle depth in asiaticocide cream group compared to control group
- reduce eye wrinkles

Anti-aging: target photoageing related collagen loss
Furthermore, asiaticoside can induce type I collagen synthesis, thus making it an effective anti-photoaging agent.
What makes up collagen?
Amino acid building blocks i.e.lysine, proline

Triterpenes
- increases lysine, proline metabolism

Wound healing
Madecassoside, asiatic acid*
- speed up wound healing
- increase antioxidative activity
- enhance collagen synthesis
- blood vessel growth (angiogenesis)

SKINCARE EXPERT LINGO
Angiogenesis is the process in which new blood vessels form from pre-existing vessels. It is a key aspect of wound healing and new tissue formation which involves collagen production.

*Most active component for wound healing
- induces expression of molecules that are responsible for tissue formation
  - extracellular matrix remodeling
- regulates inflammation

Hydration
- increases hydration of stratum corneum (outer layer of skin)
- improves epidermal barrier function
- triterpene saponins
  - hydrophilic sugar chain (glycone) that binds water within an occlusive layer
  - concentration dependent: higher the concentration of CICA, the lower transepidermal water loss (TEWL)

Cellulite reduction
- aka liposclerosis

Why cellulite forms: the role of blood vessels in tissue formation
The formation of cellulite is by an increase in the volume of fat cells which causes constriction of small blood vessels. This causes "distended" fat cells in this tissue, particularly around the hips, buttocks, thighs and arms.

How Cica works
- normalizes metabolism

- anti-inflammatory effects
- regulates microcirculation

Are there any side effects?
Application of Centella Asiatica in the recommended doses is not toxic and has no known side effects. However, excessive use of Centella asiatica may result in local allergic reactions.

Glycyrrhiza Glabra (Licorice) Leaf Extract

Licorice is derived from the plant Glycyrrhiza glabra, meaning "sweet root" in Greek, a perennial herb native to parts of Western Asia and Southern Europe. The plant is a legume, much like a bean. Within the root is where the health benefits lie.

Despite the candy form most are familiar with, licorice has been found in King Tut's tomb, was used by the Japanese geishas and is one of the essential herbs in traditional chinese medicine. Used to treat everything from the common cold to liver disease, this herb is highly esteemed for its health benefits and healing properties.

Extract from this plant boasts a plethora of active ingredients and properties that can bring many benefits to your skin, especially when it comes to brightening and repair.

The important bioactives extracted from the root are
- **glycyrrhizin acid**
  - 50 times sweeter than sugar
  - gives licorice its notable flavor
- **glabridin**
- flavonoid content i.e. **liquiritin** and **isoliquiritin**
  - yellow color
  - antioxidant-rich
  - decrease reactive oxygen species
  - anti-inflammatory properties

Anti-inflammatory agent (glycyrrhizin)
- irritation, redness
- studies: mice treated with glycyrrhizin extract from

licorice experienced reduced swelling and inflammation
- inflammatory skin conditions i.e. rosacea, atopic dermatitis, psoriasis (Journal of Drugs and Dermatology)
- distinct mechanism: glycyrrhizin does not scavenge free radicals
  - reduces inflammation by inhibiting free radical generation
  - prevents swelling and redness

UV-protection

PHOTOAGING RECAP
How UV radiation causes our skin to age
- generates free radicals

Why free radicals are damaging to skin
Free radicals are unstable molecules! When they attempt to stabilize themselves, they cause **oxidative stress** to occur, weakening living cells and tissues.

What does oxidative stress look like?

To illustrate, this process occurs when you leave an apple or avocado out on the table. After some time, the apple will turn brown – an example of the oxidation or deterioration of free radicals.

Liquiritin
UV Protection
- suppresses UVB-induced cell damage
- prevents inflammation and oxidative stress
- inhibits proteins that cause inflammation
- downregulates release of oxidants that cause oxidative stress

Glabridin
Prevents and treats dark spots
- natural lightening alternative to hydroquinone
- treat and prevent pigmentation

RAPID FIRE Q &A
How do dark spots and pigmentation develop?
Hyperpigmentation is due to the overproduction of melanin.

What is melanin?
Melanin is the pigment that gives skin its color.

How is melanin produced?
Melanocytes, a type of skin cell produces melanin with the help of an enzyme known as tyrosinase.

How does licorice root work for hyperpigmentation?
Glabridin in licorice inhibits the production of tyrosinase, the key enzyme involved in melanin production.

Why use licorice for dark spots?
No photosensitivity or toxicity risks vs hydroquinone.

Salvia Officinalis (Sage) Leaf Extract
Sage is an evergreen shrub with woody stems, grayish leaves, and blue to purple flowers. Native to the Mediterranean region, it is a member of the mint family Lamiaceae. It has a long history of culinary and medical uses, with the Romans referring to it as "holy herb" and using it in religious rituals.

With a savory, slightly peppery flavor, Sage has been listed as one of the essential herbs in Britain, along with parsley, rosemary, and thyme. It has also been distilled to form essential oils common in Europe.

Antioxidant properties
Like all plant extracts, Sage contains many antioxidant that help to defend your body against oxidative stress. Oxidative stress occurs when free radicals combine with oxygen, and the free radicals are greater than the body's ability to detoxify them. The cells in our body react badly to oxidative damage, damaging our skin cells causing premature aging.

Bioactive free radical scavengers in sage
Classification
- flavonoids
- terpenes

Specific molecules
- carnosol
- rosmarinic acid
- carnosic acid
- quercetin
- rutin
- sclareol

Effects on skin
- reduces oxidative damage
- anti-inflammatory
- increase cell renewal rates

SKIN EXPOSOME CONCEPT

The skin exposome is the amalgamation of factors that lead to aging—classified as intrinsic and extrinsic factors. The intrinsic factors relate to biological aging, the extrinsic consist of UV damage and pollution related factors. The results of aging is what we recognise as surface changes—wrinkles, sagging skin and dark spots.

What goes on under the skin is what we have discussed so far:
- oxidative stress caused by free radicals
- collagen/elastic fiber breakdown

How sage works

Multiple studies have demonstrated how *bioactives* in sage possess antioxidant and anti-inflammatory properties that help to combat skin aging.

Sclareol
- trigger cell growth
- block UVB-induced cell death
- inhibit MMP enzymes that break down the collagen and elastin
- reduce wrinkle formation

Purslane or Portulaca Oleracea L. (PO)
Bioactives
- Secondary metabolites
  - flavanoids

- alkaloids
  - saponins
  - tannins
  - terpenoids
- Wound healing
  - anti-inflammatory
  - antibacterial (saponin)
  - antioxidant
  - increase collagen production (alkaloids)

(Mugwort) Artemisia vulgaris
- perennial weed that grows in Asia, Europe and North America
- daisy family
- medicinal plant for menstrual disorders
- identified in 2022 review paper by Halina et al as a cosmetic ingredient with high potential

Bioactives
- sesquiterpenoid lactones
- coumarins
- flavanoids
- phenolic acids

Effects on skin
- antibacterial
- antifungal
- antioxidant
- bacterial ferment products

Clinical applications
- acne
- eczema/sensitivity
- sebum control
- UV protection
- perfumery

Adverse effects
- A.vulgaris well tolerated

- allergenicity of A.annua pollen
- toxicity for A.absinthium

FUN FACT
Nobel prize in 2015 for discovery of artemisinin, found in mugwort for treatment of malaria

Reduces inflammation
Mugwort helps regulate the activation of immune cells by targeting cytokine and macrophages in inflamed tissues. Cytokines are responsible for activating the growth rate of skin cells. Mugwort helps to reduce the production levels of specific proinflammatory cytokines, hence keeping inflammation under control and inhibiting excessive cell growth.

On the other hand, macrophages defend the body by digesting cellular debris, foreign substances and harmful microbes. Under normal physiological conditions, macrophages release signalling molecules to help mediate the immune system's regular responses. Inflammation occurs when an excess of signalling molecules is produced, causing immune cells to attack one's own tissues instead of foreign substances. Mugwort helps to regulate the production of signalling molecules and prevent macrophages from triggering an excessive immune response.

Mugwort also contains high levels of vitamin E, which helps to nourish and hydrate skin, creating a stronger skin barrier, protecting against further inflammation.

Acts as an antioxidant
Mugwort is a natural source of antioxidant compounds. They limit oxidative stress by scavenging the free radicals caused by an accumulation of reactive oxygen species (ROS) in the body from UV rays. They also activate the defence enzymes superoxide dismutase (SOD) and catalase. Mouse- and cell-based trials show that mugwort helps prevent damage caused by ultraviolet rays, as well as stimulates collagen, helping to reduce the appearance of fine lines. Plant-derived antioxidants can protect the human body with little or no side effects.

Antimicrobial
Mugwort also possesses antimicrobial properties that are

comparable to that of a standard antibiotic, helping prevent the growth of microorganisms such as bacteria, viruses and fungi, that cause certain skin conditions. For example, acne, is a multi-factorial skin disease linked to the presence of a bacterium, C. acnes, which generates inflammation. Microbial infection can also hinder the progress of wound healing which is particularly important for patients with acne scars. When Mugwort inhibits microorganism growth, wound healing can take place naturally and new skin cells can be regenerated, leading to tissue or scar recovery.

CHAPTER THIRTEEN

Seeds

Zea Mays (Corn) Kernel extract

- family of grasses. (Poaceae)
- cereal crop

Bioactives
- phenolics
- flavonoids
- carotenoids
- tocopherols (vitamin E, essential fatty acid)
  - four major tocopherols
  - alpha-, beta-, gamma-, delta-tocopherol

DERM'S PRO TIP:
Vitamin E cannot be synthesized by the body, hence it is considered an essential component of human diet

Amongst the grains (wheat, oat, rice), maize is considered to possess the highest antioxidant capacity.

Effects on skin
- antioxidant
- antimutagenesis
- estrogenic activities

Clinical applications
Maize or corn (Zea mays L.) is a plant belonging to the family of grasses. (Poaceae). It is cultivated globally, being one of the most important cereal crops worldwide. It is used for human consumption in the various forms of meal, cooking oil, thickener in sauces and puddings, sweetener in processed food and beverage products.

Maize contains many secondary metabolites, such as phenolics, flavonoids, and carotenoids. Corn oil is recognized as an excellent source of tocopherols. Tocopherols function as antioxidants and provide a good source of vitamin E. Like essential fatty acids, vitamin E also represents an essential component of the human diet as it cannot be synthesized by the body. The four major tocopherols found in corn oil are alpha-, beta-, gamma- and delta-tocopherol.

Cannabis Sativa (Hemp)
- herbaceous plant
- traditional Chinese Medicine to treat pain and inflammation
- first observed use in the West for itch

Bioactives
- 80 different compounds
- Leaf-derived: two key compounds
  - cannabidiol (CBD) *non-psychoactive
  - tetrahydrocannabinol (THC) *psychoactive
- CBD
- non-psychoactive cannabinoid
- found in skincare and cosmetics
- **Seed-derived (focus)**
  - Cannabis Sativa Seed oil
  - found in skincare products
  - is derived from the seed of the hemp plant
  - does not contain CBD or THC

Effects on skin
- anti-inflammatory
- antioxidant
- soothing properties
- treats inflammation, dryness, acne, and eczema

Multiple photoprotective mechanisms for treatment and prevention of photoaging

Antioxidant & Anti-inflammatory Effects
- rescue skin cells from UV-B induced damage
- stimulate production of melanin as a natural UV-protectant to reduce sun-induced inflammation and sunburn reactions
- preserve natural antioxidant proteins
- inhibit excess inflammation involved in poor wound healing
  - block critical inflammatory pathways

Eczema & Psoriasis
- anti-inflammatory effects
- eczema, psoriasis
- STUDY: 20 patients with psoriasis, eczema
  - topical CBD-enriched ointment twice daily for three months
  - improved quality of life
  - significantly improved skin elasticity, hydration, inflammation
  - improve itch symptoms
  - well tolerated no irritant or allergic reactions

Acne
- Sebum regulation
- STUDY:
  - reduce sebum production
  - decreased redness
  - reduce inflammatory markers of skin cells colonized by Propionibacterium acnes
  - direct antimicrobial effect

Oryza Sativa (Rice) Bran Extract
- Rice bran
  - outer layer of whole brown rice kernel byproduct
  - useful nutrients i.e. proteins, fats, dietary fibres, antioxidants

- rice bran oil derived for cosmetic purposes

FUN FACT: Rice bran has been used for centuries in Japan as a key ingredient in cleansers, toners, and bathing soaps to keep the skin smooth and refreshed. Historically, Japanese women have used the leftover water from washing rice in the baths to soothe and soften their skin. Turns out, we can learn a thing or two from the Japanese, as many studies show that rice bran for skin has many benefits.

Potent antioxidants
- Gamma Oryzanol
  - potent antioxidant
  - mixture of sterols and ferulic acids
  - protect from free radical damage, oxidative stress
- anti-inflammatory properties
  - reduces redness, itchiness, swelling
  - intercept UV rays
  - reduces dark spots

STUDY:
  - inhibits wrinkle formation
  - prevents TEWL

Protects from sun damage
- numerous minerals and nutrients
- prevents photoaging

Humectant: locks in moisture
- Rich in fatty acids, squalene
- oleic acid (Omega-9 fatty acid)
  - building blocks of skin barrier
  - protects from environmental stressors
  - anti-inflammatory

- Squalene
  - emollient
  - acts as a natural moisturizer
  - hydrating and maintaining the skin barrier

Avena Sativa (Oat)

- long history of use in skincare

BIOACTIVES
- Vitamin A, B, E
- avenanthramides*potent antioxidants only found in oats

Effects on skin
- anti-inflammatory
- moisturizing
- antioxidant
- skin protective

Avenanthramides (Avn)
- 30 times higher antioxidant activity than other phenolic compounds
- reduce harmful reactive oxygen species that induce oxidative stress
- STUDY: *Song et al*
  - prevent oxidative-stress-induced cell damage
  - inhibit pathways that damage skin cells

Use as cleansers
There has been a long history of using oats as a soothing treatment to cleanse irritated, inflamed skin. Oat's anti-inflammatory properties can be traced back to Avn in the skin that inhibits key inflammatory pathways and soothes skin irritation. Oatmeal saponins also help to solubilize oil, dirt, and sebaceous secretions. Used in atopic dermatitis for its ability to hydrate skin and repair the skin barrier.

How oatmeal repairs the skin barrier
- stimulates gene barrier related expression
- STUDY: 50 participants with moderate dry skin on their legs treated with a colloidal oatmeal skin protectant lotion showed significant improvement in skin moisture levels

Bakuchiol

- plant extract from Psoralea Corylifolia seeds, leaves
- ayurvedic and chinese medicine

Effects on skin
- antioxidant
- anti-inflammatory
- antibacterial
- stimulates collagen production
- reduces fine lines, wrinkles
- reduce UV-induced skin damage i.e. hyperpigmentation.

Retinol-like effects
- **Anti-ageing**

International Journal of Cosmetic Science 2014
- similar gene expression
- affect cell pathways
- stimulated collagen in cell studies
- 16 participants
- 0.5% bakuchiol
- twice daily for 12 weeks
- improvements in fine lines, wrinkles, roughness, dryness and elasticity

British Journal of Dermatology
- reduced wrinkle surface area and hyperpigmentation to similar extents

In another study, bakuchiol was found to be better than retinol at slowing down the activity of two enzymes that break down collagen and elastin.

Advantages of bakuchiol vs retinol
- **Better tolerability**
    - fewer adverse side-effects
    - less stinging, flaking
    - antioxidant + anti-inflammatory
- No photosensitivity

Antioxidant properties
Oxidative stress on skin cells results in skin ageing. Bakuchiol has been shown to activate a transcription factor that plays a major role in cellular resistance to oxidative stress. Additional antioxidant capabilities include its capacity for scavenging oxygen free radicals and its major role in preventing *mitochondrial lipid peroxidation.*

Helps with hyperpigmentation
In a study conducted, bakuchiol decreased pigment intensity and surface area over the 12-week treatment course. This may be attributable to bakuchiol's antioxidant effects, as well as its ability to disrupt melanin synthesis. Bakuchiol is able to interfere with two steps of the melanin synthesis pathway and reduce melanin production, hence being an ideal ingredient for use in both anti ageing and anti-hyperpigmentation cosmeceuticals.

Is bakuchiol the new retinol?
While the few studies published have shown that bakuchiol is a promising natural retinol alternative, we only have data of how it compares to retinol, not any other retinoids. Tretinoin, a form of retinoic acid, is a prescriptive retinoid that treats acne, hyperpigmentation, and fine lines, largely due to its potency. Tretinoin is much more potent, and does not need to be converted into an active form in the body, unlike retinol. Therefore, while bakuchiol may be a promising natural retinol alternative, it cannot replace prescription retinoids.

Side effects of bakuchiol
While in most studies, bakuchiol is generally considered to be less irritating than retinols, there is still a possibility of irritation. To illustrate, there have been 2 case reports of contact allergy to bakuchiol cosmetics since June 2019, published in the Journal of Contact Dermatitis. Therefore, it is important to perform a patch test before trying our new ingredients or skincare.

Vitis Vinifera (Grape seed extract)
- natural byproduct of the wine industry
- pressed seeds of grapes
- **antioxidant**
- **anti-inflammatory**
- antimicrobial
- polyphenols

- anthocyanins
- flavanols
- Vitamin E
- facilitate wound healing
- skin regeneration
- proanthocyanidin
    - faster healing
    - denser tissue
    - stronger
    - increased tenascin
        - protein
        - builds connective tissue
        - wound healing marker
        - antimicrobial, anti-inflammatory properties that can speed up wound healing

CHAPTER FOURTEEN

Flowers

Arnica Montana
- sunflower family
- treat inflammation by increasing circulation

FUN FACT
Its first documented medicinal use dates back to the 1500s.
According to folklore,
mountain goats and sheep were observed seeking out the plant
after stumbling and falling on hillsides.

Anti-inflammatory properties

- helenalin
- dihydrohelenalin

- modify immune response (anti-inflammatory)
- kill bacteria

Benefits:
Anti-inflammatory
- bruising
- reduces inflammation

Bruising is caused by blood vessel rupture. When applied topically, Arnica Montana increases the blood flow and aids in resolution of inflammation.

In a 2020 study conducted on the therapeutic effect of topical application of *Arnica montana* on UVB-induced skin injuries: topical treatment
- reduced the UVB-induced inflammatory response
- ameliorated oxidative damage

- **antibacterial**

- o against several strains of bacteria
- o thymol derivatives (roots)

- **antifungal**
- dandruff
- Malassezia

Side Effects
- risk of contact allergy
- avoid in pregnancy/breast feeding
- those allergic to sunflowers, marigolds, dandelions, daisies or other members of the Asteraceae family

Chamomilla Recutita (Matricaria) Flower Extract
- flowers for essential oil aka German chamomile oil
- STUDY (mice)
  - o decreased serum IgG1, IgE levels (markers of allergy)
  - o lower serum histamine
  - o less scratching
  - o immune regulation (modulate Th2 activation)
- skin calming
- risk of allergic reaction or irritation

Hamamelis Virginiana (Witch Hazel)

BIOACTIVE
- tannins
- phenolic compounds

CLINICAL EFFECTS
- **astringent**
- **anti-inflammatory**
- **antimicrobial**

Antimicrobial
STUDY:
- Cheesman et al
  - extracts from the witch hazel leaf
  - inhibits *Staphylococcus* and *Streptococcus spp* bacteria (skin infections)
  - novel antibiotic
    - overcome antibiotic resistance

Acne treatment
Witch hazel has been used topically as an astringent and anti-bacterial treatment for skin to alleviate inflammation caused by acne and eczema. This is because its high tannin content may cause astringent action. Astringents help to remove excess oil from the skin and tighten pores for individuals with oily skin. Additionally, its high antioxidant content as well as antimicrobial activity effectively fights bacteria in acne-prone skin.

Rosmarinus Officinalis (Rosemary) Flower Extract
- anti-inflammatory
- antimicrobial
- antioxidant activities

BIOACTIVE
- phenolic diterpene antioxidants (PDAs) 1–6
- carnosic acid (CA)*
- carnosol (CAL)*
- rosmanol
- rosmarinic
*responsible for antioxidant properties

Triterpenes
strongest anti-inflammatory
- ursolic
- oleancholic
- micromeric acid

Potent Nitric Oxide inhibitor
- NO
  - pro-inflammatory
- STUDY: Mice with atopic dermatitis
  - reduction in skin lesions

Anti-cancer aka chemopreventive
Wound healing
- improved skin flap survival rates

Antifungal

Cosmetic applications
- Cellulite
  - cream containing annona squamosa, zanthoxylum, rosemary
  - improved appearance
- Hair regrowth
  - mice model (androgenetic alopecia, testosterone induced)
  - inhibit DHT receptor binding
  - significant hair regrowth after 16 days
- Anti-aging
  - Rosml novel isolate
    - inhibit free radical reactions
- UV protection
  - inhibits UV induced enzymes (metalloproteinase)

Rosemary essential oil
- B-pinene
- 1,8-cineole
- borneol
- camphor
- limonene
- verbenone

Rosa Damascus (Rose Flower Extract)
- anti-inflammatory
- antimicrobial
- antioxidant activities

BIOACTIVE

- terpenes
- glycosides
- flavanoids
- anthocyanins
- carboxylic acid
- myrcene
- vitamin C
- kaempferol
- quercetin
- natural vitamin A source (retinol alternative)

Nutrient-dense

- More than 95 macro/micro constituents identified
- 18 make up 95% of oil

Key properties applicable to skincare

- antioxidant
- anti-inflammatory
- antimicrobial activity

Rosa Damask, known as Rosa damascena mill L, is one of the most important species of Rosaceae family. The damask rose in particular is crowned queen of all roses. It is well-known for being the most potent skincare active—containing a complex array of vitamins, minerals, and antioxidants that boosts skin health and resilience.

Anti-ageing

- photoageing signs i.e. fine lines, wrinkles, pigmentation
- vitamin A increases skin-cell turnover
- vitamin C skin brightening

Moisturizing effect

- skin balancing
- restore the skin's moisture level
- soothing sensitive and irritated skin

Skin barrier repair

- improve barrier function
  - reduces transepidermal water loss
  - (0.1% rose oil) increased the expression of filaggrin in tape-stripped skin of hairless mice

Antimicrobial effects
- broad spectrum antimicrobial
- Ulusoy et al (2009)
  - Escherichia coli, Pseudomonas aeruginosa, B. subtilis, Staph. aureus, Chromobacterium violaceum, Erwinia carotovora
  - gram-negative and gram-positive bacteria
  - Cutibacterium acnes (acne causing)

CHAPTER FIFTEEN

Roots

Daucus Carota Sativa (Carrot) Root Extract
Daucus Carota Sativa
- part of the Apiaceae family

Bioactives:
The four types of bioactive compounds (phytochemicals)
- phenolics
- carotenoids
- polyacetylenes
- vitamin c

Clinical effect:
- antioxidant
- anti-inflammatory
- antiproliferative

DID YOU KNOW?
Carotenoids are named after the root word "carrot" i.e. carrot accumulates an enormous quantity of carotenoids in its roots.

There are two types of carotenoids present in carrot
- carotenes
- xanthophylls

Beta-carotene makes up 80% of total carotenoids contained in domestic carrot roots. Dietary provitamin A carotenoids derived from plants are a major source of our vitamin A needs. Alpha-carotene, β-carotene, and β-cryptoxanthin obtained from carrot consumption are the carotenoids that are converted into *retinol* in the liver.

Carotenoids are high in antioxidants, thus preventing cell damage, premature skin aging and can be helpful in other skin diseases such as acne.

Retinol
- stimulates production of new skin cells
- collagen production
- reduces wrinkles

The amount and type of phytochemicals present in carrots differ based on the *colour* of the carrot. Carrots of different colours displayed a high variation in antioxidant properties. For example, purple carrots exhibited the highest antioxidant capacity due to higher phenolic compound concentration. High contents of α and β-carotene are present in orange carrots. Studies also have found that the peel has the highest phenolic contents and antioxidant activities— more than the flesh itself.

Scutellaria Baicalensis
Scutellaria Baicalensis (SB), a member of the mint family, is a purple-flowering perennial plant native to East Asia.
- key component of traditional Chinese medicine known as Huang-Qin or Golden Herb
- treats allergic and inflammatory diseases
- flavonoids such as baicalin and baicalein that confer high UV protective and antioxidant properties

Natural UV Protectant
- plant extracts containing UV-shielding and/or antioxidant properties
- alternative to potentially irritating chemical sunscreen agents

Seok et al
- sunscreen cream supplemented with extracts had a higher SPF value than a control sunscreen cream without the extract
- increases SPF value as effectively as the traditional inorganic UV blocker Zinc Oxide
  - inhibits inflammatory events

     o   absorbs UVA radiation

Prevent pigmentation formation
- inhibits melanin formation

BIOACTIVES
- baicalin
- wogonoside
- baicalein
- wogonin
- oroxylin A

Among these 5 flavones, wogonin and wogonoside were found to have an inhibitory effect on melanogenesis - the production of melanin, the pigment that causes dark spots.

Wogonin
- inhibits melanosome transport (responsible for melanin synthesis)
- color of wogonin treated cells significantly lighter from the black to dark brown color of control cells
- lightening and brightening effects

Polygonum Cuspidatum Root Extract (Knotweed)
- popular spring vegetable in Asian cultures
- traditional eastern medicine for cough, hepatitis, joint pain, asthma, cancer, hypertension
- source of trans-resveratrol
- also present in grapes, blueberries, peanuts, cocoa powder, wine
- active form as trans-resveratrol
    - o Japanese knotweed predominantly trans-isomer

Moisturising properties
In a study conducted, subjects who used cosmetic emulsions containing resveratrol showed improvement in the functioning of the hydro-lipid barrier of the skin as well as increased levels of skin hydration.

Anti-aging
- powerful antioxidant
- enhances cellular regeneration without the irritation effects of traditional retinoids
- inhibits formation of advanced glycation end-products (AGEs)
  - collagen-damaging proteins and fats
  - form in skin as a reaction from exposure to sugars

By inhibiting formation of AGEs, resveratrol helps to reduce the appearance of wrinkles and loss of firmness. Additionally, resveratrol promotes even skin tone by inhibiting tyrosinase, the key enzyme that catalyzes melanin production by oxidation.

Salvia Miltiorrhiza (Red Sage) Root Extract
- red sage or Dan Shen
- mint family, similar to common sage
- Native to China and Japan
- traditionally used for treatment of inflammatory diseases

Bioactives:
- Salvianolic acid B
- Salvianolic acid A
- Magnesium lithospermate
- Tanshinones

Clinical effects
- anti-inflammatory
- antioxidant
- antibacterial

Alternative treatment for Eczema / Psoriasis
Currently, immunosuppressive corticosteroids are one of the main treatments for eczema, or atopic dermatitis (AD). However, corticosteroids are not suitable for use for long periods as it can lead to severe side effects such as skin thinning and ulcers.

Salvianolic acid B and A have been found to have potent anti-inflammatory effects that are useful in reducing the symptoms of atopic dermatitis in mice, reducing symptoms like ear skin hypertrophy (scarring) when applied to the ears, and decreased mast cell infiltration that causes inflammation into skin lesions.

Furthermore, studies have found that when skin keratinocytes were treated with Salvianolic acid A, it significantly inhibited inflammation pathways that led to psoriasis, demonstrating that it can be developed for the treatment of psoriasis.

Acne

Tanshinones (TAN) is a class of compounds that is a major component of Salvia miltiorrhiza. Recent studies have found that TAN was able to improve the condition of facial skin by helping to reduce scarring, through improving blood circulation and promoting cell turnover. Pharmacological studies have shown that TAN also has an anti-acne effect, with inhibitory activity on *Propionibacterium acnes,* the main acne-causing bacteria. In addition, TANs have also shown to have antioxidant, anti-inflammatory and antibacterial effects, all of which are effective for acne treatment.

Anti-aging

Changes in collagen, one of the major components of the skin, have been suggested as the cause of clinical changes observed in aging skin. One major pathway of wrinkle formation is associated with the degradation of collagen in the skin. In recent years, naturally derived compounds have gained attention because of their protective effects against skin damage. Magnesium lithospermate is one of the active components of Salvia miltiorrhiza and has been found to enhance antioxidant defense mechanisms. In addition, studies have also found that it is able to significantly increase types I and III collagen in skin aging models, demonstrating that it has anti-aging effects against natural skin and aging, and UV-induced photoaging.

CHAPTER SIXTEEN

Active ingredients derived from Microorganisms

Astaxanthin
- red-orange pigment found in marine animals
- xanthophyll carotenoid
- more active than other carotenoids i.e. zeaxanthin, lutein, beta-carotene
- higher antioxidant activity

Where is it found?
- synthesized in microalgae
- bioaccumulation in plankton, crustaceans, fish
- can be synthesized by plants, bacteria, and microalgae
- primarily found in *Haematococcus pluvialis*
- dietary intake via seafood i.e. wild sockeye salmon contains 26-28mg per kg of flesh.

Antioxidant activity
The mechanisms of aging, both chronological and photoaging, include the generation of reactive oxygen species (ROS) via oxidative stress and exposure to UV light. **Astaxanthin has potent antioxidant properties**

Photoprotection
Comparative studies have examined the photoprotective properties of multiple carotenoids, and determined that astaxanthin has greater antioxidant capacity compared to other carotenoids in human skin cells. In particular, astaxanthin inhibits ROS formation and prevents oxidative stress.

Astaxanthin's antioxidant activities are not only through direct radical scavenging, but also by stimulating pathways in the body to generate our body's own natural defense against free radical damage.

Anti-inflammatory properties

It is well established that various proinflammatory markers in skin are increased as a result of UV exposure. One hypothesis that is gaining traction in fields of research is the theory of inflammaging. Inflammaging is the process of low-grade chronic inflammation in the body, and is believed to be a risk factor for many age-related diseases and mortality risk in the elderly.

Keratinocytes, the primary type of cell found in the epidermis (top layer of the skin), increase the amount of inflammation in the body as a response to UV exposure. It has been shown that **astaxanthin decreases UV-induced reactive oxygen species** in the body and inhibits inflammatory proteins in keratinocytes.

As an oral supplement

- oral astaxanthin supplementation for 12 weeks
- reduced secretion of inflammatory proteins
- decreased enzyme collagenase activity i.e. collagen breakdown

Immune-enhancing effects

Research has shown that astaxanthin enhances immunoglobulin (proteins that produce antibodies to fight infections) production. Astaxanthin also showed to increase natural killer cells that serve as our body's surveillance system in detecting tumors and viruses in our body. In one study, it was found that astaxanthin enhanced the immune response after 8 weeks of supplementation.

Effects on skin damage

Collagen and elastin are two of many proteins that help to keep your skin looking youthful and elastic. As our skin ages both chronologically and due to photodamage, changes in these proteins are observed in the formation of wrinkles, loss of elasticity, dryness, and impaired wound healing.

Studies have demonstrated that an astaxanthin extract derived from the algae *Haematococcus pluvialis* increased collagen content through the inhibition of MMPs - enzymes that break down collagen. It has also been shown that astaxanthin is an effective compound for accelerating wound healing in mice. This is done through the increase of collagen in the wound, an essential protein required in closing up the wound.

Multiple clinical studies have shown that a combination of astaxanthin and collagen hydrolysate for 12 weeks improved elasticity and skin barrier strength in humans. Furthermore, one study showed that topical application combined with oral supplementation of astaxanthin for 12 weeks resulted in significant improvements in skin wrinkle, age spot size, elasticity, and skin texture.

Effects on DNA repair

Exposing your skin to UV can cause damage to DNA. The harmful effects of exposure to UV radiation are mostly due to the errors in DNA repair, which can lead to mutations. Astaxanthin has shown to be capable of minimizing DNA damage. It also has demonstrated inhibition of UV-induced DNA damage, and increased the expression of oxidative-stress responsive enzymes, helping to combat oxidative damage.

Is it safe?

Astaxanthin from the microalgae *Haematococcus pluvialis* has been approved for dietary supplementation in Europe, Japan and USA. The Food and Drug Administration (FDA) has approved Astaxanthin from *H. Pluvialis* for human consumption of up to 12mg per day.

Davinelli S, Nielsen ME, Scapagnini G. Astaxanthin in Skin Health, Repair, and Disease: A Comprehensive Review. *Nutrients*. 2018;10(4):522. Published 2018 Apr 22. doi:10.3390/nu10040522

Corthellus Shiitake Extract (Lentinula Edodes)
- polysaccharide-rich
- long-chain molecules composed of sugar units
- immunopotentiators
- lightening benefits
- antioxidant
- anti-inflammatory
- first medicinal macrofungus to enter the realm of modern biotechnology

Anti-Aging
- antioxidant L-ergothioneine
- prevents cell breakdown
- encourages faster cellular renewal process
- stimulates collagen and elastin production
- veratric acid anti-wrinkle effect

Brightens skin tone
- kojic acid
- slows down the production of melanin
- penetrates deeply

Anti-inflammatory
- rich in B complex vitamins
  - B3, aka niacinamide
- vitamin D, selenium
  - phytonutrients defend the skin from environmental damage

Barrier Repair
- ceramides
- essential amino acids i.e. lysine, aids the balanced transport of water through the skin's layers
- boosts hydration

Spirulina
- grows in both freshwater and salt water

- cyanobacteria i.e. blue-green algae

DID YOU KNOW?
Just like plants, Spirulina produce energy and food for itself through photosynthesis. Historically, Spirulina was consumed by Aztecs centuries ago, but became popular again when NASA proposed that it could be grown in space for use by astronauts. Gram for gram, Spirulina is known to be packed with beneficial nutrients. It boasts a 60% protein content - a richer source of protein than most vegetables - and is also a good source of fatty acids, beta-carotene, and various other minerals.

How does it benefit your skin?

Rich in Antioxidants
- antioxidants
  - phycocyanin
  - allophycocyanin
- scavenges free radicals, reducing oxidative damage

Wound Healing
There are 3 steps your skin has to take in the process of wound healing:
1. Inflammation (swelling + cleansing):
The wound is closed by clotting, swelling of the injured blood vessels by which damaged cells, bacteria and other unwanted microbes leave the area

2. Proliferation (rebuilding): New tissue is made up of collagen, the wound contracts, and new tissues grow

3.Maturation (remodeling): Collagen is remodelled, reducing scar thickness, and makes the skin area of the wound stronger

Spirulina extract contains a mixture of proteins and carotenoids that work together to speed up wound healing and tissue regeneration.

BIOACTIVES
- flavonoids
- alkaloids
- triterpenoids
Promotes wound healing

- increase of collagen 1

DID YOU KNOW?
Skin protective effects
- natural defense mechanisms against UV damage
- produce mycosporin-like amino acids (MAA)
  - absorb UV rays similar to the way chemical ingredients in sunscreen work
- barrier repair
  - stratum corneum hydration

Glycine Max (Soybean) Seedcoat Extract
- vegetable oil
- reduce hyperpigmentation
- enhance skin elasticity
- control oil production
- moisturize skin

Bioactives
- Polyphenols

These are plant secondary metabolites that have shown to have beneficial biological activity such as antibacterial, anti-inflammatory, and are powerful antioxidants in vivo. Therefore, they can help to reverse and prevent signs of skin aging and UV-induced free radical damage.

- Flavonoids
- Isoflavones i.e. phytoestrogens, with estrogenic activity
  - bind to estrogen receptors in skin
  - improved skin texture, elasticity, fewer wrinkles
  - enistein *primary isoflavone

Antioxidant activity
The seed coat of black soya bean (SCBS) contains a high amount of anthocyanins —responsible for its potent antioxidant properties. Genistein, the primary isoflavone from soy products, is known to enhance the antioxidant enzyme in various mouse organs. Several studies have also shown that

isoflavones present in soybean may also exhibit anti-inflammatory activities.

Anti-inflammatory effects
Repeated exposure to UV can lead to chronic inflammation, contributing to accelerated skin aging and an increased risk of skin cancer. In another study, experiments in vivo showed that soybean-germ oil (SGO) has a remarkable protective activity against UVB-induced skin inflammation. Several studies have suggested that the topical treatment of soybean isoflavone genistein inhibits UVB-induced skin tumorigenesis in a hairless mice model

Treats skin pigmentation
Pigmentary disorders of the skin
- melasma, sun spots, age spots, post-inflammatory hyperpigmentation
- result from the overproduction and accumulation of melanin
- no known side effects

Soymilk and soymilk-derived proteins induce skin *depigmentation* by reducing melanin transfer in the skin. These proteins have been studied to have depigmenting activity, as well as the ability to prevent UV-induced pigmentation.

Anti-aging
Elastin fiber and collagen production are reduced with the aging process. Decline in skin elasticity is due to slower tissue regeneration, lower production of elastin and increased levels of enzymes elastase- which break down elastin. In studies conducted, non-denatured soybean extracts were shown to induce the synthesis of collagen and elastin, and promote the correct assembly of new elastin fibers, providing a complete protection and restoration to the skin.

Studies conducted in 30 post-menopausal women found that treatment with isoflavone-rich, concentrated soy extract caused significant increase in skin thickness and number of collagen and elastin fibres. Additionally, creams and lotions containing phytoestrogens and isoflavones in a 12-24 week study showed improvement in skin dryness, thickness, facial wrinkles, increased hyaluronic acid, and type I and III collagen production. In these studies, no significant adverse effects after topical application of these cosmeceuticals.

Betaine
- AKA Trimethylglycine, glycine betaine
- sugar beet Beta vulgaris
- synthesised from molasses
- dietary: wheat bran, wheat germ, spinach, beets
- synthesized from choline
- osmoprotectant
  - protects against osmotic stress
  - skin-lightening
  - anti-inflammatory
  - anti-aging

Salmon Roe

BIOACTIVES
- carotenoid
  - astaxanthin
    - orange-red hue
  - potent antioxidant
- vitamin E
- vitellogenin
- vitamin A
- free amino acids
- eicosapentaenoic acid (pigmentation)

Anti-inflammatory
STUDY: reduction of redness after treatment of 5% salmon roe extract after 56 days

Hydration/barrier repair
- fatty acids
- oleic and linoleic acid
- astaxanthin
- reduced water loss
- minerals sodium, phosphate, calcium

- regulate moisture levels

Anti-aging powerhouse
STUDIES:
- 5% salmon roe
  - significant reduction in wrinkles
  - decreased surface roughness, pigmentation

Olive Oil - Olea europaea
BIOACTIVES
- antioxidants
- vitamins
- fatty acids
- phenols
  - antioxidant properties higher than vitamin E
- oleic acid (83%) emollient, protective barrier

Wound Healing
STUDIES:
- promotes wound healing
  - anti-inflammatory
  - decreased oxidative damage
  - UVB radiation:
    - Ichihashi et al.
    - extra virgin olive oil delayed onset and reduced the incidence of skin cancer development

Neonatal skincare
Various types of oils have long been used for neonatal skincare regiments. These have been advocated for therapeutic use in prevention of dry skin, treatment of cradle cap as well as massage therapy. In fact, in one study, neonates treated with olive oil cream showed significantly less dermatitis with improved skin condition and appearance. Topical application of olive oil in skincare may enhance skin barrier function by protecting the stratum corneum, leading to improved skin integrity.

Sea Buckthorn
- hardy tolerates weather extremes
- *Hippophae rhamnoides*

FUN FACT Name originated in Ancient Greece when horses were fed with sea buckthorn so that they would have shiny coats (*hippos* is horses in Greek, *phaos* is shiny).

BIOACTIVES
- berries, seeds, leaves
  - carotenoids
  - vitamin C
  - flavonoids
  - polyphenols
  - polysaccharides

Vitamin C content
- 12 times higher than oranges
- UV shield
- antioxidant
- photoaging
- dark spots
- acne
- sebum control

Rich in fatty acids
- 35% palmitoleic acid
- biomimetic
  - rare acid
  - component of skin fat
  - stimulates wound healing
- lecithin
  - skin cell renewal
  - moisturizing properties
  - hair damage repair, elasticity

High amino acid content
Amino acids are the building blocks of all proteins. In the 20 amino acids we need, 9 of them are considered 'essential' as they are not produced by the body but yet are essential for survival.

18 of the 22 known amino acids have been found in sea buckthorn fruit. In particular, leucine and lysine, which are usually deficient in plants, were found in its fruit. In the skin, amino acids help to hydrate the skin, increase water retention, build collagen, as well as promote cellular repair.

Myrrh Oil
- Commiphora myrrha
- wound healing
- antimicrobial

BIOACTIVES
terpenoids

Potent antioxidant
- furanogermacradienones
- protective effect against oxidative damage
- Inhibit
    - lipid peroxidation
    - nitric oxide

Antibacterial
- acne
- rosacea
- skin infections
- myrrh resin
    - potent antibiotic activity
    - no antibiotic resistance even after repeated exposure

UV protection

The active molecules in sunscreens can be divided into inorganic and organic agents. Inorganic components of sunscreen reflect and scatter UV and visible radiation. On the other hand, organic sunscreens absorb UV radiation and then re-emit this energy as heat or light.

In addition to UV absorption properties, natural botanical compounds also act as antioxidants and anti-inflammatory agents, further protecting against the damaging effects of sun or UV radiation exposure.

Myrrh oil has been shown to provide protection against UV-induced squalene peroxidation. Squalene and its peroxide have an important role in the occurrence of sunburn. The study found that the 1:1 combination of C. myrrha oil and SPF 15 sunblock was significantly more effective than SPF 15 sunblock alone in preventing UV-induced skin damage.

Melaleuca alternifolia (Tea Tree Oil)

- essential oil
- steam distillation of the leaves, branches of M. alternifolia
- woodsy, camphorous odor

BIOACTIVES
- 100 different components
  - terpenes
    - antibacterial
    - antioxidant
      - alpha-terpinene, alpha-terpinolene, and gamma-terpinene *in order of antioxidant activity*

Acne treatment
STUDY: twice daily for 12 weeks
- decrease in acne lesions
- skin dryness and mild peeling
- no serious adverse effects.

However, it is important to note that bacteria is not the only cause of acne. Factors like hormone fluctuation, and clogged pores can also lead to acne. Hence, while tea tree oil can help, but is *not recommended as a standalone treatment for acne.*

Dandruff treatment: antifungal, anti-inflammatory
- seborrheic dermatitis
- yeast (fungus) Malassezia
- 5% tea tree oil

Essential oils are highly concentrated botanical extracts which can be irritating when used in high concentrations on the skin. Avoid in those with sensitive skin.

Cucumis Sativus (Cucumber) Fruit Extract
BIOACTIVES
- vitamin C
- beta-carotene
- manganese
- flavanoids
- triterpenes
- lignans
- silica

Hyperpigmentation
- Vitamin C
  - inhibit tyrosinase
  - block melanin
- Cucurbitacin D
- 23, 24-dihydrocucurbitacin D
  - STUDY 3% hydro-alcohol cucumber extracts
    - decreased melanin content

Antioxidant + Anti-inflammatory
- fisetin
  - flavanoid
  - free-radical scavenging

Anti-aging

- silica
- required for collagen production

lyophilized cucumber juice

- anti-hyaluronidase
- anti-elastase (elastin, collagen breakdown)
- prevents premature aging, making it a powerful anti-aging ingredient.

Plant Stem Cells
What are stem cells?

- develop into different types of cells
- reproduce in a controlled manner
- i.e. embryonic stem cells developed nerve cell, skin cells, muscle cells, etc.

Plant stem cells

- meristems
- help to regenerate after injury
- more antioxidants than human stem cells
- withstand environmental stress

Antioxidant activity

- photoaging
- reduce oxidative stress
- inhibit cell senescence

Anti-aging properties

- extract of cultured apple stem cells
  - reduce crow's feet
- Edelweiss stem cells
  - anti-collagenase
  - anti-hyaluronidase
  - collagenases

- - break collagen peptide bonds
  - hyaluronidase
    - breaks down hyaluronic acid
- Tomato stem cells
  - antioxidants
  - metal-chelating compound phytochelatins
  - prevent the damage of cellular structures
- Asian ginger plant
  - Study 22 women, 28 days
  - improvement 50% skin structure
    - pore reduction
    - 19% reduction of sebum production in the skin

CHAPTER SEVENTEEN

Natural Moisturizing Factors

Amino Acids

Amino acids are necessary for healthy skin. They form the building blocks of peptides and proteins, with each amino acid performing a specific function in the skin. Some amino acids are found naturally in the skin and work together with aquaporins to ensure adequate skin hydration and barrier functioning.

Methionine

- essential amino acid
- two types
    - L-methionine
    - D-methionine
    - building block

Benefits of methionine for skin:

1. Healthy Hair, Skin and Nails

L-methionine

- keratin
- boosts collagen production
- skin tone
- elasticity

2. Protection from Harmful Free Radicals

- potent antioxidant
- essential for glutathione synthesis
    - protect cells from free radical damage

3. Wound Healing

- tissue growth
- blood vessels
- deficiency in methionine causes poor wound healing
  - accelerated wound healing with supplementation
- also applicable to acne inflammation and healing

Serine
- non-essential amino acid
- derived from silk proteins
- produced by our body naturally from different metabolites, i.e., glycine

CLINICAL EFFECTS
- collagen production
- boost skin elasticity
- moisture retaining (natural moisturizing factor)
- immune functioning

Cosmetic preparations:
- skin conditioning
- anti-static agent
- hair conditioning
- replenish hair cysteine levels

Polyglutamic Acid
- ideal active in facial mists
- more efficient than hyaluronic acid
- carries 5X more moisture compared to hyaluronic acid
- instant optical illusory effect
  - glass skin
- water-soluble peptide
  - produced via lab fermentation
  - natto (fermented soybeans)

Studies have shown that γ-PGA has a moisturizing effect and skin elasticity more than that of collagen and hyaluronic acid.

SECTION 7

Skincare Planner

download textbook resources and printables*

*https://www.twlskin.com/dictionary/ register account and receive download access in your welcome email

SKIN EXPERT
ROUTINE PLANNER
A PRACTICAL

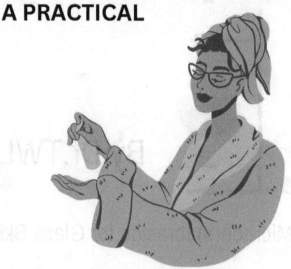

How to use this planner:

- Put knowledge into action
- Planned according to work week
  Monday-Friday
- Using knowledge you've acquired after
  completion of each module
- Build/improve existing skincare
  routine
- Choose skincare product(s)
- Make notes on actives
- Observe skin effects
- Track progress

By Dr.TWL®

MOODY MONDAY #1

Cleanse   Exfoliate   Nourish

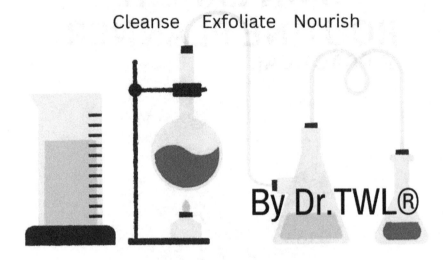

By Dr.TWL®

Home Microdermabrasion for Glass Skin

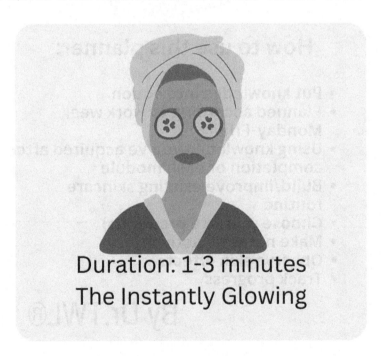

Duration: 1-3 minutes
The Instantly Glowing

MOODY MONDAY #1

Cleanse   Exfoliate   Nourish

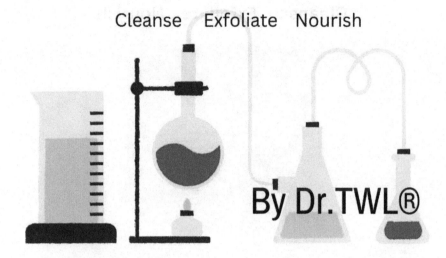

By Dr.TWL®

Home Microdermabrasion for Glass Skin

Skincare Plan:

My Hack:

My Review:

Cleanse   Exfoliate   Nourish

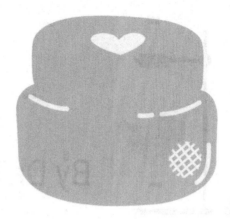

FAV PRODUCT REVIEW

Cleanse Exfoliate Nourish

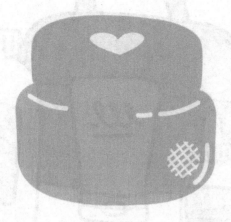

FAV PRODUCT REVIEW

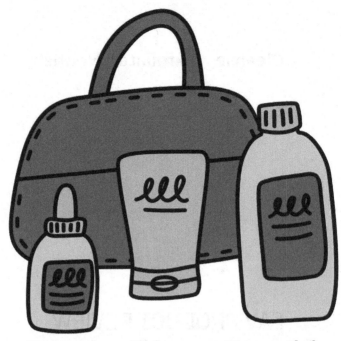

Everyday Skincare Essentials

Your Facial Mist Can Multi-Task

- On-the-go cleanser
- Pair with microfibre makeup makeup remover pad
- Moisturiser for dewy glow
- For makeup touch-ups

DERM'S CHEATSHEET

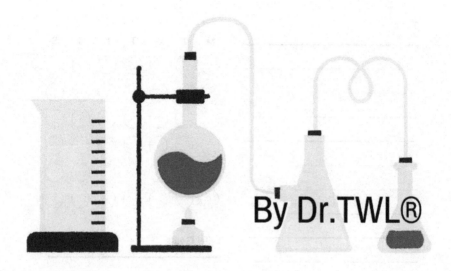

By Dr.TWL®

My Notes:

MOODY MONDAY

Today

_____

_____

_____

_____

_____

_____

_____

_____

_____

_____

_____

_____

_____

M	T	W	T	F	S	S
◯	◯	◯	◯	◯	◯	◯
◯	◯	◯	◯	◯	◯	◯
◯	◯	◯	◯	◯	◯	◯
◯	◯	◯	◯	◯	◯	◯
◯	◯	◯	◯	◯	◯	◯
◯	◯	◯	◯	◯	◯	◯

SKIN Goals

_____

_____

_____

_____

_____

_____

Notes

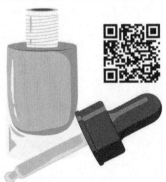

By Dr.TWL®

THOUGHTFUL TUESDAY #2

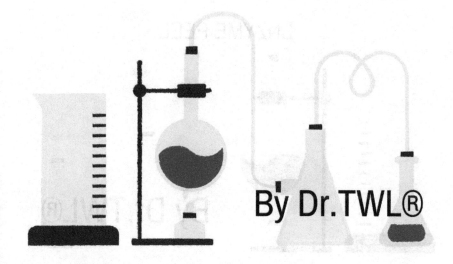

By Dr.TWL®

Chemical peel at home for universal skin types

Skincare Plan:

My Hack:

My Review:

THOUGHTFUL TUESDAY #2

ENZYME PEEL

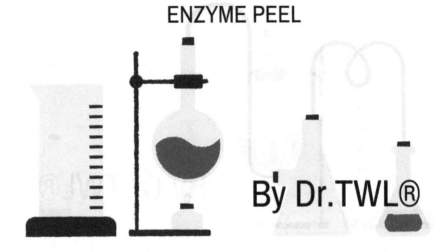

By Dr.TWL®

Chemical peel at home for universal skin types

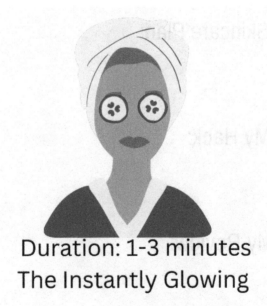

Duration: 1-3 minutes
The Instantly Glowing

Cleanse   Exfoliate   Nourish

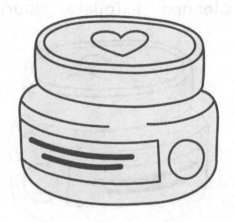

FAV PRODUCT REVIEW

Cleanse   Exfoliate   Nourish

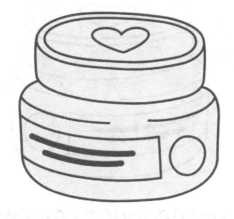

FAV PRODUCT REVIEW

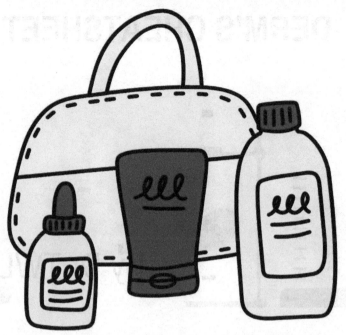

Everyday Skincare Essentials

How to choose a sunscreen

- Does not leave a white cast
- Quickly absorbed
- Smells good/neutral
- SPF 50 broad spectrum
- Dermatologist Recommended

DERM'S CHEATSHEET

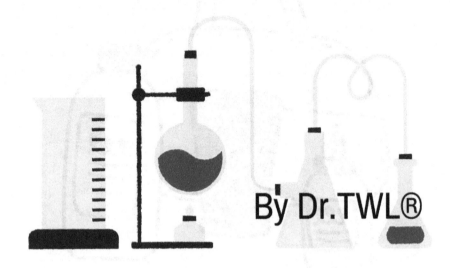

By Dr.TWL®

My Notes:

THOUGHTFUL TUESDAYS

Today

_____
_____
_____
_____
_____
_____
_____
_____
_____
_____
_____
_____

M   T   W   T   F   S   S

◯ ◯ ◯ ◯ ◯ ◯ ◯
◯ ◯ ◯ ◯ ◯ ◯ ◯
◯ ◯ ◯ ◯ ◯ ◯ ◯
◯ ◯ ◯ ◯ ◯ ◯ ◯
◯ ◯ ◯ ◯ ◯ ◯ ◯
◯ ◯ ◯ ◯ ◯ ◯ ◯

SKIN Goals

_____
_____
_____
_____
_____
_____

Notes

By Dr.TWL®

WILD WEDNESDAY #3

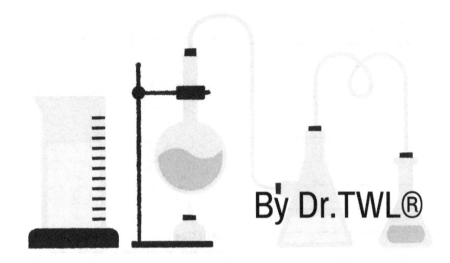

By Dr.TWL®

FACE OIL + JADE ROLLER MASSAGE

Skincare Plan:

My Hack:

My Review:

WILD WEDNESDAY #3

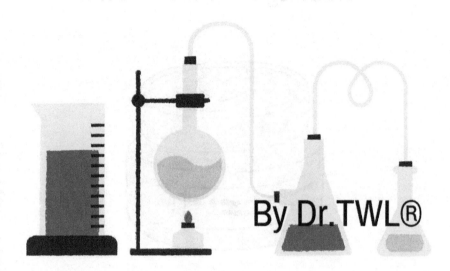

By Dr.TWL®

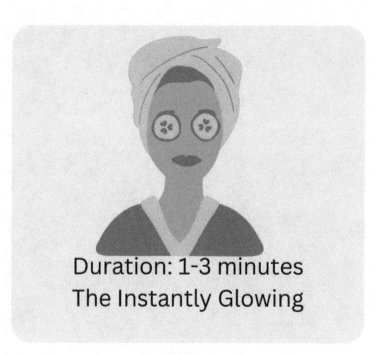

Duration: 1-3 minutes
The Instantly Glowing

Massage   Tone   Lift

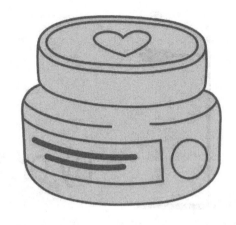

FAV PRODUCT REVIEW

Massage   Tone   Lift

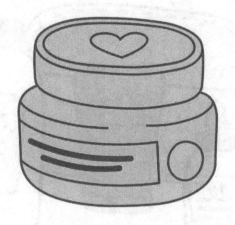

FAV PRODUCT REVIEW

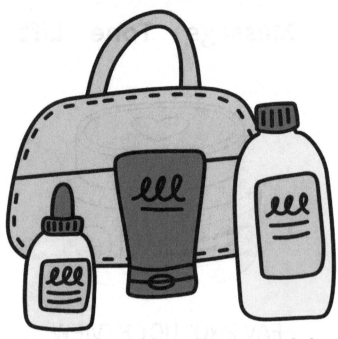

Everyday Skincare Essentials

How to choose a cleanser

- Natural emulsifiers like soy and honey
- Leaves skin hydrated not squeaky clean
- Good cleansers brighten immediately

Massage   Tone   Lift

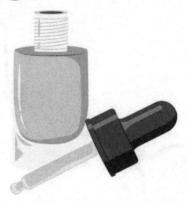

FAV PRODUCT REVIEW

Massage   Tone   Lift

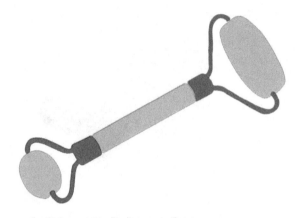

Why I love my Jade Roller

DERM'S CHEATSHEET

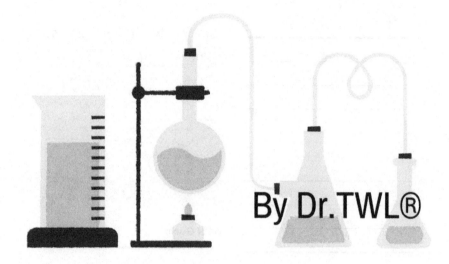

By Dr.TWL®

My Notes:

WILD WEDNESDAYS

Today

_____

_____

_____

_____

_____

_____

_____

_____

_____

_____

_____

_____

_____

M	T	W	T	F	S	S
○	○	○	○	○	○	○
○	○	○	○	○	○	○
○	○	○	○	○	○	○
○	○	○	○	○	○	○
○	○	○	○	○	○	○
○	○	○	○	○	○	○

SKIN Goals

_____

_____

_____

_____

_____

_____

Notes

By Dr.TWL®

TERRIBLE THURSDAYS #4

THE MILK CLEANSER MASK

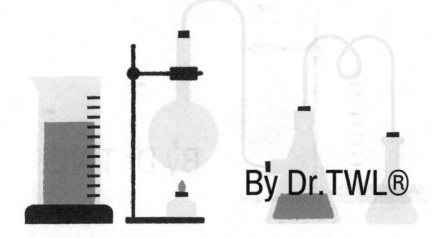

By Dr.TWL®

Feeling lazy 'cos the weekend's coming!

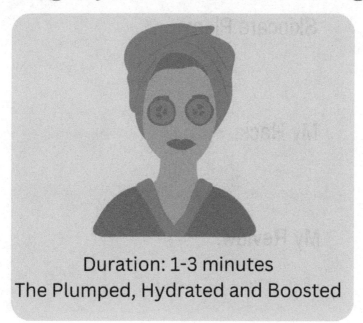

Duration: 1-3 minutes
The Plumped, Hydrated and Boosted

TERRIBLE THURSDAYS #4

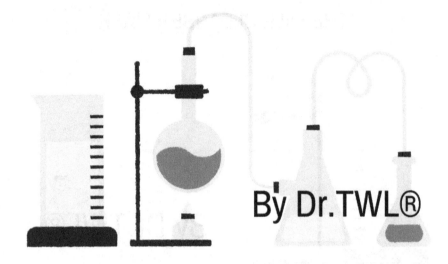

By Dr.TWL®

Skincare Plan:

My Hack:

My Review:

Plump   Glow   Boost

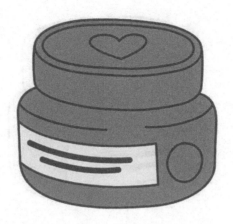

FAV PRODUCT REVIEW

Plump   Glow   Boost

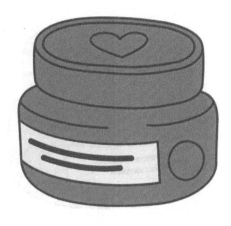

FAV PRODUCT REVIEW

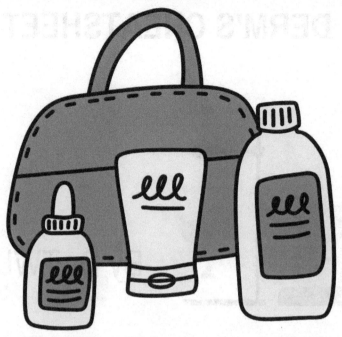

Everyday Skincare Essentials

How to cleanse thoroughly

- Double cleanse at end of day
- Use reusable cleansing microfibre pads to remove makeup
- Add sonic cleansers

DERM'S CHEATSHEET

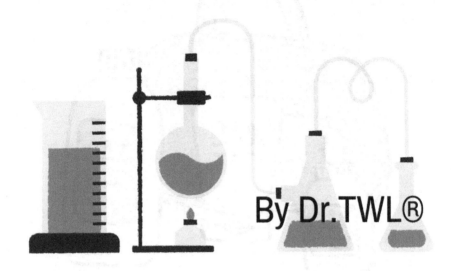

By Dr.TWL®

My Notes:

TERRIBLE THURSDAYS

Today

M	T	W	T	F	S	S
○	○	○	○	○	○	○
○	○	○	○	○	○	○
○	○	○	○	○	○	○
○	○	○	○	○	○	○
○	○	○	○	○	○	○
○	○	○	○	○	○	○

SKIN Goals

Notes

By Dr.TWL®

FERVENT FRIDAYS #5
THE FULL ON SLEEPING MASK

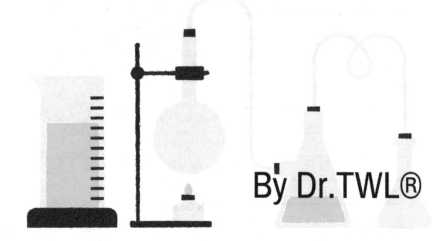

By Dr.TWL®

DIY your own sleeping mask

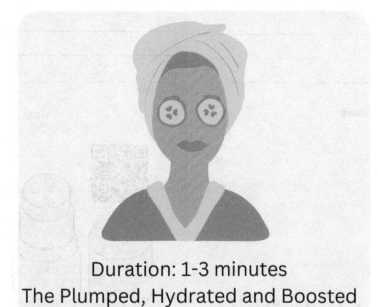

Duration: 1-3 minutes
The Plumped, Hydrated and Boosted

FERVENT FRIDAYS #5

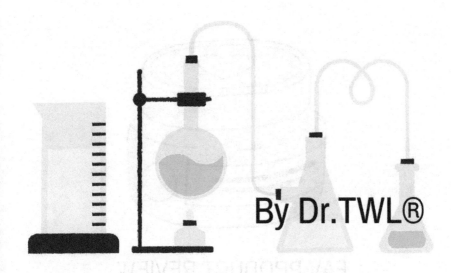

By Dr.TWL®

Skincare Plan:

My Hack:

My Review:

Plump   Glow   Boost

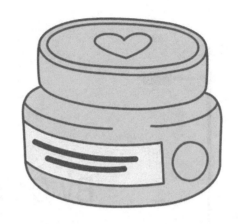

FAV PRODUCT REVIEW

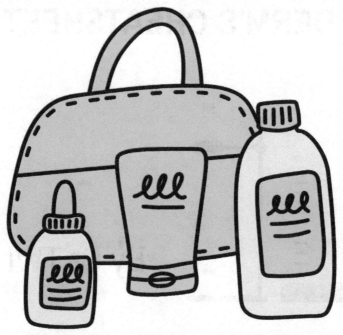

Everyday Skincare Essentials

How to DIY Sleeping Masks

- Choose your favorite emulsion or cream moisturiser formula
- Apply a palm sized amount overnight.

DERM'S CHEATSHEET

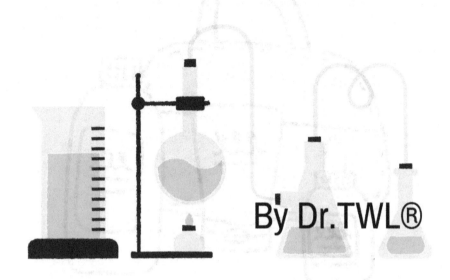

By Dr.TWL®

My Notes:

FERVENT FRIDAYS

Today

_____

	M	T	W	T	F	S	S
	○	○	○	○	○	○	○
	○	○	○	○	○	○	○
	○	○	○	○	○	○	○
	○	○	○	○	○	○	○
	○	○	○	○	○	○	○
	○	○	○	○	○	○	○

SKIN Goals

Notes

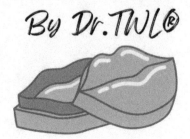

583

INGREDIENT CARD
TEMPLATES

MAKE YOUR OWN MEMORY AIDES

How to use this section:

**USE THE KEYWORD METHOD TO CREATE
VISUAL MEMORY AIDES TO HELP
REMEMBER INGREDIENTS**

By Dr.TWL®

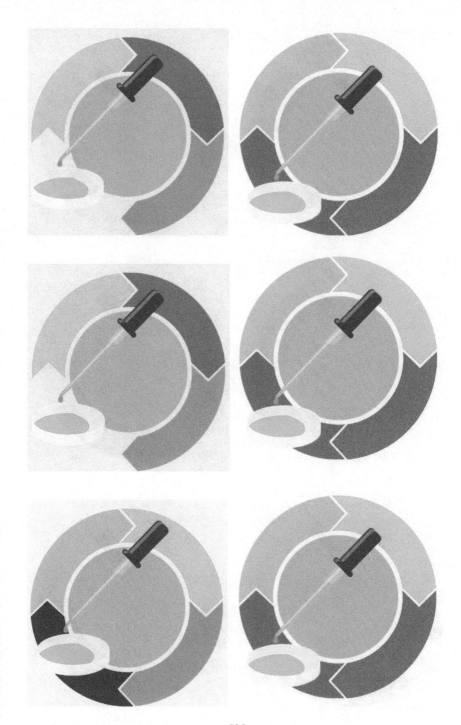

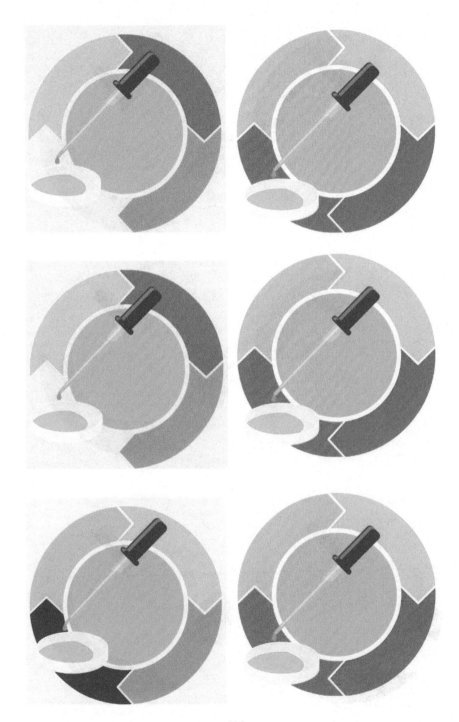

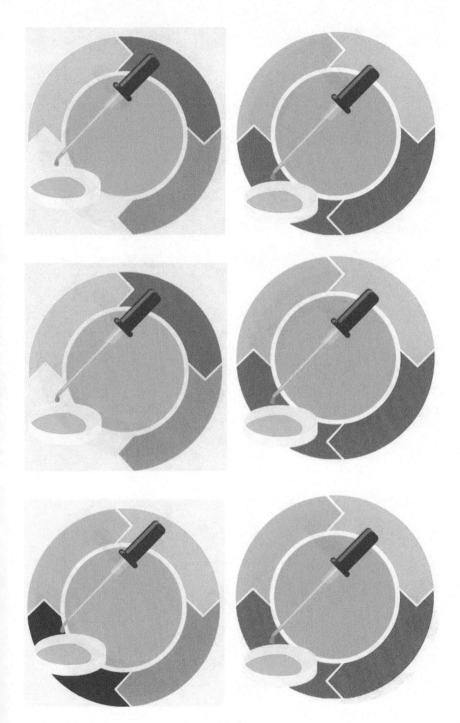

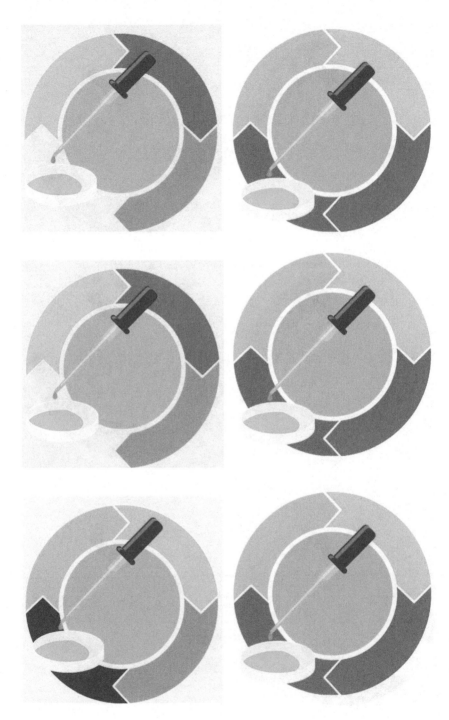

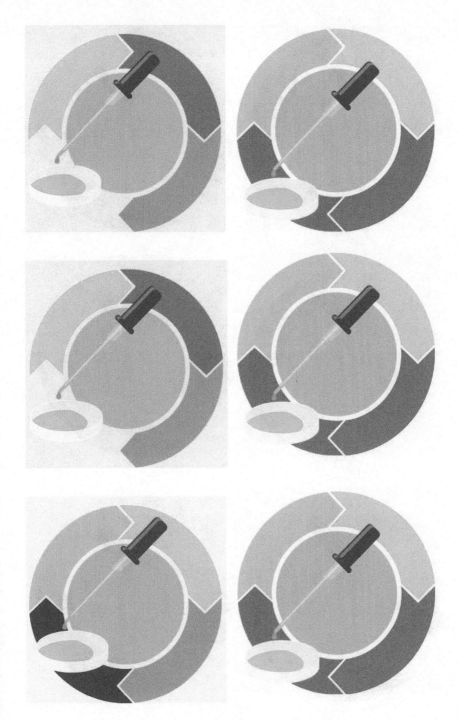

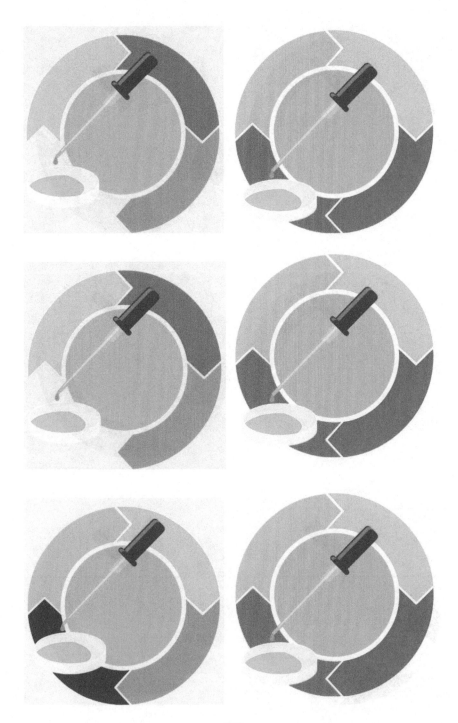

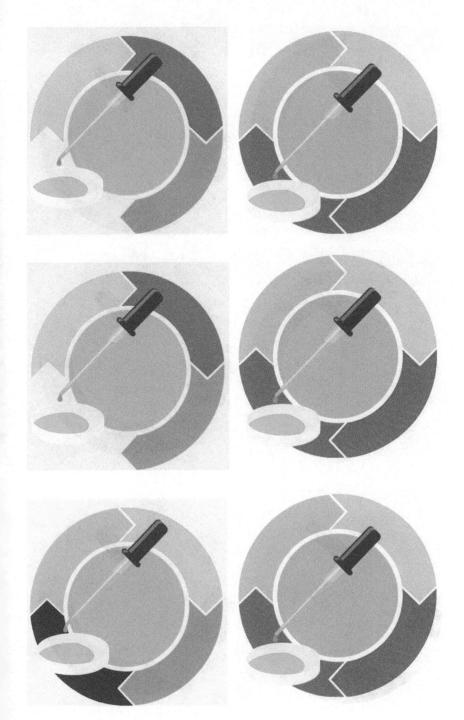

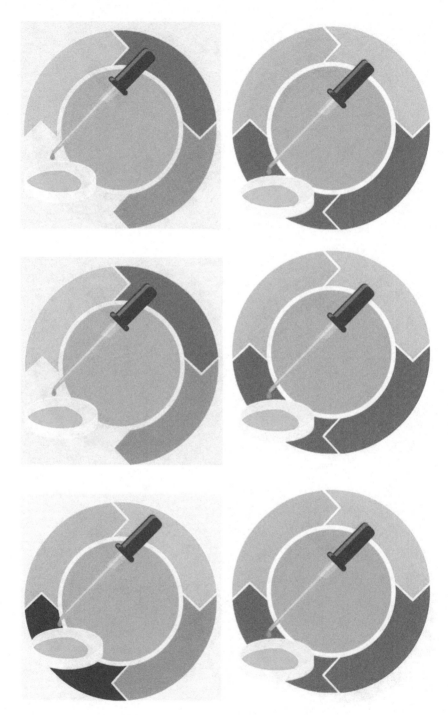

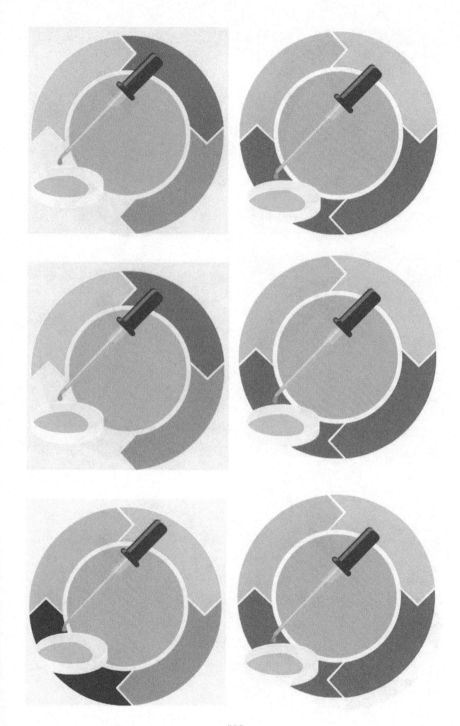

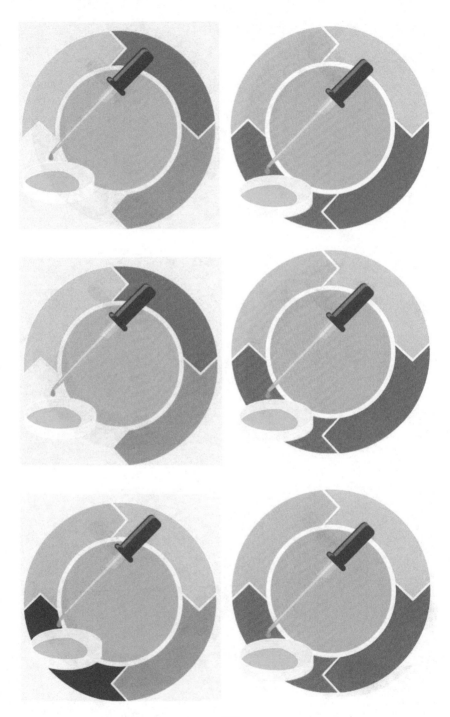

Made in the USA
Monee, IL
17 July 2024

62013697R00326